Preventive Medical Care in Psychiatry

A Practical Guide for Clinicians

Preventive Medical Care in Psychiatry

A Practical Guide for Clinicians

Edited by

Robert M. McCarron, D.O.
Glen L. Xiong, M.D.
Craig R. Keenan, M.D.
Henry A. Nasrallah, M.D.

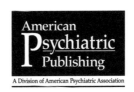

American Psychiatric Publishing
A Division of American Psychiatric Association

Washington, DC
London, England

If you would like to buy between 25 and 99 copies of this or any other American Psychiatric Publishing title, you are eligible for a 20% discount; please contact Customer Service at appi@psych.org or 800-368-5777. If you wish to buy 100 or more copies of the same title, please e-mail us at bulksales@psych.org for a price quote.

Copyright © 2015 American Psychiatric Association
ALL RIGHTS RESERVED

Manufactured in the United States of America on acid-free paper
18 17 16 15 14   5 4 3 2 1
First Edition

Typeset in Helvetica Light Standard and Warnock Pro.

American Psychiatric Publishing
A Division of American Psychiatric Association
1000 Wilson Boulevard
Arlington, VA 22209-3901
www.appi.org

Library of Congress Cataloging-in-Publication Data
Preventive medical care in psychiatry : a practical guide for clinicians / edited by Robert M. McCarron, Glen L. Xiong, Craig R. Keenan, Henry A. Nasrallah. — First edition.
    p. ; cm.
    Includes bibliographical references and index.
    ISBN 978-1-58562-479-9 (pbk. : alk. paper)
    I. McCarron, Robert M., editor. II. Xiong, Glen L., editor. III. Keenan, Craig R., editor. IV. Nasrallah, Henry A., editor. V. American Psychiatric Publishing, publisher.
    [DNLM: 1. Mental Disorders—prevention & control. 2. Preventive Psychiatry—methods. WM 31.5]
    RC454.4
    616.89—dc23   2014034613

British Library Cataloguing in Publication Data
A CIP record is available from the British Library.

To my wife, Marina, for her love and unwavering support;
to my son, Nolan Robert, for his magnificent smile and for teaching me
the indescribable joy of embracing and appreciating each and every day;
and to my patients—past, present, and future—for allowing me to be
a partner in their sometimes challenging journey to find health
and happiness.
R.M.M.

To Donna, Kara, and Addison.
G.L.X.

To my wife, Tracy, for her endless support;
to my two children, Jesse and Maya, who teach me daily
the joy of living and loving;
and to the patients, residents, and students who make my job
rewarding and challenging every single day.
C.R.K.

To my patients, who motivate and inspire me daily to discover
new knowledge to alleviate and prevent their suffering;
and to my family, whose love brings joy to my life.
H.A.N.

Contents

SECTION I
Preventive Medical Care in Psychiatry: General Principles

SECTION II
Cardiovascular and Pulmonary Disorders in the Psychiatric Patient Population

SECTION III
Endocrine and Metabolic Disorders
in the Psychiatric Patient Population

SECTION IV
Infectious Disorders
in the Psychiatric Patient Population

SECTION V
Oncological Disorders
in the Psychiatric Patient Population

SECTION VI
Special Topics

Contributors

Abdulkader Alam, M.D.
Assistant Professor of Psychiatry and Internal Medicine, University of Pittsburgh Medical Center, Pittsburgh, Pennsylvania

Robert M. Anthenelli, M.D.
Associate Chief of Staff for Mental Health, VA San Diego Healthcare System; Director, Pacific Treatment and Research Center; and Professor and Vice Chair for Veterans Affairs, Department of Psychiatry, University of California, San Diego, School of Medicine, San Diego, California

Paul Aronowitz, M.D., F.A.C.P.
Clinical Professor of Medicine, Department of Internal Medicine, University of California, Davis School of Medicine, Sacramento, California

Mili Arora, M.D.
Hematology/Oncology Fellow, Division of Hematology/Oncology, School of Medicine, University of California Davis, Sacramento, California

Soraya Azari, M.D.
Assistant Clinical Professor of Medicine, Division of General Internal Medicine, San Francisco General Hospital, University of California, San Francisco, San Francisco, California

Christopher A. Bautista, M.D.
Chief Resident, Department of Internal Medicine, University of California, Davis School of Medicine, Sacramento, California

Pravir Baxi, M.D.
Resident in Internal Medicine, Rush University Medical Center, Chicago, Illinois

Nicole M. Bekman, Ph.D.
Assistant Project Scientist, Pacific Treatment and Research Center, Department of Psychiatry, University of California, San Diego, School of Medicine, San Diego, California

Kristin Bennett, D.O.
Pain Fellow, Department of Anesthesiology and Pain Medicine, University of California, Davis Medical Center, Sacramento, California

Helen K. Chew, M.D.
Professor of Medicine, Division of Hematology/Oncology, School of Medicine, University of California Davis, Sacramento, California

Cerrone Cohen, M.D.
Resident Physician, Departments of Family and Community Medicine and Psychiatry, University of California, Davis, Sacramento, California

Stephanie Collier, M.D., M.P.H.
Resident, Department of Psychiatry, Duke University Medical Center, Durham, North Carolina

Deborah S. Cowley, M.D.
Professor, Department of Psychiatry and Behavioral Sciences, University of Washington, Seattle, Washington

Natasha Cunningham, M.D.
Instructor, Department of Psychiatry and Behavioral Sciences and Department of Medicine, Duke University, Durham, North Carolina

Elizabeth Davis, M.D.
Assistant Medical Director, General Medicine Clinic, San Francisco General Hospital; Assistant Clinical Professor, Division of General Internal Medicine, University of California, San Francisco, San Francisco, California

Dustin DeMoss, D.O.
Chief Resident, Departments of Internal Medicine and Psychiatry, Tulane Medical School, New Orleans, Louisiana

Benjamin G. Druss, M.D., M.P.H.
Professor, Graduate Faculty, and Professor and Rosalynn Carter Chair in Mental Health, Department of Health Policy and Management, Rollins School of Public Health, Emory University, Atlanta, Georgia

Jane P. Gagliardi, M.D., M.H.S., F.A.C.P., F.A.P.A.
Associate Professor of Psychiatry and Behavioral Sciences; Associate Professor of Medicine; Vice Chair for Education, Department of Psychiatry and Behavioral Sciences; Director, Psychiatry Residency Training Program, Duke University School of Medicine, Durham, North Carolina

Reena Gupta, M.D.
Assistant Clinical Professor of Medicine, Division of General Internal Medicine, San Francisco General Hospital, University of California, San Francisco, San Francisco, California

Jaesu Han, M.D.
Associate Clinical Professor, Departments of Psychiatry and Family and Community Medicine, University of California, Davis, Sacramento, California

Gwendolyn Ho, M.D.
Clinical Fellow, Department of Hematology and Oncology, University of California, Davis School of Medicine, Sacramento, California

Zachary Holt, M.D., F.A.C.P.
Director, Internal Medicine Primary Care Program, and Assistant Professor, Department of Internal Medicine, University of California, Davis, Sacramento, California

David Hsu, M.D.
Alzheimer's Disease Research Fellow, Departments of Psychiatry and Neurology, Massachusetts General Hospital, Brigham and Women's Hospital; Instructor of Psychiatry, Harvard Medical School, Boston, Massachusetts

R. Michael Huijon, M.D.
Resident, Combined Psychiatry and Family Medicine Residency, University of Pittsburgh Medical Center, Pittsburgh, Pennsylvania

Sharad Jain, M.D.
Director, UCSF/SFGH Primary Care Medicine Residency Program; Professor of Clinical Medicine, Division of General Internal Medicine, University of California, San Francisco, San Francisco, California

Dilip V. Jeste, M.D.
Estelle and Edgar Levi Chair in Aging; Director, Sam and Rose Stein Institute for Research on Aging; Distinguished Professor of Psychiatry and Neurosciences; and Director of Education, Clinical and Translational Research Institute, University of California, San Diego, San Diego, California

Wayne J. Katon, M.D.
Professor, Department of Psychiatry & Behavioral Sciences, and Director, Division of Health Services & Psychiatric Epidemiology, University of Washington School of Medicine, Seattle, Washington

Craig R. Keenan, M.D.
Professor of Medicine and Residency Program Director, Department of Medicine, University of California, Davis School of Medicine, Sacramento, California

Brooks R. Keeshin, M.D.
Assistant Professor of Pediatrics, Department of Pediatrics, University of Utah, Salt Lake City, Utah

Christopher A. Kenedi, M.D., M.P.H., F.R.A.C.P., F.A.C.P.
Consultant Physician and Psychiatrist, Departments of General Medicine and Liaison Psychiatry, Auckland City Hospital, Auckland, New Zealand; Adjunct Assistant Professor, Divisions of Internal Medicine and Psychiatry, Duke University Medical Center, Durham, North Carolina

Alan Koike, M.D., M.S.H.S.
Health Sciences Clinical Professor, Department of Psychiatry and Behavioral Sciences, University of California, Davis School of Medicine, Sacramento, California

Margaret W. Leung, M.D., M.P.H.
Palliative Care Fellow, Palliative Medicine, Harvard Medical School, Boston, Massachusetts

Lucy Lloyd, M.D.
Staff Psychiatrist, Portland VA Medical Center, Portland, Oregon

Gagan Mahajan, M.D.
Medical Director, Division of Pain Medicine, and Professor, Department of Anesthesiology and Pain Medicine, University of California, Davis Medical Center, Sacramento, California

Robert M. McCarron, D.O.
Associate Professor, Director of Integrated Medicine and Psychiatry Education, Director of Pain Psychiatry, Department of Anesthesiology, Division of Pain Medicine, Department of Psychiatry and Behavioral Sciences, Department of Internal Medicine, University of California, Davis School of Medicine, Sacramento, California

Robert K. McNamara, Ph.D.
Associate Professor of Psychiatry and Neuroscience, Department of Psychiatry and Behavioral Neuroscience, University of Cincinnati, College of Medicine, Cincinnati, Ohio

Henry A. Nasrallah, M.D.
Sydney W. Souers Professor and Chair, Department of Neurology and Psychiatry, Saint Louis University School of Medicine, St. Louis, Missouri

Virginia O'Brien, M.D.
Assistant Professor of Psychiatry and Behavioral Sciences and of Medicine, Duke University, Durham, North Carolina

John Onate, M.D.
Health Sciences Assistant Clinical Professor, Department of Psychiatry and Behavioral Sciences, University of California, Davis School of Medicine, Sacramento, California

Thuan Ong, M.D., M.P.H.
Assistant Professor, Division of Gerontology and Geriatric Medicine, University of Washington Harborview Medical Center, Seattle, Washington

Mamta Parikh, M.D.
Clinical Fellow, Department of Hematology Oncology, University of California, Davis School of Medicine, Sacramento, California

Jeffrey Rado, M.D.
Assistant Professor of Internal Medicine and Psychiatry, Rush University Medical Center, Chicago, Illinois

Y. Pritham Raj, M.D.
Clinical Associate Professor, Departments of Internal Medicine and Psychiatry, Oregon Health and Science University, Portland, Oregon

Lori E. Raney, M.D.
Owner, Collaborative Care Consulting; Medical Director, Axis Health System, Durango, Colorado

Matthew Reed, M.D., M.S.P.H.
Chief Resident, Combined Internal Medicine and Psychiatry Program, Department of Internal Medicine, Department of Psychiatry and Behavioral Sciences, University of California, Davis School of Medicine, Sacramento, California

Sarah K. Rivelli, M.D., F.A.C.P.
Program Training Director, Internal Medicine/Psychiatry Residency, and Assistant Professor of Psychiatry and Behavioral Sciences and of Medicine, Duke University, Durham, North Carolina

Chinthaka Bhagya Samaranayake, M.B.Ch.B.
Medical Registrar, Department of General Medicine, Auckland City Hospital, Auckland, New Zealand

Thomas Daniel Sapsford, M.B.Ch.B. (Hons.), M.Sc., B.Sc. (Hons.)
Medical Registrar, Department of General Medicine, Auckland City Hospital, Auckland, New Zealand

Alison Semrad, D.O., F.A.C.P.
Assistant Clinical Professor, Department of Internal Medicine, Division of Endocrinology, Diabetes and Metabolism, University of California, Davis School of Medicine, Sacramento, California

Jeffrey R. Strawn, M.D.
Assistant Professor of Psychiatry and Pediatrics, Department of Psychiatry and Behavioral Neuroscience, University of Cincinnati, College of Medicine, Cincinnati Children's Hospital Medical Center, Cincinnati, Ohio

Hendry Ton, M.D., M.S.
Director of Education, Center for Reducing Health Disparities; Medical Director, Transcultural Wellness Center; and Health Sciences Associate Clinical Professor, Department of Psychiatry and Behavioral Sciences, University of California, Davis School of Medicine, Sacramento, California

Erik R. Vanderlip, M.D., M.P.H.
Assistant Professor, Departments of Psychiatry and Medical Informatics, University of Oklahoma School of Community Medicine, Tulsa, Oklahoma

Radha Verman, M.D.
Hematology/Oncology Fellow, Division of Hematology/Oncology, School of Medicine, University of California Davis, Sacramento, California

Anna M. Wehry, B.S.
ROSE Scholar, Department of Psychiatry and Behavioral Neuroscience, University of Cincinnati, College of Medicine, Cincinnati, Ohio

Xixi Wong, M.D.
Resident, Combined Psychiatry and Family Medicine Residency, University of Pittsburgh Medical Center, Pittsburgh, Pennsylvania

Lawson Wulsin, M.D.
Professor of Psychiatry and Family Medicine and Training Director, Family Medicine Psychiatry Residency Program, Department of Psychiatry and Behavioral Neuroscience, University of Cincinnati, Cincinnati, Ohio

Glen L. Xiong, M.D., F.A.P.A., F.A.C.P.
Associate Clinical Professor, Department of Psychiatry and Behavioral Sciences, University of California, Davis School of Medicine, Sacramento, California

Disclosure of Competing Interests

The following contributors to this book have indicated a financial interest in or other affiliation with a commercial supporter, a manufacturer of a commercial product, a provider of a commercial service, a nongovernmental organization, and /or a government agency, as listed below:

Robert M. Anthenelli, M.D.—Dr. Anthenelli provides consultancy and/or advisory board services to Pfizer Inc. The Pacific Treatment and Research Center (PAC-TARC) receives research funding support from the National Institute on Alcohol Abuse and Alcoholism, National Institute on Drug Abuse, Department of Veterans Affairs, and Pfizer Inc.

Robert K. McNamara, Ph.D.—*Research support:* Inflammation Research Foundation (IRF), Martek Biosciences Inc., Ortho-McNeil Janssen, NARSAD, National Institutes of Health. Dr. McNamara was a member of the IRF Scientific Advisory Board.

Henry A. Nasrallah, M.D.—*Research grants:* Otsuka, Roche, Shire; *Consulting/speaking honoraria:* Boehringer Ingelheim, Janssen, Lundbeck, Merck, Novartis, Otsuka, Sunovion.

Jeffrey Rado, M.D.—*Research grant support:* Alkermes, Eli Lilly, Ortho-McNeil Janssen, Sunovion.

Y. Pritham Raj, M.D.—*Speaker:* AstraZeneca Pharmaceuticals.

Alison Semrad, D.O., F.A.C.P.—Dr. Semrad has been paid for her participation in Advisory Boards for Corcept Pharmaceuticals as well as for Onyx Pharmaceuticals Inc.

Jeffrey R. Strawn, M.D.—*Research support:* American Academy of Child and Adolescent Psychiatry, Forest Research Laboratories, Lundbeck, Shire, Eli Lilly.

Xixi Wong, M.D.—*Shareholder:* Merck.

The following contributors to this book have indicated no competing interests to disclose during the year preceding manuscript submission:

Abdulkader Alam, M.D.
Paul Aronowitz, M.D., F.A.C.P.
Mili Arora, M.D.
Soraya Azari, M.D.
Christopher A. Bautista, M.D.
Pravir Baxi, M.D.
Nicole M. Bekman, Ph.D.
Kristin Bennett, D.O.
Helen K. Chew, M.D.
Cerrone Cohen, M.D.

Stephanie Collier, M.D., M.P.H.

Deborah S. Cowley, M.D.

Natasha Cunningham, M.D.

Elizabeth Davis, M.D.

Dustin DeMoss, D.O.

Jane P. Gagliardi, M.D., M.H.S., F.A.C.P., F.A.P.A.

Reena Gupta, M.D.

Jaesu Han, M.D.

Gwendolyn Ho, M.D.

Zachary Holt, M.D., F.A.C.P.

David Hsu, M.D.

R. Michael Huijon, M.D.

Sharad Jain, M.D.

Dilip V. Jeste, M.D.

Craig R. Keenan, M.D.

Brooks R. Keeshin, M.D.

Christopher A. Kenedi, M.D., M.P.H., F.R.A.C.P., F.A.C.P.

Alan Koike, M.D., M.S.H.S.

Margaret W. Leung, M.D., M.P.H.

Lucy Lloyd, M.D.

Robert M. McCarron, D.O.

Virginia O'Brien, M.D.

John Onate, M.D.

Thuan Ong, M.D., M.P.H.

Mamta Parikh, M.D.

Lori E. Raney, M.D.

Matthew Reed, M.D., M.S.P.H.

Sarah K. Rivelli, M.D., F.A.C.P.

Chinthaka Bhagya Samaranayake, M.B.Ch.B.

Thomas Daniel Sapsford, M.B.Ch.B. (Hons.), M.Sc., B.Sc. (Hons.)

Hendry Ton, M.D., M.S.

Erik R. Vanderlip, M.D., M.P.H.

Radha Verman, M.D.

Anna M. Wehry, B.S.

Lawson Wulsin, M.D.

Glen L. Xiong, M.D., F.A.P.A., F.A.C.P.

Foreword

The term *integration* comes from the Latin root *integrare,* "to make whole." For psychiatrists and other mental health providers, *integration* means a frame shift from treating mental disorders to treating the whole-person needs of people with mental disorders. Studies since the early 1900s have documented the poor health and early mortality of people with serious mental illnesses; in a 2006 report, "Morbidity and Mortality in People With Serious Mental Illnesses," the National Association of State Mental Health Directors stated that we, as professionals in the field of mental health, own this problem. Now, the 2010 Patient Protection and Affordable Care Act, commonly called the Affordable Care Act (P.L. 111-148), is providing new opportunities to develop models of care that are integrated both within individuals and across populations.

For us to take on this challenge, we will need to have the knowledge and skills to understand how to prevent and detect common medical conditions in our patients. The task is not trivial; it involves new approaches to training psychiatrists and other mental health practitioners, and to retraining providers who may be years or decades beyond their original clinical degrees, in how to provide population-based, whole-person care.

Preventive Medical Care in Psychiatry provides a key resource for clinicians and mental health systems looking to provide the highest-quality integrated services to patients. It provides evidence-based approaches to care across the prevention spectrum, from primary prevention (how to keep people healthy), to secondary prevention (how to detect early signs of common illnesses), through tertiary prevention (how to prevent disability and adverse outcomes once patients develop medical problems). Practitioners can use this information to more effectively interface with general medical practitioners, to provide screening for common medical problems in their patients, and to ensure that patients receive immunizations and treatments for common medical problems. How they use the manual will depend on their scope of practice within their organization, on their personal level of comfort in providing medical treatments, and on the medical resources available in their communities.

Our field has a once-in-a-generation opportunity to help our patients live longer and healthier lives. This book will serve as an invaluable guide as we move down this new and exciting path.

Benjamin G. Druss, M.D., M.P.H.

Preface

Psychiatric research has focused for many years on prevention of suicide and accidents in patients with mental illness in order to decrease premature mortality. Over the last decade, however, research has found that only about 10% of the increased mortality in patients with severe mental illness is due to suicide or accidents. The other 90% of premature deaths are due to chronic medical illnesses, such as cardiovascular disease, chronic obstructive pulmonary disease (COPD), cancer, and infectious diseases.

Another issue that has led to concern about increased medical mortality rates in patients with mental illness is that many psychiatric medications, especially atypical antipsychotics, can lead to weight gain, metabolic syndrome, development of type 2 diabetes, and increased cardiovascular disease risk. These potential outcomes have led to development of guidelines for psychiatrists to enhance monitoring of weight, blood pressure, lipid levels, and glycemic control.

Patients with chronic mental illness also have higher rates of adverse health risk behaviors, such as smoking, poor diet, and lack of physical activity, which put them at high risk for the development of obesity, type 2 diabetes, and cardiovascular disease. Despite these high risks, many patients with chronic mental illness do not have a primary care doctor. Studies have shown that they experience disparities in care, such as receiving fewer vaccinations, preventive screens such as Pap smears, and cardiac interventions.

Extensive data now show bidirectional interactions between chronic medical illnesses and mental disorders. For example, mental disorders such as depression are risk factors for early development of diabetes and coronary artery disease, and complications of these illnesses can worsen or provoke depression. If psychiatrists are going to truly practice patient-centered medicine, additional training in helping patients to decrease adverse health behaviors and to enhance their self-care of chronic medical disorders will be essential to good medical care.

This timely book edited by Dr. McCarron and colleagues provides valuable information for psychiatrists who are concerned about potential premature mortality in their patients. This book is not aimed at training psychiatrists to have the skills of primary care doctors but instead focuses on the types of tools psychiatrists can use to help their patients take better care of their health by reducing health risk behaviors, such as smoking; approaches to monitoring and treating weight gain caused by psychiatric medications; and ways to help patients with improving self-care of chronic medical illnesses that have developed.

This volume provides state-of-the-art information for psychiatrists on health risk behaviors; chronic medical disorders such as diabetes, coronary artery disease, hyperlipidemia, osteoporosis, COPD, and thyroid disease; infectious illnesses such as sexually transmitted disease, HIV/AIDS, and viral hepatitis; and common cancers such as breast and prostate cancer. The book is written by experts in the field, many of whom have dual training in psychiatry and medicine. Most have extensive experience with medical student and resident education and with providing continuing medical education to experienced clinicians. This book should be required reading for psychiatry residents and can help update the practice of experienced psychiatrists.

Wayne J. Katon, M.D.

Introduction

Compared with the general population, people who have serious mental illness have increased general medical comorbid conditions, receive minimal preventive medical services, and have a reduction in life span of up to 30 years. Although there are many reasons for these variations, the stigma associated with psychiatric disorders and decreased awareness of the inherent vulnerability in this patient population likely play critical roles. In recent years, mental health professionals have been called on to perform physical health monitoring for patients with mental illness who do not receive primary or preventive medical care. This task is difficult without targeted, longitudinal training in this area.

Preventive Medical Care in Psychiatry: A Practical Guide for Clinicians is written for psychiatrists in training and in clinical practice, as well as other health care providers, who wish to learn an evidence-based and user-friendly approach to preventing commonly encountered, treatable, and potentially lethal illnesses in their patients. This is *not* a textbook for clinicians who wish to provide in-depth medical care. In this volume we focus on clinical care that is within the scope of psychiatrists and other mental health providers who work in outpatient mental health and integrated clinics. Therefore, if you wish to learn about the latest indications for pacemaker placement or about how to work up acute abdominal pain, read no further. However, if you wish to learn about ways to prevent or reduce the physical burden from heart attacks, stroke, common cancers, infectious disease, pulmonary problems, and endocrine disorders in patients with mental illness, you have found the right resource.

We hope that as policy makers and clinical directors start to see the importance of integrating medicine and psychiatry, this text will serve as a valuable resource for those who wish to develop diagnostic and treatment protocols for community mental health programs, mental health homes, and other integrated clinical programs. We firmly believe that systemic changes must be made in the education of students and clinicians at the interface of medicine and psychiatry before any large-scale policy changes can be made to the health care system. Put another way, it is nearly impossible to legislate changes to clinical care without providing a curriculum to support those changes.

Section I presents the rationale for why mental health providers need to provide effective primary and preventive health care for people with serious mental illness. In this section, the authors review preventive medicine principles, discuss important information on how to create a system that supports integrated care, present a framework whereby cultural considerations can be woven into everyday practice, and provide a framework for educators who wish to include integrated and preventive care in their existing curriculum. Section II addresses the heightened risk for cardiovascular and pulmonary disease in those who have mental illness. Section III covers important topics related to endocrine and metabolic disorders, such as diabetes, obesity, metabolic syndrome, osteoporosis, and thyroid disorders. In Section IV, the authors review primary and secondary preventive strategies for infectious diseases such as common sexually transmitted infections, viral hepatitis, and HIV/AIDS. An overview on suggested immunizations for those with psychiatric illness is also included. Section V includes current diagnostic, preventive, and treatment guidelines for the most common cancers found in those who have serious mental illness. Section VI, which addresses special topics, includes up-to-date preventive medical and psychiatric care information related to geriatrics, child and adolescent health, and pain medicine.

The appendix to this book includes a guideline for preventive medicine in psychiatry (PMaP) for providers. This age-based chart gives guidance to clinicians on how best to prevent common medical conditions in those who have mental illness.

We hope that this book serves as a useful resource for mental health clinicians and trainees. If you have any ideas on how we can improve the next edition, please let us know. Thank you for your many efforts to improve the quality of life and longevity for your patients who suffer from serious mental illness.

Robert M. McCarron, D.O.
Glen L. Xiong, M.D.
Craig R. Keenan, M.D.
Henry A. Nasrallah, M.D.

Acknowledgments

We would like to acknowledge the Association of Medicine and Psychiatry (AMP) for its leadership and support in the area of integrated training and clinical care. We give a special thanks to Roger G. Kathol, M.D. (inaugural AMP president), Lawson Wulsin, M.D. (immediate past AMP president), and Sarah K. Rivelli, M.D. (AMP president).

We would also like to acknowledge David J. Patron for his tireless efforts as assistant editor.

SECTION I

Preventive Medical Care in Psychiatry: General Principles

CHAPTER 1

Medical Comorbidities and Behavioral Health

Glen L. Xiong, M.D., F.A.P.A., F.A.C.P.
Lori E. Raney, M.D.

Medical Morbidity and Mortality

In a landmark study published by the Centers for Disease Control and Prevention, Colton and Manderscheid (2006) reported that people with serious mental illness (SMI) have an average life expectancy that is 25 years less than that of the general population. Figure 1–1 shows the years of potential life lost, which ranges from 13 to 30 years, across seven states in the United States in 1999 or 2000. The shorter life expectancy is astounding and is related in part to a lack of primary and preventive medical care for those who have mental illness. People with SMI not only face the stigma of having a mental illness but also experience higher medical morbidity and mortality. Decades of research have repeatedly demonstrated that people with SMI experience increased mortality and medical morbidities compared with the general population. Contributors to this book hope to advance the notion that longitudinal "cross-education" between primary care providers (PCPs) and behavioral health providers (BHPs) is paramount when considering ways to effectively address this growing problem. Education of mental health providers and train-

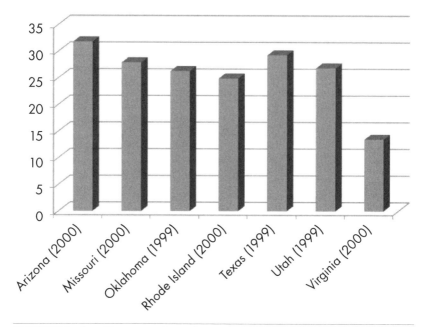

FIGURE 1–1. Mean number of years of potential life lost (1999–2000) across seven states in the United States.

Note. People with serious mental illness receiving services in public mental health systems. Data are from the latest year reported by each state in the study.
Source. Data are from Colton and Manderscheid 2006.

ees in the area of preventive care must be part of the solution (see Chapter 4, "Preventive Medicine and Psychiatric Training Considerations").

The *standardized mortality ratio* is often used in research to approximate (or indirectly predict) mortality risks. This ratio is defined as the ratio of death due to a specific cause for a specific population (in this case, people with SMI) to death from the same cause in the general population. Table 1–1 provides estimates of standardized mortality ratios for different medical causes in people with schizophrenia and bipolar disorder, based on systematic reviews (Roshanaei-Moghaddam and Katon 2009; Saha et al. 2007) and a population-based cohort study that provided data on more specific diseases for people with schizophrenia (Carney et al. 2006). As is evident in Table 1–1, persons with SMI are at higher risk of dying from chronic medical conditions compared with the general population. Conditions such as cardiovascular disease, diabetes, chronic obstructive pulmonary disease, and hepatitis C can be managed by contemporary primary and preventive medical interventions. These conditions, as well as others, are often not diagnosed or effectively managed in those who have SMI.

TABLE 1–1. **Standardized mortality ratios for people with schizophrenia and bipolar disorder**

	Standardized mortality ratios	
	Schizophrenia[a]	Bipolar disorder[b]
Cardiovascular	2	1.9–3.5
Cerebrovascular	0.87	1.4–1.7
Endocrine (e.g., diabetes)	5.28	2.5
Hypothyroidism[c]	1.8	
Infectious	4.6	7–14.8
Hepatitis C[c]	7.5	
Neoplastic	1.4	1.5
Respiratory (COPD)	4	3.1–3.2

Note. COPD = chronic obstructive pulmonary disease.
Source. Data from [a]Saha et al. 2007; [b]Roshanaei-Moghaddam and Katon 2009; [c]Carney et al. 2006.

In a report by the Medical Directors Council of the National Association of State Mental Health Program Directors (NASMHPD), Parks et al. (2006) estimated that although suicide and injury accounted for 40% of the excess mortality of patients with schizophrenia, 60% of the excess mortality can be attributed to cardiovascular disease, diabetes (including kidney-related deaths), respiratory diseases (pneumonia and influenza), and other infections. People with SMI have at least two to three times the risk of diabetes, dyslipidemia, hypertension, and obesity (McEvoy et al. 2005; Newcomer and Hennekens 2007). Additionally, 50%–80% of people with SMI are tobacco smokers and consume more than one-third of available tobacco products (Compton et al. 2006). Of note, use of inhaled tobacco is one of the most important reversible risk factors for vascular disease.

The individual medical conditions that contribute to metabolic syndrome, in addition to tobacco dependence, accelerate the development of cardiovascular disease. In a Spanish cohort of patients with schizophrenia, schizophreniform disorder, or schizoaffective disorder, researchers found that cardiovascular risk scores (using the Framingham Cardiovascular Risk Score) and metabolic syndrome prevalence were similar to those of individuals in the Spanish general population who were 10–15 years older (Bobes et al. 2007). Thus, people with SMI appear to "age" and die prematurely. Using the United

Kingdom's General Practice Research Database, Osborn et al. (2007) further demonstrated that people with SMI who were between ages 18 and 49 had a higher risk of death from coronary heart disease, stroke, and lung cancer, compared with an age-matched general population (Figure 1–2). Therefore, the delivery of primary and preventive medical care, early on, in people with SMI who are younger than 50 years may be critical to address the staggering health disparity.

Second-Generation Antipsychotics: Monitoring Treatment

In addition to biological, social, and environmental risk factors, treatment of psychotic and severe affective disorders with second-generation antipsychotics may worsen cardiovascular and metabolic conditions. There is robust evidence to support the causal effect of some second-generation antipsychotics on risk of weight gain, insulin resistance, and dyslipidemia. Although not all antipsychotics may worsen metabolic profiles, the currently available antipsychotics that are generally considered to be more effective for refractory illness (e.g., clozapine and olanzapine) seem to cause the highest risk. The most direct evidence found a dose-response relationship between olanzapine and clozapine serum concentrations and worsening metabolic outcomes (Simon et al. 2009). Sodium valproate, one of the most commonly used mood stabilizers, is also associated with significant weight gain. Although much less attention has been devoted to its potential metabolic adverse effects, sodium valproate may likely require monitoring similar to that of second-generation antipsychotics.

Despite consensus guidelines from the American Psychiatric Association, American Diabetes Association, and other groups on the monitoring of antipsychotic-induced obesity and diabetes (American Diabetes Association et al. 2004), evidence shows that adoption of the monitoring guidelines has been slow. In the United Kingdom, Mackin et al. (2007) found that recognition of elevated baseline rates of obesity and dyslipidemia is low in antipsychotic-treated community psychiatric patients, possibly due to "an alarmingly poor rate of monitoring of metabolic parameters" (p. 4), and treatment of adverse metabolic outcomes also appears to be less than that of the general population. In their cohort, which spanned 106 community treatment programs, physical health parameters continued to worsen despite notification of relevant health care professionals. The rates of lack of treatment for diabetes, dyslipidemia, and hypertension were 30%, 60%, and 88%, respectively, in patients with schizophrenia in the Clinical Antipsychotic Trials of Intervention Effectiveness (CATIE) study at baseline (Nasrallah et al. 2006).

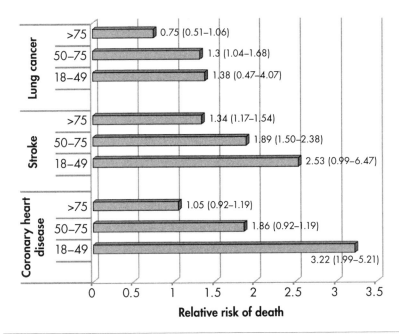

FIGURE 1–2.   Relative risk of death stratified by age in people with serious mental illness, ages 18–49.

Data are from the United Kingdom's General Practice Research Database (Osborn et al. 2007). Risk of death is adjusted for age, sex, and calendar period. Values are expressed as mean with 95% confidence interval. Note that 95% confidence intervals that cross unity (1.00) are statistically insignificant.

Although randomized controlled studies have demonstrated that lifestyle and pharmacological approaches can be used to effectively manage obesity and metabolic syndrome in patients taking antipsychotics (Álvarez-Jiménez et al. 2008; Maayan et al. 2010), more research is needed to test the long-term effectiveness and incorporation of these interventions in real-world settings. Additionally, switching antipsychotics has received emerging research attention. Gradual switching of an antipsychotic with high risk of metabolic side effects to one with lower risk may work in reducing weight and metabolic outcomes; however, some patients find the new medication ineffective and may discontinue it and return to the prior one (Newcomer et al. 2013). For now, careful consideration of the benefits versus the risk of antipsychotic switching must occur on an individual basis. The frequency of initiating antipsychotic switching strategies to reduce metabolic side effects in routine clinical settings has received little attention.

Barriers to Primary and Preventive Health Services

The limited access to primary and preventive health care by patients with SMI has received extensive attention and research (Druss and Rosenheck 1998). Ample empirical research has demonstrated that people with SMI underutilize preventive and screening health services, especially in the areas of blood pressure monitoring, vaccinations, mammography, cholesterol monitoring, and osteoporosis screening (Lord et al. 2010). Some of the barriers to use of preventive services may be due to demographic factors and medical insurance coverage (Xiong et al. 2010). People with SMI are also less likely to receive secondary preventive health care and invasive medical procedures. Patients with SMI who experience acute myocardial infarction are significantly less likely to receive proven drug therapies such as thrombolytic medications, aspirin, β-blockers, and angiotensin-converting enzyme inhibitors (Druss et al. 2001). Using administrative data from the Cooperative Cardiovascular Project (1994–1995), Druss et al. (2000) found that people with mental disorders are less likely to receive invasive cardiovascular procedures (i.e., cardiac catheterization, angioplasty, coronary artery bypass grafting).

Role of Psychiatrists in Medical Care

The Group for the Advancement of Psychiatry, an organization of psychiatrists dedicated to shaping psychiatric thinking, public programs, and clinical practice in mental health, has examined the responsibility of psychiatrists for patients' medical conditions (Dixon et al. 2007). The authors reported that the responsibility lies on a continuum, with the following responsibilities in order of priority:

1. Medical conditions that occur as a result of psychiatrists' actions
2. Medical conditions that can cause, trigger, or exacerbate psychiatric conditions or interfere with treatment
3. Preventive monitoring, screening, and education for medical conditions that disproportionately affect psychiatric patients

Additionally, "service or practice settings" are an important determinant of how the responsibilities will be fulfilled.

Consideration of the larger health care environment is also necessary in conceptualizing the role of psychiatrists and mental health professionals. PCPs, including primary care physicians and mid-level practitioners (nurse practitioners and physician assistants), are increasingly recognizing the importance of screening and initiating treatment for psychiatric disorders in their practices. At the same time, access to primary care services has been challenged by the increasing population growth and additional enrollment of patients into the health care marketplace, especially in the United States with implementation of the 2010 Patient Protection and Affordable Care Act (P.L. 111-148), often referred to as the Affordable Care Act, combined with a shortage of PCPs. In many settings, a psychiatrist may be the patient's only consistent care provider, essentially becoming a "primary care psychiatrist." This tension between increasing population growth (and need for primary care services) and limited access to primary care providers will likely further increase the health disparities experienced by people with SMI. Psychiatrists and mental health professionals not only need to recognize the unique medical conditions faced by people with SMI but also may need to provide treatment for the more common medical conditions, either directly or through collaborative arrangements.

Primary care and specialist providers have recognized that improving management of psychiatric conditions also improves outcomes of medical conditions. Psychiatrists who are capable of managing core medical issues will likely demonstrate improved psychiatric and overall health outcomes for their patients, further heightening the rationale for improved medical care for people with SMI. Therefore, psychiatrists and mental health professionals at the local, regional, and national levels will be called on increasingly to serve as advocates to improve access to medical services for people with SMI and as participants in health systems reform.

Medicine and Psychiatry Interface

The Four Quadrant Clinical Integration Model described by NASMHPD (Center for Integrated Health Solutions 2014) has helped conceptualize the interdependency of medical and psychiatric illnesses (Parks et al. 2006) (Figure 1–3). Quadrants I and III represent people with mild to moderate mental health disorders who are served mainly by the primary health care system. Quadrants II and IV represent people with SMI who primarily see psychiatrists and receive services in the mental health system. In Quadrant II, people with SMI have either limited or early chronic medical conditions. Over time, the same individual may develop more complex medical disorders and thus progress to Quadrant IV. For individuals in Quadrant IV, who have severe psychiatric and medical conditions, the severe medical condition is likely to interfere with management of the severe psychiatric disorder, and therefore interacts adversely to increase overall disability. Those individuals in Quadrant IV are also the most likely to require frequent medical and psychiatric hospitalizations and the least likely to make decisions or function independently. Individuals in Quadrant II are those who would benefit

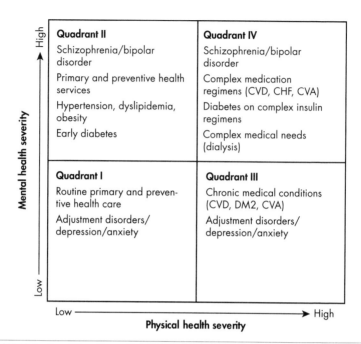

FIGURE 1–3. The Four-Quadrant Clinical Integration Model.

Note.   See text for explanation. CHF = congestive heart failure; CVA = cerebrovascular accident; CVD = cardiovascular disease; DM2 = diabetes mellitus type 2.

Source.   Adapted from Center for Integrated Health Solutions 2014; Mauer 2006; Parks et al. 2005.

the most from primary and preventive medical services to reduce their progression to Quadrant IV.

As alluded to by the Group for the Advancement of Psychiatry (Dixon et al. 2007), the exact delivery of medical services is determined by practice settings and available support services. Because the availability of health care resources is unlikely to outpace demand, service delivery must rely on more efficient reorganization of existing resources as the principal driver of innovation. Collaborative care models have emerged to meet this challenge.

Collaborative Care Models

Since the publication of the NASMHPD report detailing reasons for the decrease in life expectancy in the SMI population (Parks et al. 2006), new models to improve the physical health status of this group have emerged. These models are being tested nationwide and, although lacking the robust evidence base of other collaborative models such as those in primary care settings, offer the promise of improving health and prolonging life by addressing common conditions leading to increased cardiovascular disease risk in particular. Typically, the models currently being tested have at least three key components (Kern 2015):

1. Locating primary care services in or near behavioral health organizations
2. Care coordination activities to link patients to services
3. Health promotion or wellness activities to address maladaptive health behaviors

Primary and Behavioral Health Care Integration Grantees

More than 100 sites across the United States have received federally funded grants for Primary and Behavioral Health Care Integration (PBHCI) projects since the program's inception in 2009 (Substance Abuse and Mental Health Services Administration 2009). Many of these efforts include partnerships between community mental health centers and federally qualified health centers to provide onsite primary care services. Care management services are required to help link patients to services, identify and overcome barriers to receiving care, and track clinical outcomes in a registry format. A unique and creative aspect of this program is the variety of approaches the PBHCI grantee sites are taking to helping patients identify and engage in healthy approaches to improve their overall health. One early publication identifies some of the challenges these programs have faced in working to merge the cultures of primary care and behavioral health (Scharf et al. 2013b), and clinical outcome data so far have shown only modest improvements in a few clinical outcomes (Scharf et al. 2013a).

Medicaid State Plan Amendments

Funded by the 2010 Affordable Care Act, the State Plan Amendment for Medicaid Health Homes allows for the establishment of a health home in which the criteria for participation can include one serious and persistent mental illness. The health home service can be in a behavioral health setting (whereas most health homes are located in primary care settings). Although direct primary care services are not permitted with this funding (in contrast to the PBHCI grants), funding for six core health home services can be added to improve health outcomes. These include comprehensive care management, care coordination, health promotion, comprehensive transitional care services between facilities, individual and family support, and referral to community and social support services. The most established behavioral health home type nationwide is the Missouri model, developed by Joe Parks, M.D. (Parks 2015), which includes a primary care physician consultant to help establish priorities for disease management and improving health status. The consultant also provides a ready ally for the psychiatric medical staff and a source of collaboration for those providers who may wish to provide some direct care for medical conditions (Raney 2013).

Finally, some behavioral health sites are choosing to apply for and become federally qualified health centers themselves or are simply adding primary care facilities in their clinics, with the hope that sustainable funding models will become available. Without adequate additional funding to cover the limited reimbursement provided by public payers such as Medicaid and Medicare, these models may not be sustainable. There is hope that current innovations in health care funding reform will offer solutions so community mental health centers can provide care in the natural "medical home" of the SMI population.

Final Thoughts

Behavioral health providers are in a unique position to develop and oversee a plan to partner with patients and PCPs, with the goal of addressing significant and often lethal health disparities found in individuals with mental illness. For such changes to occur, BHPs must use an evidence-based practice pattern that includes assessment and prevention of common cardiopulmonary, metabolic, and oncological disorders and infectious diseases. True integration of primary care and behavioral health must include longitudinal cross-education—as well as large-scale changes in health care policy—with an emphasis on decreasing morbidity and all-cause mortality in individuals who have mental illness.

References

Álvarez-Jiménez M, Hetrick SE, González-Blanch C, et al: Non-pharmacological management of antipsychotic-induced weight gain: systematic review and meta-analysis of randomised controlled trials. Br J Psychiatry 193:101–107, 2008

American Diabetes Association, American Psychiatric Assocation, American Association of Clinical Endocrinologists, et al: Consensus development conference on antipsychotic drugs and obesity and diabetes. Diabetes Care 27:596–601, 2004

Bobes J, Arango C, Garcia-Garcia M, Rejas J: Healthy lifestyle habits and 10-year cardiovascular risk in schizophrenia spectrum disorders: an analysis of the impact of smoking tobacco in the CLAMORS schizophrenia cohort. Schizophr Res 9(1–3):101–109, 2010

Carney CP, Jones L, Woolson RF: Medical comorbidity in women and men with schizophrenia: a population-based controlled study. Gen Intern Med 21(11):1133–1137, 2006

Center for Integrated Health Solutions: Four Quadrant Model. Washington, DC, National Council for Community Behavioral Healthcare. Available at: http://www.integration.samhsa.gov/resource/four-quadrant-model. Accessed July 7, 2014.

Colton CW, Manderscheid RW: Congruencies in increased mortality rates, years of potential life lost, and causes of death among public mental health clients in eight states. Prev Chronic Dis 2:A42, 2006

Compton MT, Daumit GL, Druss BG: Cigarette smoking and overweight/obesity among individuals with serious mental illnesses: a preventive perspective. Harv Rev Psychiatry 14:212–222, 2006

Dixon LB, Adler DA, Berlant JL, et al: Psychiatrists and primary caring: what are our boundaries of responsibility? Psychiatr Serv 58:600–602, 2007

Druss BG, Rosenheck RA: Mental disorders and access to medical care in the United States. Am J Psychiatry 155:13:1775–1777, 1998

Druss BG, Bradford DW, Rosenheck RA, et al: Mental disorders and use of cardiovascular procedures after myocardial infarction. JAMA 283:506–511, 2000

Druss BG, Bradford WD, Rosenheck RA, et al: Quality of medical care and excess mortality in older patients with mental disorders. Arch Gen Psychiatry 58:565–572, 2001

Kern JS: Providing primary care in behavioral health settings, in Integrated Care: Working at the Interface of Primary Care and Behavioral Health. Edited by Raney LE. Washington, DC, American Psychiatric Publishing, 2015, pp 169–192

Lord O, Malone D, Mitchell AJ: Receipt of preventive medical care and medical screening for patients with mental illness: a comparative analysis. Gen Hosp Psychiatry 32:519–543, 2010

Maayan L, Vakhrusheva J, Correll CU: Effectiveness of medication used to attenuate antipsychotic-related weight gain and metabolic abnormalities: a systematic review and meta-analysis. Neuropsychopharmacology 35:1520–1530, 2010

Mackin P, Bishop DR, Watkinson HMO: A prospective study of monitoring practices for metabolic disease in antipsychotic-treated community psychiatric patients. BMC Psychiatry 7:28:1–6, 2007

Mauer J: Behavioral Health/Primary Care Integration: The Four Quadrant Model and Evidence-Based Practices. Rockville, MD, National Council for Community Behavioral Healthcare, February 2006

McEvoy JP, Meyer JM, Goff DC, et al: Prevalence of the metabolic syndrome in patients with schizophrenia: baseline results from the Clinical Antipsychotic Trials of Intervention Effectiveness (CATIE) schizophrenia trial and comparison with national estimates from NHANES III. Schizophr Res 80:19–32, 2005

Nasrallah HA, Meyer JM, Goff DC, et al: Low rates of treatment for hypertension, dyslipidemia and diabetes in schizophrenia: data from the CATIE schizophrenia trial sample at baseline. Schizophr Res 86:15–22, 2006

Newcomer JW, Hennekens CH: Severe mental illness and risk of cardiovascular disease. JAMA 298:1794–1796, 2007

Newcomer JW, Weiden PJ, Buchanan RW: Switching antipsychotic medications to reduce adverse event burden in schizophrenia: establishing evidence-based practice. J Clin Psychiatry 74:1108–1120, 2013

Osborn DP, Levy G, Nazareth I, et al: Relative risk of cardiovascular and cancer mortality in people with severe mental illness from the United Kingdom's General Practice Research Database. Arch Gen Psychiatry 64:242–249, 2007

Parks J: Behavioral health homes, in Integrated Care: Working at the Interface of Primary Care and Behavioral Health. Edited by Raney LE. Washington, DC, American Psychiatric Publishing, 2015

Parks J, Pollack D, Bartels S, et al: Integrating Behavioral Health and Primary Care Services: Opportunities and Challenges for State Mental Health Authorities. Alexandria, VA, National Association of State Mental Health Program Directors (NASMHPD) Medical Directors Council, 2005

Parks J, Svendsen D, Singer P, et al: Morbidity and Mortality in People With Serious Mental Illness. Alexandria, VA, National Association of State Mental Health Program Directors (NASMHPD) Medical Directors Council, 2006

Patient Protection and Affordable Care Act of 2010, Pub. L. No. 111-148, 124 Stat. 119, 109–1024

Raney LE: Integrated care: the evolving role of psychiatry in the era of health care reform. Psychiatr Serv 64:1076–1078, 2013

Roshanaei-Moghaddam B, Katon W: Premature mortality from general medical illnesses among persons with bipolar disorder: a review. Psychiatr Serv 60:147–156, 2009

Saha S, Chant D, McGrath J: A systematic review of mortality in schizophrenia. Arch Gen Psychiatry 64:1123–1131, 2007

Scharf D, Eberhart N, Hackbarth N, et al: Evaluation of the SAMHSA Primary and Behavioral Health Care Integration (PBHCI) Grant Program: Final Report. Rand Corporation, December 2013a. Available at: http://aspe.hhs.gov/daltcp/reports/2013/PBHCIfr.shtml. Accessed May 20, 2014.

Scharf D, Eberhart N, Schmidt N, et al: Integrating primary care into community behavioral health settings: programs and early implementation experiences. Psychiatr Serv 64:660–665, 2013b

Simon V, van Winkel R, De Hert M: Are weight gain and metabolic side effects of atypical antipsychotics dose dependent? A literature review. J Clin Psychiatry 70:1041–1050, 2009

Substance Abuse and Mental Health Services Administration, Request for Applications (RFA) No. SM-09-011. Rockville, MD, Substance Abuse and Mental Health Services Administration, 2009

Xiong GL, Iosif AM, Bermudes RA, et al: Preventive medical services use among community mental health patients with severe mental illness: the influence of gender and insurance coverage. Prim Care Companion J Clin Psychiatry 12:e1–e6, 2010

CHAPTER 2

Fundamentals of Preventive Care

Craig R. Keenan, M.D.

Clinical Overview

Preventive care is care intended to prevent illnesses and injuries as opposed to curing them or treating their symptoms. Laypersons usually consider preventive care in its purest form: as something that prevents illness in healthy persons. Examples include vaccinating children against polio and recommending seat-belt use. For practicing clinicians, however, the umbrella of preventive care covers many other scenarios, such as risk reduction counseling for individuals taking on unhealthy behaviors (e.g., suggesting condom use for patients with many sexual partners), early identification of existing diseases (e.g., performing mammography to find early breast cancer), or prevention of further disease events in persons who already carry a diagnosis (e.g., recommending aspirin use after a myocardial infarction to prevent a next infarct). Also, preventive care generally falls into one of four types of clinical activities: screening, counseling on lifestyle changes, immunizations, or preventive medications.

Categories of Preventive Care

Preventive care activities are categorized as primary, secondary, or tertiary prevention.

Primary prevention is focused on preventing new disease from occurring by removing its causes. Examples include childhood immunizations, smoking cessation to prevent lung cancer, and taking antihypertensive medications to prevent myocardial infarction or stroke.

Secondary prevention involves detecting diseases in early stages while individuals are asymptomatic and when treatment can prevent disease progression. In secondary prevention, screening is used to find the disease. Screening can include laboratory tests (e.g., blood tests to assess cholesterol levels), history taking (e.g., questions about smoking status), physical examination (e.g., measuring blood pressure), or imaging (e.g., mammography). If screening test results are positive, more testing is often done to definitively diagnose the disease, and then treatment is implemented to prevent worsening of disease. A classic example of secondary prevention is breast cancer screening: if mammography finds suspicious breast microcalcifications, it is followed by a diagnostic biopsy and then, if indicated, definitive treatment of breast cancer for potential cure.

Tertiary prevention involves taking actions to prevent worsening of disease or complications after a person has already been diagnosed with a disease. These interventions make up a large part of the daily practice of adult medicine providers under the umbrella of "chronic disease management." Examples include prescribing statins for lowering lipids in a patient with coronary artery disease and ordering a repeat colonoscopy after colon cancer treatment to look for recurrence.

The terms used to describe preventive care are often confused and misused in practice. For example, the comment that "secondary prevention after myocardial infarction requires statins, aspirin, and β-blockers to prevent future events" is technically referring to tertiary prevention. In addition, testing for a disease in someone with symptoms is no longer called screening, but instead is referred to as *diagnostic testing*; however, many clinicians still refer to such testing as screening. Further contributing to the confusion is the fact that the same test or intervention may be used for any category of prevention and for diagnosis. For example, a computed tomography scan of the chest can be used for primary diagnosis of lung cancer in a symptomatic patient with a cough, for secondary prevention to find asymptomatic lung cancer in a smoker, and for tertiary prevention in a patient already treated for lung cancer to look for a cancer recurrence.

Many of the preventive services covered in this book are secondary prevention screening tests in asymptomatic patients, for conditions such as hy-

TABLE 2–1.	**Essential criteria for an effective screening program**

The screening test must identify a disease that becomes clinically significant if left untreated.

The screening test must be able to detect the disease in a preclinical stage.

The disease in question must be treatable, so that finding it and treating it early will lead to reduced morbidity or mortality.

The test must have acceptable sensitivity and specificity in order to avoid high false-positive rates (to avoid unnecessary testing) and false-negative test results (to be effective at finding early disease).

The ideal screening test is reasonably priced, so it can be applied widely, and poses minimal harm or discomfort to the patient.

pertension, cancer, and diabetes. For a screening program to be effective, it must meet some minimum standards, which are listed in Table 2–1. Of course, not all diseases or tests meet these criteria. For example, potential screening tests have yet to identify pancreatic cancer early enough such that early treatment can make a difference in outcome. Other screening tests can result in significant harms. For example, false-positive screening tests for cancer can lead to invasive diagnostic biopsies, repeat imaging and radiation exposure, and significant mental stress. Other tests have significant costs, such as colonoscopy, which may limit their usefulness across a large population. Usually, randomized controlled trials are necessary to prove that screening tests lead to reduced morbidity and mortality without excessive harms. It is important for mental health providers to consider these principles as they apply them to a large population.

Recommended Guidelines for Preventive Care

To find preventive practice recommendations, a practicing provider can perform a simple Web or PubMed search for the condition in question. Widely used clinical preventive guidelines are published by government organizations, specialty groups (e.g., American College of Physicians, American Psychiatric Association), disease-specific organizations (e.g., American Cancer Society), care systems or insurance plans (e.g., Veterans Affairs, Blue Cross), and many other groups (e.g., Institute for Clinical Systems Improvement, National Quality Forum). The National Guideline Clearinghouse, which was created by the Agency for Healthcare Research and Quality, provides a searchable database for evidence-based guidelines on thousands of conditions (www.guideline.gov). This site requires guidelines to have been developed, reviewed, or revised in the past 5 years, which helps avoid using outdated recommendations.

There are often many and differing preventive guidelines for a given condition. Selecting the "best" guideline can be a challenge and often is up to a given clinician based on perspective and practice style. One important consideration is the grading of recommendations that should be included in any evidence-based guidelines. The grading system should take into account the quality and amount of evidence supporting an intervention, as well as an assessment of the likelihood that the benefits of an intervention will outweigh the undesirable effects.

One example of a grading system, that of the U.S. Preventive Services Task Force (USPSTF), is shown in Table 2–2, but other grading systems are also available. The USPSTF, created in 1984, produces many recommendation statements over the broad spectrum of preventive care. The USPSTF tends to be conservative in its recommendations, meaning that it requires solid scientific evidence of benefit before it recommends a given service. Specialty- or disease-specific groups (e.g., American Cancer Society) tend to be less conservative in this regard and sometimes will recommend preventive services based on expert opinion but without definitive supportive evidence. Table 2–3 provides some common resources for preventive practice guidelines.

Models for Implementing Preventive Care in Practice

A final topic that bears discussion is how to implement a multitude of preventive care activities in a busy practice. Two models commonly used by primary care practices could be adopted by psychiatric care providers. The first is the comprehensive annual physical examination, in which the patient has a visit once per year and all preventive services are provided, including history and examinations in the office, ordering of screening tests, and counseling on lifestyle measures. This often is a long visit, but it saves time on subsequent office visits, because prevention issues are postponed until the next annual examination.

In the second model, the clinician systematically does a small amount of preventive care at each visit. For example, a pneumococcal vaccine may be given at one visit, a referral for a screening colonoscopy at the second visit, and a referral for a diabetic eye examination at the third. This model works well for patients with conditions for which they must see their doctor regularly, such as diabetes or heart disease. Because patients with significant men-

TABLE 2–2. U.S. Preventive Services Task Force (USPSTF) grading system

Grade	Definition	Suggestions for practice
A	The USPSTF recommends the service. There is high certainty that the net benefit is substantial.	Offer or provide this service.
B	The USPSTF recommends the service. There is high certainty that the net benefit is moderate or there is moderate certainty that the net benefit is moderate to substantial.	Offer or provide this service.
C	The USPSTF recommends selectively offering or providing this service to individual patients based on professional judgment and patient preferences. There is at least moderate certainty that the net benefit is small.	Offer or provide this service for selected patients depending on individual circumstances.
D	The USPSTF recommends against the service. There is moderate or high certainty that the service has no net benefit or that the harms outweigh the benefits.	Discourage the use of this service.
I Statement	The USPSTF concludes that the current evidence is insufficient to assess the balance of benefits and harms of the service. Evidence is lacking, of poor quality, or conflicting, and the balance of benefits and harms cannot be determined.	Read the clinical considerations section of the USPSTF recommendation statement. If the service is offered, patients should understand the uncertainty about the balance of benefits and harms.

Source. U.S. Preventive Services Task Force Grade Definitions. July 2012. http://www.uspreventiveservicestaskforce.org/uspstf/grades.htm.

TABLE 2–3. **Commonly used resources for preventive care recommendations**

Advisory Committee on Immunization Practices: Immunization recommendations for adults and children from the Centers for Disease Control and Prevention

  http://www.cdc.gov/vaccines/hcp/acip-recs/index.html

  Adult immunization schedules: http://www.cdc.gov/vaccines/schedules/hcp/adult.html

American Cancer Society: Recommendations for cancer screening

  http://www.cancer.org/healthy/findcancerearly/cancerscreeningguidelines/american-cancer-society-guidelines-for-the-early-detection-of-cancer

American Diabetes Association: Clinical Practice Recommendations for treatment of diabetic patients, including multiple preventive measures

  http://professional.diabetes.org/ResourcesForProfessionals.aspx?cid=84160

American Heart Association: Guidelines for treating common cardiovascular diseases, including many prevention guidelines.

  http://my.americanheart.org/professional/StatementsGuidelines/ByTopic/ByTopics_UCM_316895_Article.jsp

Institute for Clinical Systems Improvement: Evidence-based recommendations for preventive services and disease-specific guidelines

  Preventive services for adults: https://www.icsi.org/_asset/gtjr9h/PrevServAdults.pdf

  Guidelines: https://www.icsi.org/guidelines__more

U.S. Preventive Services Task Force: Rigorous evidence-based recommendations for screening, counseling, preventive medications, and immunizations

  http://www.uspreventiveservicestaskforce.org/recommendations.htm

tal illness see their psychiatric providers quite regularly, this system would potentially work well for them. It does not work as well for healthy patients who may not see their physician regularly. They may go years between visits and miss many opportunities for preventive care. For such infrequent visitors, a reminder system is a must to get people to periodic prevention visits. Regardless of the model used, a preventive care reminder tool in the patient's chart (paper or electronic) listing age- and disease-appropriate primary, secondary, and tertiary preventive care measures is an essential quick-reference tool to keep tabs on what is done and what needs to be done.

Final Thoughts

Behavioral health providers (BHPs) for patients with significant mental illness often have more contact with their patients than do non-BHPs. In many instances, BHPs may be their patients' only contact with the health system. Thus, they can be a key part of helping patients receive essential preventive care.

BHPs and the clinics or systems where they work should determine what preventive care they can do and what care they are going to defer to another provider. Even if the BHPs will not be doing the preventive care themselves, a process should be implemented to connect patients with providers who can do it. This often entails using or establishing networks with primary care providers or systems that cater to underserved populations (e.g., county clinic systems). If a BHP is performing preventive care, a system to track the information must be in place. Lastly, there must be excellent communication between primary providers and the BHPs to avoid duplication of efforts and ensure appropriate follow-up of abnormal results. This improved communication is a big, but achievable, challenge. It lies at the core of integrated care.

BHPs are in a unique position to develop and oversee a plan to partner with patients and primary care providers, with the goal of addressing significant and often lethal health disparities found in those with mental illness. For this to happen, BHPs must use an evidence-based practice pattern that includes assessment and prevention of common cardiopulmonary, metabolic, and oncological disorders and infectious diseases. True integration of primary care and behavioral health must include longitudinal cross-education (as well as large-scale changes in health care policy), with an emphasis on decreasing morbidity and all-cause mortality in those who have mental illness.

CHAPTER 3

Cultural Considerations in Psychiatry

Alan Koike, M.D., M.S.H.S.
Hendry Ton, M.D., M.S.

Case Discussion

Mr. X, a 40-year-old English-speaking Chinese man with schizophrenia and poorly controlled diabetes mellitus undergoing insulin treatment, was admitted to an inpatient psychiatric facility for disorganized thoughts and aggressive behavior toward his parents. On admission, his hemoglobin A_{1c} was 8.7 (≤ 7.0 is a target for diabetic management). Over the course of his hospital stay, his psychotic symptoms improved, but he had poor adherence to his diabetic treatment. The treatment team managed his diabetes with education, oral medications, and insulin, in consultation with an internist. These interventions had limited efficacy because the patient adamantly maintained that he did not have diabetes. He refused to take diabetic medications, and his blood glucose remained poorly controlled.

Clinical Overview

Knowing the cultural context of patients' illnesses and experiences is fundamental to effective prevention strategies. Ethnic minority populations are growing rapidly in the United States (Smedley et al. 2004). According to the Institute of Medicine's report *Unequal Treatment* (Smedley et al. 2002), racial and ethnic minorities receive lower quality of care than nonminorities, resulting in worse outcomes and increased mortality. The Surgeon General, in *Mental Health: Culture, Race, and Ethnicity* (U.S. Department of Health and Human Services 2001), reported that minorities have less access to and receive a lower quality of mental health services.

Ignoring a patient's cultural perspective can result in adverse consequences in areas of prevention, such as less preventive screening and delayed immunizations (Flores et al. 2002). Comas-Díaz (2012) recommends adopting a multicultural care perspective. A multicultural approach starts with the desire to work with patients of diverse cultural backgrounds. It requires understanding the patient's perspective, developing the therapeutic relationship, and adapting one's approach to meet the patient's needs. It is a reciprocal learning experience that requires self-reflection and continuous assessment. This perspective incorporates the concept of *cultural humility,* which starts not with the patient's belief system but rather with the health care provider's beliefs and assumptions about and goals related to the encounter (Trevalon and Murray-Garcia 1998). The mnemonic "CREATE cultural competence" may be helpful to clinicians who wish to consistently improve clinical skills at the intersection of culture and medicine (Table 3–1).

The Outline for Cultural Formulation

Many mental health providers recognize the importance of cultural issues but feel ill equipped to address these concerns in adopting preventive health measures. Mere factual knowledge about cultural groups has limited utility without a framework to understand that information. The Outline for Cultural Formulation (OCF), first introduced in DSM-IV (American Psychiatric Association 1994) and revised for DSM-5 (American Psychiatric Association 2013), provides a systematic approach for assessing the impact of culture on illness and treatment. Although designed for the psychiatric encounter, the OCF may be used for preventive strategies as well. The OCF comprises five components: 1) cultural identity of the patient, 2) cultural conceptualizations of distress, 3) psychosocial stressors and cultural features of vulnerability and resilience, 4) cultural features of the relationship between the individual and the clinician, and 5) overall cultural assessment.

Cultural Identity of the Patient

Cultural identity describes the multiple overlapping sets of identities that contribute to an individual's understanding of who he or she is and how he or she fits into the world. Although race and ethnicity are often considered important parts of cultural identity, other factors such as religious and spiritual views, gender, sexual orientation, disabilities, and socioeconomic status may be as or more important in any given person. Clinicians can gain a greater

---
TABLE 3–1.   CREATE cultural competence

Collaborate with a cultural broker when encountering complex, culturally influenced medical situations.

Reflect on your own cultural beliefs and how they may affect the treatment plan.

Empathize with the patient's cultural belief system, even if you do not fully understand or agree with a particular belief or related behavior.

Ancillary staff should be trained about CREATE, as they are often the first and last to interact with patients at each medical encounter.

Timing of specific culturally related stressors to illness may help the provider conceptualize and diagnose the clinical problem more accurately.

Educate yourself about commonly encountered cultures (e.g., religions and ethnicities).

---

understanding of the patient as a whole person by learning about cultural identities.

Cultural Conceptualizations of Distress

Cultural conceptualizations of distress describe the constructs that shape the person's understanding and experience of his or her problems or symptoms. These constructs affect how an individual's symptoms are expressed and communicated. Individuals may have explanations for their illnesses that differ greatly from traditional or mainstream medical practice. Mental health providers should attempt to elicit each patient's beliefs about and understanding of his or her illness (Kleinman 1989).

Psychosocial Stressors and Cultural Features of Vulnerability and Resilience

Psychosocial stressors and cultural features of vulnerability and resilience are the key stressors and supports in an individual's life. Patients do not exist in a vacuum, and it is important to understand the role that family, religion, and other social groups play in the individual's functioning.

Cultural Features of the Relationship Between the Individual and the Clinician

Cultural misunderstandings, stereotyping, and conflicting views of illness and treatment can affect the patient-provider relationship. Identifying differences in language, culture, and social status can help avoid breakdowns in communication. Past experiences of racism and discrimination can affect trust and the therapeutic relationship. The clinician needs to honestly examine his or her own cultural identity, beliefs, assumptions, and biases.

Overall Cultural Assessment

The overall cultural assessment summarizes the clinical implications of the issues identified in the previous four sections of the OCF. Preventive strategies should identify and address culturally related problems and build on cultural strengths.

The DSM-5 OCF can help identify the cultural factors that interplay with a person's health. An important addition in DSM-5 is the Cultural Formulation Interview (CFI), a set of 16 questions that providers may use during an assessment. The CFI has been field-tested for practicality and for acceptability with patients. From our experience, we have found the CFI to be a bit long and unwieldy. Therefore, in Table 3–2, we provide a shorter version of the CFI, consisting of what we believe to be eight high-yield questions.

Case Discussion (*continued*)

A cultural consultation was obtained in the hopes of improving Mr. X's management of his diabetes. The cultural consultant, a psychiatrist, used the OCF to assess the situation.

Cultural Identity of the Patient. The consultant determined that Mr. X identified with being ethnically Chinese. His family lived in the mountains of southern China until they immigrated to the United States in 1981. As an immigrant in a U.S. community with limited diversity, the patient was bullied and socially ostracized because of his ethnicity, heavily accented speech, and small stature during adolescence. He coped psychologically by distancing himself from self-concepts of frailty and defended himself physically by learning martial arts. Hence, when confronted with the diagnosis of diabetes, particularly during a hospitalization when he felt vulnerable and isolated, the patient became defensive and disengaged.

Cultural Conceptualizations of Distress. The cultural consultant explored Mr. X's health maintenance beliefs, which appeared to be strongly consistent with traditional Chinese beliefs. The patient relied heavily on concepts of martial discipline, including daily practice of technically challenging physical maneuvers and attention to diet to maintain physical balance. Although he recognized the important role of psychotropics for the treatment of his mental health condition, he disputed that Western medicine had any role in the maintenance of what he argued to be good physical health.

Psychosocial Stressors and Cultural Features of Vulnerability and Resilience. Mr. X experienced significant sociocultural isolation in the community and during hospitalization in a psychiatric facility. His parents had informed the treatment team that they had relocated to a different city

TABLE 3–2. **Cultural Formulation Interview**

Cultural Definition of the Problem

1. What troubles you most about your problem?

Cultural Perceptions of Cause, Context, and Support

2. Why do you think this is happening to you? What do you think are the causes of your [PROBLEM]?

3. Are there any kinds of supports that make your [PROBLEM] better, such as from family, friends, or others?

4. Are there any kinds of stresses that make your [PROBLEM] worse, such as difficulties with money, or family problems?

Role of Cultural Identity

Sometimes, aspects of people's background or identity can make the [PROBLEM] better or worse. By *background* or *identity*, I mean, for example, the communities you belong to, the languages you speak, where you or your family are from, your race or ethnic background, your gender or sexual orientation, and your faith or religion.

5. For you, what are the most important aspects of your background or identity?

Cultural Factors Affecting Self-Coping and Past Help Seeking

6. Sometimes people have various ways of dealing with problems like [PROBLEM]. What have you done on your own to cope with your [PROBLEM]?

7. Has anything prevented you from getting the help you need?

8. What kinds of help would be most useful to you at this time for your [PROBLEM]?

Source. Adapted from American Psychiatric Association 2013.

and no longer wished to have contact with their son. Because of his mental illness, the patient was also shunned in his ethnic community—a challenge experienced by many mental health patients, but particularly by ethnic minorities, who also experience barriers connecting to mental health consumer groups. While hospitalized, the patient had limited contact with others of similar cultural background, compounding his sense of isolation and vulnerability. However, the patient was clearly proud of his martial arts background and used this to relate to others in the unit, albeit superficially.

Cultural Features of the Relationship Between the Individual and the Clinician. Given his strong connection to his culture of origin, the prior history of racial bullying, and his current experiences of sociocultural isolation, it was not surprising that Mr. X brightened and readily engaged with the cultural consultant, an Asian American psychiatrist. The patient eagerly inquired about the consultant's cultural background. The consultant chose to disclose this, recognizing the patient's need to feel culturally connected and understanding the important role that this would have in building a therapeutic relationship. The consultant subsequently began to explore the patient's health and health maintenance beliefs.

Overall Cultural Assessment. Using the OCF, the cultural consultant recognized that Mr. X's denial of his diabetes appeared to be strongly influenced by several factors: 1) The patient had had limited exposure to Western health concepts, such as diabetes, and by default tended to understand health using a more traditional Chinese framework. 2) Attempts to educate the patient about the Western concept of diabetes might unintentionally force the patient to confront his own physical frailty, particularly in light of his having been physically bullied and now being abandoned by his family and community. 3) He seemed to regard the providers who had tried to educate him as outsiders who were uninterested in his perspectives, and hence he was disinclined to consider theirs. Based on this formulation, the consultant postulated that he needed to introduce a health maintenance model that would meaningfully draw on Western and Eastern concepts of health, while also drawing on the patient's recognized strengths. He also believed that the cultural confluences in their relationship, although not essential, would nevertheless facilitate this process.

Mr. X was encouraged to adhere to a diabetic diet by associating it with traditional Chinese health beliefs. Hyperglycemic symptoms are often associated with "hot symptoms" (i.e., dry mouth, loss of water due to polyuria), which are more culturally understandable. Diabetic diets can be framed as foods that promote coolness. In many Asian cultures, sugars are associated with hot or drying effects. In this case, the patient responded much more favorably to the following comment from the provider: "When your blood sugar is too high, your body becomes hotter and drier, causing you to feel weak and dry and to lose too much water through your urine. The recommended foods help to naturally promote a cooler body, and avoiding the less healthy foods will also help the body keep a healthy balance between hot and cold." Insulin was introduced as another way to effectively promote coolness, but the consultant explained that it needed to be used with skill and discipline to avoid causing too much coolness, resulting in weakness, lethargy, and shaking, and even permanent harm. Mr. X came to regard the attributes needed for self-injection as similar to those needed for martial arts practice. After the consultation, the patient became amenable to self-injection of subcutaneous insulin at night. At follow-up 4 months later, the patient's hemoglobin A_{1c} was 5.5, and he was still able to self-administer his insulin injections.

Final Thoughts

Culturally competent medical care involves all patient encounters, as each patient is unique and has multiple cultural identities that do not exclusively relate to race or ethnicity. The diagnosis and treatment plan should consistently reflect important cultural considerations for each patient. The mnemonic CREATE cultural competence can be routinely used by the provider to effectively address cultural issues in the medical or psychiatric setting.

Resources

The Joint Commission: Advancing Effective Communication, Cultural Competence, and Patient- and Family-Centered Care: A Roadmap for Hospitals. Oakbrook Terrace, IL, April 2014. Available at: http://www.jointcommission.org/roadmap_for_hospitals.

Perin B: Phrases of Courtesy in Nine Languages: A Tool for Medical Providers. Seattle, WA, University of Washington School of Medicine, 2013. Available at: http://ethnomed.org/clinical/communication/phrases-of-courtesy-in-nine-languages-a-tool-for-providers.

Think Cultural Health: http://www.thinkculturalhealth.org.

U.S. Department of Health and Human Services Office of Minority Health: http://minorityhealth.hhs.gov.

References

American Psychiatric Association: Diagnostic and Statistical Manual of Mental Disorders, 4th Edition. Washington, DC, American Psychiatric Association, 1994

American Psychiatric Association: Diagnostic and Statistical Manual of Mental Disorders, 5th Edition. Washington, DC, American Psychiatric Association, 2013

Comas-Díaz L: Multicultural Care: A Clinician's Guide to Cultural Competence. Washington, DC, American Psychological Association, 2012, pp 4–5

Flores G, Rabke-Verani J, Pine W, et al: The importance of cultural and linguistic issues in the emergency care of children. Pediatr Emerg Care 18:271–284, 2002

Kleinman A: The Illness Narratives: Suffering, Healing, and the Human Condition. New York, Basic Books, 1989, pp 43–44

Smedley BD, Stith AY, Nelson AR (eds): Unequal Treatment: Confronting Racial and Ethnic Disparities in Health Care. Washington, DC, National Academies Press, 2002

Smedley BD, Butler AS, Bristow LR (eds): In the Nation's Compelling Interest: Ensuring Diversity in the Health Care Workforce. Committee on Institutional and Policy-Level Strategies for Increasing the Diversity of the U.S. Health Care Workforce. Washington, DC, National Academies Press, 2004

Trevalon M, Murray-Garcia J: Cultural humility versus cultural competence: a critical distinction in defining physician training outcomes in multicultural education. J Health Care Poor Underserved 9:117–125, 1998

U.S. Department of Health and Human Services: Mental Health: Culture, Race, and Ethnicity: A Supplement to Mental Health: A Report of the Surgeon General. Rockville, MD, US Department of Health and Human Services, Public Health Service, Office of the Surgeon General, 2001

CHAPTER 4

Preventive Medicine and Psychiatric Training Considerations

Deborah S. Cowley, M.D.
Robert M. McCarron, D.O.

Clinical Overview

Psychiatric patients with severe, chronic mental illness have higher rates of medical comorbidity and lower life expectancies than the general population. Many such individuals are seen in community mental health settings and have poor access to or do not seek effective primary and preventive health care. The treating psychiatrist becomes the de facto primary care physician for these patients and is well positioned to ensure that they receive preventive health screenings, as well as diagnosis and treatment of medical conditions.

In this chapter we discuss the current state of psychiatric education in primary medical and preventive health care, review outcomes of existing training experiences that integrate primary medical care rotations into the psychiatric curriculum, and suggest possible curricular changes in psychiatry residency and fellowship education in order to teach psychiatrists how to optimize the medical care of their patients.

The evidence for the need for improved medical care for people with severe, chronic mental illnesses is compelling. For example, a 17-year follow-up
study of more than 80,000 people in the United States showed that those with
mental disorders died an average of 8.2 years earlier than the rest of the population, with excess mortality due primarily to socioeconomic factors, poor
access to effective primary care and preventive health care, and chronic health
conditions (Druss et al. 2011). Individuals diagnosed with schizophrenia die
20–30 years earlier than other people (Saha et al. 2007), whereas those with bipolar disorder have a twofold higher mortality rate (Crump et al. 2013). Earlier mortality in these studies is not attributable to higher rates of suicide alone,
with most deaths being due to natural causes, primarily cardiovascular disease. Patients with depression are also at higher risk of medical illness and have
a significantly increased risk of myocardial infarction (Van der Kooy et al.
2007). Of note, earlier detection of medical illness in psychiatric patients has
been shown to decrease mortality (Crump et al. 2013).

Integrated Training Experiences

Such findings of lower life expectancies for people with severe, chronic mental illnesses have led to calls for psychiatrists to use their medical skills. However, the Accreditation Council for Graduate Medical Education (ACGME)
requires that psychiatry residents complete only 4 months of "primary care"
(medicine, family medicine, or pediatrics) training and that this be in the first
year of training. Residents frequently complete all or part of this requirement
on inpatient services, with little experience in preventive care or common
outpatient medical conditions. Even when outpatient rotations are included,
trainees are unlikely to remember what they have learned later in residency
or after graduation. Practicing psychiatrists rarely perform medical evaluations or physical examinations on their patients. At the same time, the ACGME
psychiatry milestones for residency training include specific milestones regarding performing physical and neurological examinations and screening
for, evaluating, diagnosing, and ensuring treatment of medical illnesses in psychiatric patients (Accreditation Council for Graduate Medical Education and
American Board of Psychiatry and Neurology 2013).

To date, clinical rotations for psychiatry residents that focus on providing primary medical care for patients with chronic mental illness have been
located primarily in Veterans Affairs (VA) settings. Two such rotations have
reported outcomes. Patients at the Portland VA receiving both medical and
psychiatric care from a single senior psychiatry resident reported high levels
of satisfaction with their care. Compared with control patients matched for
age, gender, psychiatric diagnosis, and medical burden, there were no differences in psychiatric symptom burden, active medical problems, or screen-

ing rates for preventive health over the course of a year (Snyder et al. 2008). Residents completing this elective psychiatry–primary medical care rotation, providing both medical and psychiatric care for patients, reported feeling more prepared than their peers to address medical problems in their patients and greater comfort in knowing when to refer patients for medical care. However, they were not more likely to perform medical evaluations or treat medical problems after graduation (Dobscha et al. 2005). For residents working in another VA psychiatry–primary care program, heightened awareness of the importance of medical comorbidities in psychiatric patients and collaboration with primary care providers (PCPs) did not translate into incorporating primary care practices or electing to provide medical as well as psychiatric care to a panel of patients (Rohrbaugh et al. 2009).

The fact that residents who chose elective rotations, and were presumably particularly interested in the psychiatry-medicine interface, did not go on to perform medical evaluations or provide primary care for their psychiatric patients raises questions: How realistic is it to expect psychiatrists to take on this role? What educational goals should be required for psychiatry residents, in order to improve medical care for chronically mentally ill individuals? These questions lead to more questions: Should psychiatry residencies and public psychiatry fellowships aim to train psychiatrists to deliver primary medical care? Should the goal be instead to teach trainees to screen for and identify medical illness and coordinate care with PCPs? Or should psychiatrists be trained to work in interdisciplinary teams providing integrated mental health and medical care, with a role focusing more on enhancing patient motivation for seeking and adhering to medical care, collaborating with medical providers, and providing team leadership and oversight?

Residents in combined training programs—that is, internal medicine–psychiatry, family medicine–psychiatry, or pediatrics–psychiatry–child and adolescent psychiatry residencies—are ideally prepared to provide primary medical care to patients with chronic, severe mental illness and to lead teams delivering integrated mental health and medical care. Despite earlier concerns that physicians with combined training were practicing only one specialty, more recent data show that the majority of graduates practice both specialties, and over two-thirds of internal medicine–psychiatry and family medicine–psychiatry graduates are active in integrated mental health and primary medical care (Jain et al. 2012). Combined training and board certification in both psychiatry and a primary care field provides the background and expertise for these physicians to treat psychiatric and medical conditions within their scope of practice. However, given the limited number of combined training programs and graduates, it is not possible for these physicians to meet the demand for medical treatment for patients with chronic mental illness.

Research studies have demonstrated success in improving medical outcomes in the mental health sector using a variety of approaches that may inform how psychiatrists should be trained. For example, in a study of 407 patients at an urban community mental health center, those assigned a nurse care manager were more likely to have a PCP, received a higher percentage of recommended preventive and cardiometabolic services, and had better scores on the Framingham Cardiovascular Risk Index after 12 months (Druss et al. 2010). Nurse care managers provided health education, motivational interviewing, coaching about how to interact effectively with PCPs, referrals, communication with PCPs, and assistance with systems barriers. A number of studies within the VA system have shown improved health outcomes when medical services are colocated within mental health clinics. For example, having a PCP present within a mental health service for seriously mentally ill VA patients with poor or no engagement with primary care resulted in an increase in primary care visits and improved goal attainment for blood pressure, lipids, and body mass index after 6 months (Pirraglia et al. 2012). In another model, patients with depression and chronic illness (coronary heart disease, diabetes, or both) were managed by a team that included a nurse care manager, primary care physician, consulting psychiatrist, and psychologist. Compared with control patients receiving usual care, patients in the intervention group had significantly improved glycosylated hemoglobin, lipids, blood pressure, depression scores, and satisfaction with care at 12 months (Katon et al. 2010).

Targeted Integrated Training for Residents

There appear to be several potential targets for training psychiatrists to ensure adequate medical care for their patients. These include education about preventive care, screening, and identification of common medical problems; training in collaboration with PCPs and interdisciplinary care teams; and education about systems issues and barriers so that psychiatrists can provide or oversee advocacy and assistance to patients in navigating the health care system. With the implementation of the 2010 Patient Protection and Affordable Care Act (P.L. 111-148), as well as the increasing focus on integration of mental health and primary medical care, it has become especially important that psychiatry residents learn to work in integrated care systems as members or leaders of interdisciplinary teams with the common goal of improving mental health and medical outcomes in an evidence-based and cost-effective manner.

Currently, there is no evidence regarding the best way to provide this training to psychiatry residents and fellows, and the effectiveness of curricular changes will need to be studied. However, there are several possible approaches that could be considered, including clinical rotations, didactics, interdisciplinary case conferences, and projects. These are summarized in Table 4–1.

Some educators (e.g., Wright 2009) have suggested distributing primary care rotations throughout residency instead of limiting them to the first postgraduate year. This change in training could lead to improved retention of skills and knowledge, especially if residents applied knowledge of prevention and primary care medicine to their own patients, ideally in settings such as community mental health centers or other clinical services for chronically and severely mentally ill patients who are most in need of medical attention. Such longitudinal primary care rotations would require supervision either by both psychiatry and primary care faculty or by supervisors with combined training. In addition, implementing such a rotation would require faculty development for psychiatry faculty, both to update their knowledge of preventive and basic primary care and to provide a rationale for the training model. Such a longitudinal primary care rotation might be especially valuable for residents planning a career in public psychiatry or integrated care.

Joint didactics, case conferences, and/or quality improvement projects with residents in primary care specialties and with other mental health and primary care trainees could increase awareness and understanding of the perspectives, expertise, and roles of other providers in an interprofessional team.

Most integrated care clinical rotations currently offered within psychiatry residencies do not focus on providing medical care within the mental health sector but instead train psychiatry residents to work as consultants within primary care settings. Usually, residents are colocated in a primary care clinic and see patients who are referred by PCPs for evaluation and recommendations regarding mental health conditions, under the supervision of the consulting faculty psychiatrist. In some cases, trainees work in population-based models such as collaborative care, where their primary goal is to serve as a consultant to a population of patients. Collaborative care includes systematic screening for mental health conditions, initial interventions by nonpsychiatrist mental health care managers, systematic tracking of clinical outcomes, and increasing intensity of mental health interventions with the severity of the disorder and nonresponse to initial interventions. For example, patients responding well to antidepressant treatment for depression would not be seen by a psychiatrist or psychologist, whereas those not responding would receive progressively more time- and cost-intensive interventions, such as in-person consultation with a psychiatrist, pharmacological augmentation strategies, and evidence-based psychosocial interventions. Multiple studies have shown that collaborative care improves depressive

TABLE 4–1. Proposed educational experiences in preventive and primary care for psychiatry residents

Type of experience	Description	Educational goals
Clinical rotations in preventive and primary care	Change some or all of PGY-1 primary care requirement to outpatient settings	Knowledge and skills in preventive and outpatient primary care
	Longitudinal outpatient preventive and primary care rotation in some or all of PGY-3 and PGY-4 in community mental health or other mental health setting treating chronically, severely ill psychiatric patients	Knowledge and skills in preventive and outpatient primary care Application of knowledge and skills to care of chronically and severely ill psychiatric patients
Clinical rotations in integrated care	Psychiatric consultation colocated in primary care outpatient clinic	Skills in collaboration and communication with primary care providers, working as a clinical and educational consultant
	Collaborative care rotation	Knowledge and skills in population-based care, supervising care managers, and working as a member and leader of an interprofessional team
Didactics	Didactics about preventive care; screening, diagnosis, and treatment of common medical problems	Knowledge of preventive care; screening, diagnosis, and treatment of common medical problems
	Didactics about the health care system; access and barriers to effective medical care for psychiatric patients	Knowledge of systems issues affecting access to and quality of medical care for psychiatric patients

TABLE 4–1. Proposed educational experiences in preventive and primary care for psychiatry residents (*continued*)

Type of experience	Description	Educational goals
Case conferences	Joint case conferences with primary care residents and/or other mental health and primary care providers and trainees	Case-based collaboration and communication with primary care providers and interprofessional team members
Projects	Quality improvement projects focusing on improving medical care for psychiatric patients	Knowledge and skills in quality improvement and addressing systems issues and barriers to care
Other training	Motivational interviewing	Skill in enhancing patient motivation to seek medical care and make lifestyle changes
	Advocacy	Skill in helping patients navigate the health care system, advocating for overall system change

Note. PGY = postgraduate year.

symptoms, treatment adherence, remission rates, quality of life, functional status, and patient satisfaction with care in primary care settings. Rotations as a psychiatric consultant within a primary care clinic or collaborative care model do not address medical care for patients seen primarily within the mental health sector but do provide valuable experience working with PCPs and interprofessional teams.

Other educational experiences might include didactics about systems issues, such as the need for a common electronic medical record to facilitate communication between mental health and primary care, financial barriers, referral sources, and access to care. Education in motivational interviewing and advocacy would likely help residents to motivate patients to seek primary medical care and assist them with systems barriers. Table 4–2 provides a more detailed example of how integrated care may be included in the 4-year psychiatric curriculum.

Final Thoughts

Given the significantly increased mortality among psychiatric patients as a result of medical conditions, it is important to educate psychiatry residents so that they can ensure that their patients receive needed and effective medical care. This effort may involve teaching residents to perform preventive medical care, help patients with lifestyle changes such as tobacco cessation or weight management, and/or diagnose and treat common medical problems. Alternatively, psychiatrists may be called on to oversee medical care delivery within mental health settings and collaborate with PCPs as part of interprofessional teams. As a basic goal, psychiatrists can improve medical care for their patients through screening for and recognition of conditions requiring medical care and through effective coordination with PCPs. With the implementation of integrated care and increasing attention to medical comorbidity and mortality in psychiatric patients, educators have an opportunity to develop and study curricula to best train future psychiatrists and benefit patients.

It is essential to make evidence-based changes to the psychiatric educational infrastructure that correspond to and support significant changes to the mental health delivery system. Psychiatry trainees must receive training that better approximates current and real-world clinical practice. We believe the best way to accomplish this is to require learners to have longitudinal clinical and didactic experiences that emphasize the importance of behavioral health–primary care integration by using a multidisciplinary, team-based approach to patient care.

TABLE 4–2.	Integrated curriculum for residency training
Postgraduate year	Proposed integrated curriculum for psychiatry residents
PGY-1	Minimum of 4 months of primary care medicine.
	• Intensive care clinical experiences are not recommended.
	• Preferred experiences include complexity intervention or "med-psych units," primary care or urgent care sites serving patients with high BH needs, and primary care sites with strong multidisciplinary teams.
	During all 4 years of training, initial physical examinations and assessments of all general medical complaints made by patients in a psychiatric hospital should be done by the psychiatry resident.
	Longitudinal didactics related to primary and secondary prevention of common general medical disorders.
PGY-2	One half-day per week of brief psychotherapy and psychiatric medication management in the primary care setting.
	• Focus on a practical introduction to supportive psychotherapy, motivational interviewing, and cognitive behavioral therapy is recommended.
	• Setting may include colocated BH services in primary care, collaborative care sites, or (less preferably) physically separate BH and primary care sites with enhanced access and communication.
	Longitudinal didactics related to primary and secondary prevention of common general medical disorders.
	Longitudinal didactics related to performing "primary care psychiatry" consultation-liaison and/or collaborative care in the primary care setting.
	• Clinical assessments based on AMPS screening.
	Didactics in quality- and practice-based improvement.
	• Completion of a quality improvement project related to BH care in a primary care setting is recommended.

TABLE 4–2.   Integrated curriculum for residency training (continued)

Postgraduate year	Proposed integrated curriculum for psychiatry residents
PGY-3	One half-day per week of primary care medicine, with a focus on providing primary and secondary prevention of common disorders.
	• The setting may be a colocated primary care site for the SPMI population, or a primary care site with a substantial BH population; select specialty sites might be considered depending on interests (such as HIV, geriatric, correctional medicine).
	• May include 2–4 hours per week as a consultant psychiatrist to primary care, development of education and training for primary care in psychiatry, or a collaborative care rotation.
	All or a portion of the 1 year of psychotherapy training can be done in the primary care or medical setting, with a focus on brief psychotherapies, such as motivational interviewing, cognitive-behavioral therapy, or problem-solving therapy.
	Longitudinal didactics related to primary and secondary prevention of common general medical disorders.
	Longitudinal didactics related to performing "primary care psychiatry" consultation–liaison and collaborative care in the primary care setting.
	• Clinical assessments based on AMPS screening are recommended.
	Didactics in quality- and practice-based improvement are recommended.
	• Completion of a quality improvement project related to improving primary care among BH patient panel is recommended.

TABLE 4–2. Integrated curriculum for residency training (*continued*)

Postgraduate year	Proposed integrated curriculum for psychiatry residents
PGY-4	One half-day per week of primary care medicine, with a focus on providing primary and secondary prevention of common disorders.
	• Preferred sites would include strong multidisciplinary teams, patient-centered care, and quality improvement. Two months of elective time in pain medicine, sleep medicine, or other specialties that have a strong interface with general psychiatry.
	Didactics in quality- and practice-based improvement.
	• Completion of a quality improvement project on improving BH–medical care integration with focus on the system of care and improving access, delivery, or transitions is recommended.

Note. AMPS = AMPS Psychiatric Assessment (**A**nxiety, **M**ood, **P**sychosis, **S**ubstance abuse) (see Chapter 27, "Pain Medicine in the Psychiatric Patient Population," for more discussion); BH = behavioral health; PGY = postgraduate year; SPMI = severe and persistently mentally ill.

References

Accreditation Council for Graduate Medical Education, American Board of Psychiatry and Neurology. The Psychiatry Milestone Project. November 2013. Available at: http://www.acgme.org/acgmeweb/Portals/0/PDFs/Milestones/PsychiatryMilestones.pdf. Accessed August 11, 2014.

Crump C, Sundquist K, Winkleby MA, et al: Comorbidities and mortality in bipolar disorder: a Swedish national cohort study. JAMA Psychiatry 70:931–939, 2013

Dobscha SK, Snyder K, Corson K, et al: Psychiatry resident graduate comfort with general medical issues: impact of an integrated psychiatry–primary medical care training track. Acad Psychiatry 29:448–451, 2005

Druss BG, von Esenwein SA, Compton MT, et al: A randomized trial of medical care management for community mental health settings: the Primary Care Access, Referral, and Evaluation (PCARE) study. Am J Psychiatry 167:151–159, 2010

Druss BG, Zhao L, von Esenwein S, et al: Understanding excess mortality in persons with mental illness: 17-year follow up of a nationally representative US survey. Med Care 49:599–604, 2011

Jain G, Dzara K, Gagliardi JP, et al: Assessing the practices and perceptions of dually trained physicians: a pilot study. Acad Psychiatry 36:71–73, 2012

Katon WJ, Lin EHB, Von Korff M, et al: Collaborative care for patients with depression and chronic illness. N Engl J Med 363:2611–2620, 2010

Patient Protection and Affordable Care Act of 2010, Pub. L. No. 111-148, 124 Stat. 119, 109–1024

Pirraglia PA, Rowland E, Wu W-C, et al: Benefits of a primary care clinic co-located and integrated in a mental health setting for veterans with serious mental illness. Prev Chronic Dis 9:E51, 2012

Rohrbaugh RM, Felker B, Kosten T: The VA psychiatry–primary care education initiative. Acad Psychiatry 33:31–36, 2009

Saha S, Chant D, McGrath J: A systematic review of mortality in schizophrenia: is the differential mortality gap worsening over time? Arch Gen Psychiatry 64:1123–1131, 2007

Snyder K, Dobscha SK, Ganzini L, et al: Clinical outcomes of integrated psychiatric and general medical care. Community Ment Health J 44:147–154, 2008

Van der Kooy K, van Hout H, Marwijk H, et al: Depression and the risk for cardiovascular diseases: systematic review and meta-analysis. Int J Geriatr Psychiatry 22:613–626, 2007

Wright MT: Training psychiatrists in nonpsychiatric medicine: what do our patients and our profession need? Acad Psychiatry 33:181–186, 2009

SECTION II

Cardiovascular and
Pulmonary Disorders
in the Psychiatric
Patient Population

CHAPTER 5

Coronary Artery Disease

Jane P. Gagliardi, M.D., M.H.S., F.A.C.P., F.A.P.A.
Lawson Wulsin, M.D.

Case Discussion

Ms. S is a 57-year-old black woman who has had infrequent contact with primary care providers but has been treated since age 25 for schizophrenia, for which she has been hospitalized multiple times and is now followed by an Assertive Community Treatment team. She smokes at least two packs of cigarettes per day and is obese. She is "mildly depressed" and says she would "sometimes rather not be on this earth."

Clinical Overview

In this chapter we discuss some of the direct and indirect associations between mental health and coronary artery disease (CAD), including an association between depression and CAD, mental stress, and cardiac ischemia. The development of CAD and CAD risk factors may arise directly or indirectly from mental illness or the treatment of mental illness. Cigarette smoking, obesity, hyperlipidemia, and decreased adherence to primary and secondary preventive measures may develop as part of the behavioral or biological features of a chronic mental illness or as side effects of its treatment.

Heart disease is the leading cause of death among men and women in the United States. Death rates from heart disease are shown in Figure 5–1 for

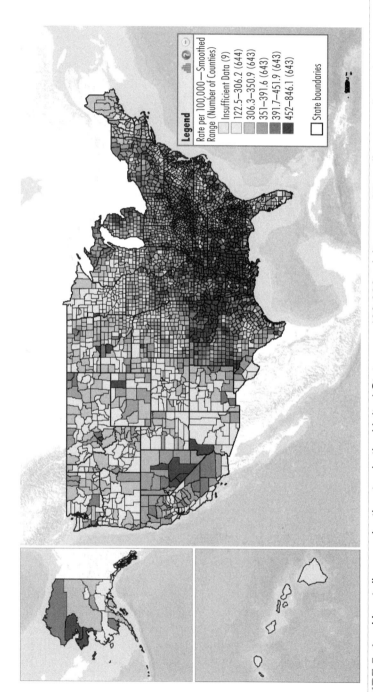

FIGURE 5–1. Heart disease death rates in the United States per 100,000 adults, ages 35+, all races, all genders, 2008–2010, by county.

Source. This map was created using the Interactive Atlas of Heart Disease and Stroke, a Web site developed by the Centers for Disease Control and Prevention, Division for Heart Disease and Stroke Prevention. Available at: http://www.cdc.gov/dhdsp/maps.

U.S. counties. CAD is the most common form of heart disease and was responsible for a reported one in six deaths in 2008 (Go et al. 2013) and a total of 385,000 deaths in the United States in 2009 (Centers for Disease Control and Prevention 2013). More than 770,000 deaths will be impacted by myocardial infarctions (fatal or nonfatal) on an annual basis (Moyer and U.S. Preventive Services Task Force 2012). Risk factor modification is widely recognized as an important strategy for decreasing morbidity and mortality from CAD (Bikdeli et al. 2013).

Health care providers may estimate 10- and 30-year CAD risks using various tools (e.g., the 10-year Framingham risk calculator, shown in Figure 5–2). Some risk factors, including gender, age, and family history, are not modifiable. Modifiable risks for CAD include hypertension, hypercholesterolemia, diabetes mellitus (DM), obesity, smoking, and sedentary lifestyle. Diabetes and absolute systolic blood pressure have the greatest impact on CAD risk.

Prognosis for CAD can be variable, ranging from full asymptomatic recovery to the development of ischemic cardiomyopathy, disability, and death. There are mixed reports on the impact of ethnicity and gender, although women are noted to present more frequently with atypical symptoms and small vessel disease. Patients with risk factors such as smoking, hypertension, hyperlipidemia, family history of early CAD, obesity, and sedentary lifestyle are at higher risk of complicated outcomes. Other medical problems, including DM, chronic kidney disease, chronic lung disease, and malignancy, have a negative impact on CAD outcomes (Fihn et al. 2012). Hypertension is linked to the development of left ventricular hypertrophy and diastolic heart failure, which have been associated with worse outcomes and coronary events (Desai et al. 2013). Other comorbid vascular diseases, such as peripheral arterial disease and cerebrovascular disease, confer increased risk of mortality for patients with CAD, as do physical limitations associated with symptomatic angina. Symptoms, functional capacity, and quality of life also are associated with survival and subsequent acute coronary events.

Psychiatric illness intersects with CAD in a number of ways. CAD and certain mental illnesses share risk factors; it is not clear whether there is a common underlying pathological process manifesting in both CAD and mental illness or whether there is a causal association (and, if so, in what direction it operates). Some mental illnesses, such as panic or anxiety disorders, share symptomatic features with angina and acute coronary syndrome (ACS). Clinical symptoms characteristic of depression (apathy, amotivation) and schizophrenia (disorganization, paranoia) may lead to poor self-care or impaired adherence to programs designed to lower CAD risk factors. Some mental illnesses, such as psychotic disorders, are associated with higher rates of smoking.

Risk Assessment Tool for Estimating Your 10-Year Risk of Having a Heart Attack

The risk assessment tool below uses information from the Framingham Heart Study to predict a person's chance of having a heart attack in the next 10 years. This tool is designed for adults aged 20 and older who do not have heart disease or diabetes. To find your risk score, enter your information in the calculator below.

Age:	☐ years
Gender:	⊙ Female ○ Male
Total Cholesterol:	☐ mg/dL
HDL Cholesterol:	☐ mg/dL
Smoker:	⊙ No ○ Yes
Systolic Blood Pressure:	☐ mmHg
Are you currently on any medication to treat high blood pressure?	⊙ No ○ Yes

[Calculate Your 10-Year Risk]

FIGURE 5–2.   The Framingham risk calculator.

Source.   National Heart, Lung, and Blood Institute: Risk Assessment Tool for Estimating Your 10-Year Risk of Having a Heart Attack, 2013. Available at: http://cvdrisk.nhlbi.nih.gov/calculator.asp. Accessed July 7, 2014.

Lower socioeconomic status in general is associated with poorer prognosis for CAD, as are specific individual risk factors of poor social support, poverty, and stress (Fihn et al. 2012). Lower socioeconomic status also is a risk factor for the development of depression (Gilman et al. 2002)—an interesting observation, especially in light of the growing body of evidence that links depression with CAD. In fact, some experts consider depression to be a stronger risk factor for myocardial infarction (MI) than traditional medical risk factors such as obesity, hypertension, and secondhand smoke (Pozuelo et al. 2009). In patients with ACS, clinical or subclinical depression has been found to be a strong independent predictor of worse survival, and anxiety may also play a role in poorer outcomes (Fihn et al. 2012). Patients with depression or anxiety may also experience more medical symptoms from the same degree of illness, and their quality of life may be worse than anticipated due to purely physical symptoms or limitations.

Up to 60% of premature deaths in patients with schizophrenia are attributable to medical illnesses (Griswold et al. 2010). Individuals with schizophrenia have a higher risk of coronary events than the general population (Darba et al. 2013). Patients with bipolar affective disorder die 8–9 years earlier than control subjects, with cardiovascular disease being one of the leading causes of death (Crump et al. 2013). Many attribute the exaggerated rate to impaired access to or underutilization of primary care; the very presence of mental illness may impair patients' adherence to evidence-based treatment recommendations or preventive strategies. Patients with severe chronic mental illness are more likely to experience higher morbidity and mortality related to CAD than are their counterparts without mental illness, and data demonstrate that individuals with mental illness have higher death rates and die younger than other members of the age-matched general population (Colton and Manderscheid 2006; Wildgust and Beary 2010). The impact of mental illness and the medications used to treat it are important areas for public health interventions (Newcomer and Hennekens 2007).

More than 30% of American adults are officially obese, as defined by a body mass index (BMI) greater than 30; rates of DM are rising; the incidence of metabolic syndrome (obesity, dyslipidemia, hypertension, and diabetes) exceeds 30%; and many Americans have a sedentary lifestyle (Lloyd-Jones et al. 2010). The rates of these same risk factors may be significantly higher among patients with severe and chronic persistent mental illness; for example, patients with schizophrenia smoke more, eat less healthfully, and participate less in behavioral modification that targets risk factors than do patients without schizophrenia (Davidson 2002; Dipasquale et al. 2013). Patients with chronic mental illness may be less physically active and more prone to developing obesity, other risk factors, and complications of CAD (Wildgust and Beary 2010). Improving the exercise capacity and overall physical fitness of patients with schizophrenia is an important strategy for modifying CAD risk (Strassnig et al. 2011).

The association between mental stress and cardiac symptomatology has been long known. Takotsubo cardiomyopathy, also known as "stress cardiomyopathy" or the "broken heart syndrome," is clinically indistinguishable from ACS except that Takotsubo cardiomyopathy usually resolves without sequelae (Prasad et al. 2008). Some studies suggest that the stress of mental illness contributes to pathogenesis of CAD (Osborn et al. 2008). Mechanisms implicated in the mind-heart connection include sympathetic activation, vagal deactivation, platelet activation, hypothalamic-pituitary-adrenocortical activity, and inflammatory mediators including cytokines and anticholinergic mechanisms. Mental stress itself has the capacity to induce coronary ischemia and may prompt coronary events at a rate that exceeds that of exercise-induced coronary ischemia. Mental stress–induced myocardial ischemia is reported to occur in as many as three-quarters of individuals with CAD and is associated with poorer outcomes (Jiang et al. 2013). Mental illness itself may, through mental stress, have an important pathophysiological role in CAD.

CAD is associated with a high rate of depression (Wheeler et al. 2013). Up to 40% of patients with CAD have clinically significant symptoms, and upwards of 20% of patients with CAD have symptoms that meet criteria for major depressive disorder; in contrast, 5%–10% of persons without CAD are estimated to have major depressive disorder (Huffman et al. 2013). Post-MI depression has been associated with higher rates of sudden cardiac death and worse outcomes (Khawaja et al. 2009). Anxiety also may portend worse outcomes from CAD (Wang et al. 2013), including higher all-cause mortality (Watkins et al. 2013). There is some hope but limited evidence that treatment of depression and anxiety, whether with antidepressant medications or behavioral therapies aimed at improving coping, may improve CAD outcomes (Chiavarino et al. 2012; Jiang et al. 2013).

Panic disorder may pose a particular challenge to health care providers, because symptoms of a panic attack closely mimic angina or ACS, and patients who present frequently with chest pain but for whom MI is ruled out are at risk of being categorized as having "noncardiac chest pain" any time they present. Although it can be tempting to disregard chest pain in a patient with known panic disorder, the patient experiencing panic-related chest pain may also be experiencing stress-induced myocardial ischemia (Soares-Filho et al. 2012).

Practical Pointers

- Many of the comorbidities associated with severe mental illness, such as smoking and low socioeconomic status, are also risk factors for coronary artery disease (CAD) events or a worse prognosis for CAD.
- Patients with CAD have a higher rate of major depressive disorder, with up to 40% having significant symptoms of depression.
- Atypical antipsychotic medications can cause metabolic syndrome, which increases CAD risk.

Diagnosis

CAD can present in a variety of ways, ranging from unrecognized or "silent" CAD through stable angina, unstable angina, ACS, or MI, to sudden cardiac death. Patients with silent CAD will present with electrocardiograms (ECGs) showing Q waves, indicating a prior MI, and account for up to 20% of MIs. There is an association between DM, hypertension, and unrecognized CAD. Stable patients may present with episodic chest pain or dyspnea on exertion. Subsequent diagnosis is usually made with a stress test (i.e., exercise ECG stress test, stress nuclear imaging, and stress echocardiogram). Patients with acute, active symptoms often present to the emergency room or physician's office, and CAD is diagnosed on the basis of electrocardiographic findings and/or cardiac enzyme elevations. Cardiac angiography is the gold standard for demonstrating atherosclerotic stenosis on imaging. Cardiac computed tomography (CT) can provide CT angiographic images showing stenosis or provide coronary artery calcium scores that can predict CAD risk.

Preventive Guidelines

Low (<10%), moderate (10%–20%), or high (>20%) 10-year risk of CAD can be ascertained using risk calculators, such as that available through the National Heart, Lung, and Blood Institute (http://cvdrisk.nhlbi.nih.gov/calculator.asp; Figure 5–2). The U.S. Preventive Services Task Force (USPSTF) recommends against screening with either resting or exercise ECGs for individuals suspected to be at low risk for CAD because the information provided by this testing does not add to the clinical risk assessment (Moyer and U.S. Preventive Services Task Force 2012). The USPSTF does not recommend for or against CAD screening in patients at moderate or elevated CAD risk because there is insufficient evidence that such screening would improve outcomes (Moyer and U.S. Preventive Services Task Force 2012). Many patients with CAD risk factors may benefit from risk factor reduction via lifestyle modifications and medication.

Lifestyle modification and attention to modifiable coronary risk factors are important primary prevention strategies. Dietary modifications, exercise, not smoking, and maintenance of normal BMI (<25) are associated with lower risk of CAD (Chiuve et al. 2011; Hartley et al. 2013). The Mediterranean diet has been associated with better cardiovascular outcomes, although patients do not always adhere to a high-fiber diet rich in omega-3 fatty acids, fruits, and vegetables.

Medications may also be helpful in primary prevention strategies. The evidence-based practice guidelines of the American College of Chest Physicians (Vandvik et al. 2012) recommend that individuals over age 50 without symptomatic CAD take low-dose aspirin (75–100 mg/day); however, low-risk patients who dislike taking medications over the long term may elect not to follow this recommendation. Taking low-dose aspirin is more beneficial for individuals at moderate to high risk of CAD. Statin agents are also effective at primary prevention of cardiovascular events in higher-risk persons. Full details on their recommended use can be found in Chapter 7, "Dyslipidemia." Blood pressure reduction via diet, exercise, and medications also reduces primary CAD events.

Once a patient develops CAD, ongoing risk factor modification is important for secondary prevention of future CAD events. Evidence is strong for medications in secondary prevention; adherence to antiplatelet agents, β-blockers, statins, and angiotensin-converting enzyme (ACE) inhibitors is associated with improved outcomes in patients with CAD (Kumbhani et al. 2013). Many psychiatrists and primary care providers may have been cautioned against the use of β-blockers in patients with depression; however, prospective data have not borne out an association between depression and β-blocker prescription. Evidence supporting the use of β-blockers in patients with CAD is much stronger than the aggregate evidence supporting possible harm (Muzyk and Gagliardi 2010). Recommendations for specific antiplatelets and for single versus combination antiplatelet therapy depend on chronicity and type of revascularization of CAD (Vandvik et al. 2012). In general, patients without coronary stents should take aspirin, whereas patients with stents, especially drug-eluting stents, should receive combination therapy.

Treatment Recommendations

Treatment guidelines published in the National Guideline Clearinghouse include a number of recommendations regarding the treatment of CAD in the primary care setting (Kaiser Permanente Care Management Institute 2008). The reader is referred to the entire document for complete information. In brief, the guidelines address depression; CAD screening; specific therapies, including ACE inhibitors or angiotensin receptor blockers (ARBs), oral anticoagulants, antiplatelet therapy, and β-blocker therapy; and specific recommendations for lifestyle modification.

Primary Prevention: Treatment in an Effort to Prevent the Development of CAD

Lifestyle modification is recommended to improve cardiovascular health.

- Smoking cessation is a strongly evidence-based recommendation for patients with established or increased risk of CAD.
- Exercise, in the form of 30–60 minutes at least 3–4 days per week, is recommended.
- A diet rich in fruits, vegetables, legumes, nuts, whole grains, and omega-3 fatty acids is recommended. Whenever possible, patients should work to increase "good" polyunsaturated fats from nuts, fish, fish oil supplements, flaxseed, and canola and soybean oils. Trans fats should be eliminated.
- The use of supplemental folic acid, β-carotene, or vitamin B_6, B_{12}, C, or E is not recommended.
- Routine stress testing or coronary calcium scoring in an effort to detect asymptomatic CAD is not recommended.

Secondary Prevention: Treatment After Diagnosis With CAD

- Blood pressure targets for patients with CAD can vary by guideline but should at a minimum be lower than 140/90 mmHg in patients younger than 75 years (James et al. 2014). Other guidelines recommend less than 130/80 mmHg.
- Lipid lowering should be undertaken with statins (not lifestyle modification), with a goal of reducing low-density lipoprotein (LDL) cholesterol. The most recent guidelines recommend high-potency statin therapy for secondary prevention in patients with established CAD (Stone et al. 2013). A moderately potent statin is recommended for primary prevention in patients without CAD but with LDL cholesterol greater than 190 mg/dL or with significant 10-year risk of cardiovascular events. (See Chapter 7, "Dyslipidemia," for further details.)
- ACE inhibitor therapy is recommended for patients who have CAD. For patients who are unable to tolerate ACE inhibitors, ARB therapy can be an alternative for patients with diabetes and hypertension or left ventricular systolic dysfunction.
- β-Blocker therapy is recommended for patients in whom it is not contraindicated. Guidelines list chronic obstructive pulmonary disease but not depression as a possible contraindication. β-Blockers are proven to improve mortality risk in patients after MI and also are effective antianginal agents.
- Other than amlodipine and felodipine, which may be helpful for the treatment of angina or hypertension in patients with left ventricular systolic dysfunction, calcium channel blockers are not routinely recommended for patients with CAD.
- Depression is a recognized risk for worse cardiovascular outcomes in patients with CAD, but the evidence for specific modalities of treatment is insufficient to make recommendations for or against using antidepressant medications in an effort to impact cardiovascular health.
- A variety of recommendations exist regarding platelet inhibition; in patients without elevated risk for embolism, aspirin is recommended as monotherapy over oral anticoagulants (e.g., warfarin) or combination antiplatelet therapy. If patients cannot tolerate aspirin, clopidogrel is a reasonable alternative.
- The addition of antiplatelet therapy to oral anticoagulation increases bleeding risk without clear benefit with regard to other outcomes and is not recommended.
- Patients with left ventricular thrombus or other elevated risk for embolism should be treated with oral anticoagulants.

- Patients who have undergone coronary artery stent placement should be treated either with combination aspirin and clopidogrel or with a newer antiplatelet agent (i.e., ticagrelor or prasugrel) for 4 weeks (bare metal stent) to 12 months (drug-eluting stent). During the recommended period of combination antiplatelet therapy, elective procedures that would necessitate discontinuing antiplatelet therapy should be postponed to permit uninterrupted completion of the antiplatelet therapy.
- Hormone therapy is not recommended as a CAD risk–mitigating strategy and should be discontinued if CAD risk is the main indication for its use.

When to Refer

Psychiatrists should be comfortable with the use of antihypertensive therapies and the implementation and appropriate monitoring of ACE inhibitors, statins, β-blockers, and lifestyle modification. In situations prompting referral, the psychiatrist ideally will collaborate with the primary care provider to help enhance patient adherence to recommended treatment strategies.

Situations warranting referral to a primary care provider and/or cardiologist include the following:

- Recent MI, with a goal of optimizing medications
- New symptoms of possible CAD (e.g., chest pain, dyspnea on exertion)
- New symptoms of left ventricular systolic dysfunction (e.g., dyspnea, exercise intolerance, edema, paroxysmal nocturnal dyspnea, orthopnea)
- Any history of syncope, which could be indicative of arrhythmia or medication intolerance
- Inability to reach target blood pressure or lipid levels within 6 months of initiation of appropriate therapies
- New identification of DM, in which case the patient will benefit from comprehensive education and ongoing monitoring, including referrals to ophthalmology, yearly sensory examinations, and management of other cardiovascular risk factors

Special Treatment Considerations for the Psychiatric Patient Population

It is important for the psychiatrist to be aware of patients' underlying medical conditions as well as all of the medications recommended to treat their conditions; ideally, an integrated care strategy or at the very least clear communication between mental health and primary care providers will take place. There are recommended monitoring parameters for some of the medications used in the treatment and prevention of CAD. There are also possible drug-drug interactions between some of the medications used to treat psychiatric disorders and guideline-recommended medications for CAD.

Medications: Increased Risk of Adverse Effects

Second-generation antipsychotic medications used in the treatment of primary psychotic disorders and bipolar disorders, as well as the off-label treatment of some cognitive disorders, are associated with significant weight gain and the development of metabolic syndrome.

Medications used to treat depression, particularly selective serotonin reuptake inhibitors, are associated in epidemiological studies with doubled odds of bleeding through mechanisms related to platelet inhibition and gastric effects. This risk increases with the use of additional platelet inhibitors such as aspirin or clopidogrel (Andrade 2012).

Lithium, used for the treatment of bipolar disorder and for augmentation of antidepressant therapy, is excreted solely by the kidney. As stated in the previous section, "Treatment Recommendations," patients with CAD or DM should be prescribed an ACE inhibitor or ARB medication. However, the addition of an ACE inhibitor, ARB therapy, or diuretic therapy (common in patients for symptomatic relief in congestive heart failure) can impair lithium excretion and lead to lithium toxicity. In one nested case-control study, 3% of observed cases of lithium toxicity were attributable to newly initiated ACE inhibitor or ARB medications (Juurlink et al. 2004). It is essential that patients taking lithium and their psychiatrists be aware of the need to monitor levels more frequently and to be vigilant for the development of lithium toxicity if ACE or ARB therapy is prescribed.

An association between β-blockers and clinical depression has been reported in multiple textbooks, although the empirical evidence supporting the link is not available in nested cohorts within prospective randomized trials of patients with CAD (Muzyk and Gagliardi 2010). Patients with CAD should be tried on β-blockers in an effort to achieve optimal medical management and, because they have CAD and are at increased risk of depression in the first place, all patients with CAD should undergo monitoring for depressive symptomatology.

Medication Interactions

Clopidogrel is activated through the cytochrome P450 (CYP) 2C19 isoenzyme. Medications such as fluoxetine or fluvoxamine, which inhibit the function of CYP2C19, can impair the effectiveness of clopidogrel (Andrade 2012). Prasugrel and ticagrelor are newer antiplatelet agents that are often used in place of clopidogrel, especially after stent placement. Ticagrelor is metabolized by the CYP3A4 enzyme. Potent inducers, such as carbamazepine, can reduce its effectiveness. Prasugrel is metabolized by the same enzyme, but inducers and inhibitors have minimal effect on its effectiveness.

Monitoring for Metabolic Syndrome

In 2004, a consensus conference was convened to address the association between antipsychotic medications (particularly the atypical or second-generation medications) and the development of metabolic syndrome (American Diabetes Association et al. 2004). Baseline monitoring should include obtaining a personal and family history of diabetes, hyperlipidemia, hypertension, or cardiovascular disease; ascertainment of weight and height for accurate BMI calculation; waist circumference; blood pressure; and fasting plasma glucose and lipid profile. Patients with baseline obesity, hyperlipidemia, or glucose intolerance may be better off taking alternative medications but at a minimum should be initiated on appropriate therapy to address these problems (see Table 5–1). Patients starting these medications should also be counseled on healthy diet, lifestyle, and exercise, and patients and families should be counseled about risks and about symptoms of new-onset DM and diabetic ketoacidosis.

Other Considerations

Although official recommendations have been published for depression screening strategies (Lichtman et al. 2008) and psychosocial risk screening in patients identified with CAD, it is harder to find official screening strategies for CAD in patients with psychiatric illness.

Given the increased risk of metabolic syndrome among certain psychiatric patients and the risk of silent CAD in others, it stands to reason that risk factor screening and modification should be undertaken in patients with psychiatric illness. One challenge, not unique to but certainly enhanced in the presence of certain psychiatric illnesses, is that of motivation and adherence. Patients who are apathetic or unmotivated (as is common with major depressive disorder) may lack the energy or drive to follow recommendations. There is evidence that a comprehensive approach to the care of patients using a collaborative care strategy, including attention to the mental health diagnosis (in this case depression) along with the medical diagnoses (in this case CAD and associated risk factors), results in improvement in both mental and physical health (Katon et al. 2010).

Perhaps more challenging is enlisting patients with paranoia or an inherent distrust of medications and health care providers (as is frequently the case with chronic paranoid schizophrenia) to adhere to either medication or lifestyle modification. Commonsense strategies such as enlisting a multidisciplinary team with the psychiatrist coordinating care and optimizing antipsychotic treatment may provide some benefit (Heald et al. 2010).

TABLE 5–1. Baseline and ongoing monitoring for patients prescribed second-generation antipsychotics

Parameter and timing	Weight (BMI)	Waist circumference	Blood pressure	Fasting plasma glucose	Fasting lipid profile
Before prescribing second-generation antipsychotics, confirm personal and family history of obesity, diabetes mellitus, dyslipidemia, hypertension, and cardiovascular disease.					
If patient is overweight or obese, consider referral for nutrition and physical activity counseling.					
Educate patients and family members regarding signs and symptoms of diabetes mellitus.					
Baseline	X	X	X	X	X
4 weeks	X				
8 weeks	X				
12 weeks	X		X	X	X
Quarterly	X				
Annually		X	X	X	
Every 5 years					X
Treat or refer for treatment if obesity, diabetes mellitus, dyslipidemia, hypertension, or cardiovascular disease is identified.					
If parameters worsen, consider tapering or switching antipsychotic medication.					

Note. BMI=body mass index. *Source.* Adapted from American Diabetes Association et al. 2004.

Although primary CAD prevention with medications is not routinely recommended for the general population, increased risks associated with psychiatric diagnoses, particularly schizophrenia (and the medications used to treat it), may warrant consideration of aggressive primary prevention strategies (Srihari et al. 2013). For example, some experts recommend initiation of metformin therapy for patients started on the second-generation antipsychotic medications olanzapine and clozapine, regardless of baseline fasting blood glucose level (Brooks et al. 2009).

Physicians and researchers have long observed an association between emotional stress and coronary events, but evidence demonstrating that treating the emotional distress benefits coronary outcomes has been elusive. Treatment of underlying psychiatric conditions improves depression, adherence to drug therapy, and quality of life, but impact on mortality and cardiovascular health has not consistently been demonstrated (Kaiser Permanente Care Management Institute 2008; Pozuelo et al. 2009). Researchers recently demonstrated a decreased incidence of mental stress–induced myocardial ischemia in a group of subjects randomized to 6 weeks of therapy with the antidepressant escitalopram compared with subjects randomized to 6 weeks of placebo (Jiang et al. 2013). Clinicians are more likely to achieve effective risk reduction for CAD if they effectively manage the psychiatric illness that contributes to those risks.

Case Discussion (*continued*)

Ms. S, who has lived for 32 years with schizophrenia, is at risk of cardiovascular morbidity and mortality from her mental illness and metabolic syndrome. Although she is followed by an Assertive Community Treatment team and receives close psychiatric monitoring, she has not been systematically assessed or treated for CAD risk factors. Ms. S should undergo routine and periodic monitoring of her BMI, fasting lipids, and fasting glucose. She would benefit from an exercise program, counseling for smoking cessation, and integrated care to facilitate adherence to treatments to optimize her cardiovascular risk factors. Lastly, the treatment of her schizophrenia should be optimized. Her long-standing history of schizophrenia increases risk of suicide. This risk should be assessed routinely.

Clinical Highlights

- Patients with coronary artery disease (CAD) are at increased risk of developing clinical and subclinical depression.
- Depression and anxiety are associated with worse outcomes in CAD.

- Patients with severe and persistent mental illness may not participate fully in primary care or may not engage in preventive health care. Mental health providers are well positioned to participate in the cardiovascular care of their patients.
- Patients with severe and persistent mental illness may engage in behaviors that increase CAD risk, such as smoking or unhealthy eating.
- Medications prescribed to treat psychiatric disorders, including antidepressants, antipsychotics, and stimulant medications, can pose direct and indirect risk to cardiovascular health.
- Patients' CAD risk may be calculated using the Framingham risk calculator.
- CAD events may be reduced with primary or secondary prevention strategies.

Resources

For Patients

American Heart Association: Consumer and patient education materials, 2011. Available at: http://www.heart.org/HEARTORG/General/Consumer-and-Patient-Education-Materials_UCM_314813_Article.jsp.

Centers for Disease Control and Prevention: Heart Disease: Educational Materials for Patients, 2013. Available at: http://www.cdc.gov/heartdisease/materials_for_patients.htm.

For Clinicians

Find guidelines for management of CAD (Kaiser Permanente Care Management Institute 2008): Available at: https://www.framinghamheartstudy.org/risk-functions/cardiovascular-disease/10-year-risk.php

Framingham Heart Study: http://www.framinghamheartstudy.org

National Heart, Lung, and Blood Institute: Risk Assessment Tool for Estimating Your 10-Year Risk of Having a Heart Attack, 2013. Available at: http://cvdrisk.nhlbi.nih.gov/calculator.asp.

References

American Diabetes Association, American Psychiatric Association, American Association of Clinical Endocrinologists, North American Association for the Study of Obesity: Consensus development conference on antipsychotic drugs and obesity and diabetes. Diabetes Care 27:596–601, 2004

Andrade C: Drug interactions in the treatment of depression in patients with ischemic heart disease. J Clin Psychiatry 73:e1475–e1477, 2012

Bikdeli B, Ranasinghe I, Chen R, et al: Most important outcomes research papers on treatment of stable coronary artery disease. Circ Cardiovasc Qual Outcomes 6:e17–e25, 2013

Brooks JO 3rd, Chang HS, Krasnykh O: Metabolic risks in older adults receiving second-generation antipsychotic medication. Curr Psychiatry Rep 11:33–40, 2009

Centers for Disease Control and Prevention: Heart disease facts. 2013. Available at: http://www.cdc.gov/heartdisease/facts.htm. Accessed June 24, 2013.

Chiavarino C, Rabellino D, Ardito RB, et al: Emotional coping is a better predictor of cardiac prognosis than depression and anxiety. J Psychosom Res 73:473–475, 2012

Chiuve SE, Fung TT, Rexrode KM, et al: Adherence to a low-risk, healthy lifestyle and risk of sudden cardiac death among women. JAMA 306:62–69, 2011

Colton CW, Manderscheid RW: Congruencies in increased mortality rates, years of potential life lost, and causes of death among public mental health clients in eight states. Prev Chronic Dis 3:A42, 2006

Crump C, Sundquist K, Winkleby MA, et al: Comorbidities and mortality in bipolar disorder: a Swedish national cohort study. JAMA Psychiatry 70:931–939, 2013

Darba J, Kaskens L, Aranda P, et al: A simulation model to estimate 10-year risk of coronary heart disease events in patients with schizophrenia spectrum disorders treated with second-generation antipsychotic drugs. Ann Clin Psychiatry 25:17–26, 2013

Davidson M: Risk of cardiovascular disease and sudden death in schizophrenia. J Clin Psychiatry 63 (suppl 9): 5–11, 2002

Desai CS, Colangelo LA, Liu K, et al: Prevalence, prospective risk markers, and prognosis associated with the presence of left ventricular diastolic dysfunction: the Coronary Artery Risk Development in Young Adults Study. Am J Epidemiol 177:20–32, 2013

Dipasquale S, Pariante CM, Dazzan P, et al: The dietary pattern of patients with schizophrenia: a systematic review. J Psychiatr Res 47:197–207, 2013

Fihn SD, Gardin JM, Abrams J, et al: 2012 AACF/AHA/ACP/AATS/PCNA/SCAI/STS guideline for the diagnosis and management of patients with stable ischemic heart disease. J Am Coll Cardiol 60:e44–e164, 2012

Gilman SE, Kawachia I, Fitzmaurice GM, et al: Socioeconomic status in childhood and the lifetime risk of major depression. Int J Epidemiol 31:359–367, 2002

Go AS, Mozaffarian D, Roger VL, et al; American Heart Association Statistics Committee and Stroke Statistics Subcommittee: Heart disease and stroke statistics—2014 update: a report from the American Heart Association. Circulation 129(3):e28–e292, 2014

Griswold KS, Pastore PA, Homish GG: Access to primary care: are mental health peers effective in helping patients after a psychiatric emergency? Primary Psychiatry 17(6):42–45, 2010

Hartley L, Igbinedion E, Holmes J, et al: Increased consumption of fruit and vegetables for the primary prevention of cardiovascular diseases. Cochrane Database Syst Rev 6:CD009874, 2013

Heald A, Montejo AL, Millar H, et al: Management of physical health in patients with schizophrenia: practical recommendations. Eur Psychiatry 25(suppl):S41–S45, 2010

Huffman JC, Celano CM, Beach SR, et al: Depression and cardiac disease: epidemiology, mechanisms, and diagnosis. Cardiovasc Psychiatry Neurol Apr 7, 2013 [Epub ahead of print]

James PA, Oparil S, Carter BL, et al: 2014 evidence-based guideline for the management of high blood pressure in adults. Report from the panel members appointed to the Eighth Joint National Committee (JNC 8). JAMA 311:507–520, 2014

Jiang W, Velazquez EJ, Kuchibhatla M, et al: Effect of escitalopram on mental stress–induced myocardial ischemia: results of the REMIT trial. JAMA 309:2139–2149, 2013

Juurlink DN, Mamdani MM, Kopp A, et al: Drug-induced lithium toxicity in the elderly: a population-based study. J Am Geriatr Soc 52:794–798, 2004

Kaiser Permanente Care Management Institute: Coronary Artery Disease (CAD) Clinical Practice Guidelines. Oakland, CA, Kaiser Permanente Care Management Institute, 2008

Katon WJ, Lin EH, Von Korff M, et al: Collaborative care for patients with depression and chronic illness. N Engl J Med 363:2611–2620, 2010

Khawaja IS, Westermeyer JJ, Gajwani P, et al: Depression and coronary artery disease: the association, mechanisms, and therapeutic implications. Psychiatry (Edgmont) 6:38–51, 2009

Kumbhani DJ, Steg PG, Cannon CP, et al: Adherence to secondary prevention medications and four-year outcomes in outpatients with atherosclerosis. Am J Med 126:693–700, 2013

Lichtman JH, Bigger T, Blumenthal JA, et al: Depression and coronary heart disease: recommendations for screening, referral, and treatment: a science advisory from the American Heart Association Prevention Committee of the Council on Cardiovascular Nursing, Council on Clinical Cardiology, Council on Epidemiology and Prevention, and Interdisciplinary Council on Quality of Care and Outcomes Research: endorsed by the American Psychiatric Association. Circulation 118:1768–1775, 2008

Lloyd-Jones D, Adams RJ, Brown TM, et al: Executive summary: heart disease and stroke statistics—2010 update: a report from the American Heart Association. Circulation 121:948–954, 2010

Moyer VA; U.S. Preventive Services Task Force: Screening for coronary heart disease with electrocardiography: U.S. Preventive Services Task Force recommendation statement. Ann Intern Med 157:512–518, 2012

Muzyk AJ, Gagliardi JP: Do beta blockers cause depression? Curr Psychiatry 9:50–52, 2010

Newcomer JW, Hennekens CH: Severe mental illness and risk of cardiovascular disease. JAMA 298:1794–1796, 2007

Osborn DP, Wright CA, Levy G, et al: Relative risk of diabetes, dyslipidaemia, hypertension and the metabolic syndrome in people with severe mental illnesses: systematic review and metaanalysis. BMC Psychiatry 8:84, 2008

Pozuelo L, Zhang J, Franco K, et al: Depression and heart disease: what do we know, and where are we headed? Cleve Clin J Med 76:59–70, 2009

Prasad A, Lerman A, Rihal CS: Apical ballooning syndrome (Tako-Tsubo or stress cardiomyopathy): a mimic of acute myocardial infarction. Am Heart J 155:408–417, 2008

Soares-Filho GL, Mesquita CT, Mesquita ET, et al: Panic attack triggering myocardial ischemia documented by myocardial perfusion imaging study. A case report. Int Arch Med 5:24, 2012

Srihari VH, Phutane VH, Ozkan B, et al: Cardiovascular mortality in schizophrenia: defining a critical period for prevention. Schizophr Res 146:64–68, 2013

Stone NJ, Robinson J, Lichtenstein AH, et al: 2013 ACC/AHA guideline on the treatment of blood cholesterol to reduce atherosclerotic cardiovascular risk in adults: a report of the American College of Cardiology/American Heart Association Task Force on Practice Guidelines. J Am Coll Cardiol Nov 7, 2013 [Epub]

Strassnig M, Brar JS, Ganguli R: Low cardiorespiratory fitness and physical functional capacity in obese patients with schizophrenia. Schizophr Res 126:103–109, 2011

Vandvik PO, Lincoff AM, Gore JM, et al: Primary and secondary prevention of cardiovascular disease: antithrombotic therapy and prevention of thrombosis, 9th ed: American College of Chest Physicians evidence-based clinical practice guidelines. Chest 141(suppl):e637s–e668s, 2012

Wang G, Cui J, Wang Y, et al: Anxiety and adverse coronary artery disease outcomes in Chinese patients. Psychosom Med 75:530–536, 2013

Watkins LL, Koch GG, Sherwood A, et al: Association of anxiety and depression with all-cause mortality in individuals with coronary heart disease. J Am Heart Assoc 2:e000068, 2013

Wheeler A, Schrader G, Tucker G, et al: Prevalence of depression in patients with chest pain and non-obstructive coronary artery disease. Am J Cardiol 112:656–659, 2013

Wildgust HJ, Beary M: Are there modifiable risk factors which will reduce the excess mortality in schizophrenia? J Psychopharmacol 24(suppl):37–50, 2010

CHAPTER 6

Hypertension

Robert M. McCarron, D.O.

David Hsu, M.D.

Dustin DeMoss, D.O.

Case Discussion

Mrs. B is a 47-year-old white woman who presents to the clinic to establish psychiatric care. She has had two previous psychiatric hospitalizations for "mania"; the most recent was 6 months prior to presentation. The patient states that she has tried taking multiple psychotropic medications but has found little to no relief from her mood symptoms. She was most recently discharged on lithium and venlafaxine and reports mild improvement with her depression.

She has a past medical history significant for hypertension and chronic kidney disease, for which she takes lisinopril, an angiotensin-converting enzyme (ACE) inhibitor. The patient describes having read on the Internet that she should not be taking lithium and lisinopril together. She appears somewhat distraught over this and is asking for further guidance.

Clinical Overview

Hypertension is a major risk factor for cardiovascular disease, directly contributing to one-quarter of all heart attacks and one-third of all strokes (U.S. Department of Health and Human Services 2004). For every 20 mmHg of systolic blood pressure above 115 mmHg, there is a twofold increase in death from stroke and coronary artery disease (Lewington et al. 2002). Still, almost 30% of Americans are diagnosed with hypertension each year, and only half of all Americans with hypertension have controlled blood pressure (Egan et al. 2010). The most common diagnosis in the primary care clinic is hypertension, and about 65 million individuals in the United States have this diagnosis. Hypertension is one of the four main criteria of metabolic syndrome, along with diabetes mellitus, dyslipidemia, and obesity. From a public health perspective, it is imperative that clinicians—including mental health clinicians—focus on hypertension as a goal for prevention of vascular-related morbidity and mortality.

Psychiatrists are in a good position to institute preventive measures with regard to blood pressure control. Hypertension has been associated with stress and poor social support (Bosworth et al. 2003), major depression (Carroll et al. 2010), bipolar disorder (Goldstein et al. 2009; Johannessen et al. 2006), and generalized anxiety disorder (Carroll et al. 2010). Similarly, patients with schizophrenia had increased 10-year cardiac mortality when compared with control subjects in the Clinical Antipsychotic Trials of Intervention Effectiveness (CATIE) schizophrenia trial (Goff et al. 2005). These patients had higher rates of hypertension, diabetes, and smoking, as well as lower levels of high-density lipoprotein (HDL) cholesterol. In a follow-up study, researchers found that the rate of nontreatment for hypertension in patients with schizophrenia was 62.4% (Nasrallah et al. 2006).

The most important skill that psychiatrists need in order to enhance the medical health of their patients is *empathy*. According to the Seventh Report of the Joint National Committee on Prevention, Detection, Evaluation, and Treatment of High Blood Pressure (JNC 7), "The most effective therapy prescribed by the most careful clinician will control hypertension only if patients are motivated. Motivation improves when patients have positive experiences with, and trust in, the clinician. Empathy builds trust and is a potent motivator" (U.S. Department of Health and Human Services 2004, p. 61).

There is a trend toward more integrated or collaborative care, in which psychiatrists work closely with other physicians, nurses, social workers, and therapists. Monitoring of blood pressure can be performed directly by the psychiatrist or other members of the treating team. Informed consent for psychotropic medications may involve discussions about hypertension, and the psychiatrist will need to follow up on the potential side effects. Clinics and hospitals that care for patients with mental health diagnoses should be equipped with devices that accurately measure blood pressure.

Practical Pointers

- Patients diagnosed with mental illness are less likely to be assessed or treated for hypertension.
- Patients who have mental illness are more likely to have hypertension and other related metabolic derangements that may increase risk for vascular injury and premature death.
- Hypertension is a largely modifiable cardiac risk factor. Mental health care providers are well positioned to monitor and initiate treatment for patients who have hypertension.
- Psychotropic medications may adversely influence blood pressure. Therefore, vital signs should be monitored at each visit.

Diagnosis

The JNC 7 committee developed diagnostic criteria for hypertension in 2003 (Table 6–1) (U.S. Department of Health and Human Services 2004). The JNC 8 committee did not change these criteria and focused more on specific targets for treatment (James et al. 2014). Normal blood pressure is defined as less than 120/80 mmHg. Prehypertension is defined as blood pressure between 120/80 mmHg and 139/89 mmHg. Antihypertensive medication therapy is not indicated for prehypertension. Stage 1 hypertension is defined as blood pressure between 140/90 mmHg and 159/99 mmHg, and stage 2 hypertension is above 160/100 mmHg. A diastolic blood pressure greater than 120 mmHg with end-organ damage (e.g., retinal hemorrhage, hypertensive encephalopathy) is classified as malignant hypertension or emergent, and without end-organ damage is classified as hypertensive urgency.

Hypertension is diagnosed based on the average of two or more seated blood pressure readings (U.S. Department of Health and Human Services 2004). Self-monitoring with home blood pressure machines is also a valid method for measuring blood pressure. Patients should be encouraged to bring their blood pressure measuring device to clinic visits if they have any questions about accuracy of home measurements. Because blood pressure varies throughout the day, it is important to measure it in a standard fashion. Blood pressure should be measured in both arms while the person is sitting comfortably with the arm at heart level. A medical history should be obtained, followed by a physical examination to see if the patient has any identifiable secondary causes of hypertension (e.g., stimulant or alcohol misuse, sleep apnea, steroid use, thyroid disease, chronic kidney disease, pheochromocytoma, obesity, coarctation of the aorta).

Although most diagnoses of hypertension are categorized as essential hypertension (also termed primary or idiopathic hypertension), consider-

TABLE 6–1. Diagnostic classification of blood pressure

Classification	Systolic blood pressure		Diastolic blood pressure
Normal	<120 mmHg	AND	<80 mmHg
Prehypertension	120–139 mmHg	OR	80–89 mmHg
Stage 1 hypertension	140–159 mmHg	OR	90–99 mmHg
Stage 2 hypertension	≥160 mmHg	OR	≥100 mmHg

Source. Adapted from U.S. Department of Health and Human Services 2004.

ation of a broad differential diagnosis is indicated when patients are taking multiple medications with suboptimal results. Table 6–2 details the most common causes of hypertension.

Preventive Guidelines

The U.S. Preventive Services Task Force (2007) recommends screening for high blood pressure in adults age 18 years and older. This recommendation is the evidence-based standard of care for the prevention of hypertension (Wolff and Miller 2007). Patients with normal blood pressure should be screened at least every 2 years, whereas those with prehypertension should be screened annually. We suggest that blood pressure be measured at each mental health care visit, particularly if psychotropic medications are prescribed.

Treatment Recommendations

The main goals of treating hypertension are to prevent strokes, heart attacks, and serious renal insults. For those with stage 1 hypertension, a reduction of systolic blood pressure by 12 mmHg over 10 years will prevent one death for every 11 patients treated. For those with cardiovascular disease, the number needed to treat to prevent one death is only nine (U.S. Department of Health and Human Services 2004). The two most important treatment strategies are lifestyle modification and pharmacotherapy.

Lifestyle Modification

Psychiatrists should be comfortable helping patients with lifestyle modification because it involves the use of cognitive, behavioral, and motivational therapies. Behavioral interventions, such as counseling, self-monitoring, and structured training courses, have been validated as helping to lower blood

TABLE 6–2. Common causes of hypertension
Essential or idiopathic hypertension (>90%)
Kidney disease
Medications (e.g., oral contraceptives, some antidepressants, chronic nonsteroidal anti-inflammatory agents, anabolic steroids)
Chronic alcohol abuse
Primary aldosteronism
Sleep apnea
Coarctation of the aorta
Pheochromocytoma

pressure (Boulware et al. 2001). Other lifestyle modifications that have proven to be effective in lowering blood pressure include weight reduction, dietary sodium restriction, physical activity, moderation of alcohol consumption, and adoption of the Dietary Approaches to Stop Hypertension (DASH) eating plan (U.S. Department of Health and Human Services 2004). Incorporation of each lifestyle modification can decrease systolic blood pressure by 5–20 mmHg (Table 6–3).

Pharmacotherapy

The JNC 8 committee considered three questions while determining thresholds for pharmacological treatment. The diagnostic criteria for hypertension have not been changed since 2003. Three questions are used as a focal point for treatment (James et al. 2014):

1. When adults with hypertension are being treated, does medication management at specific blood pressure thresholds improve health outcomes?
2. When adults with hypertension are being treated, does treatment of blood pressure to a specified blood pressure threshold improve health outcomes?
3. Which medications are most effective for the treatment of hypertension and specific comorbid medical conditions (i.e., kidney disease, diabetes) and subgroups (i.e., high-risk ethnicities)?

As shown in the JNC 8 guidelines in Figure 6–1, for adults under age 60, blood pressure above 140/90 mmHg should be treated with antihypertensive medication. In this age group, a diastolic blood pressure less than 90 mmHg is probably more important than a systolic pressure less than 140 mmHg.

TABLE 6–3. Lifestyle modification for the treatment of hypertension

Modification	Recommendation	Approximate systolic blood pressure reduction
Weight reduction	Maintain body mass index of 18.5–24.9.	5–20 mmHg/10-kg weight reduction
Adopt DASH eating plan	Eat diet rich in fruits, vegetables, and low-fat dairy products with a reduced content of saturated and total fat.	8–14 mmHg
Dietary sodium reduction	Reduce dietary sodium intake to no more than 100 mEq/L (2.4 g sodium or 6 g sodium chloride).	2–8 mmHg
Physical activity	Engage in regular aerobic physical activity such as brisk walking (at least 30 minutes per day, most days of the week).	4–9 mmHg
Moderation of alcohol consumption	Limit consumption to no more than **two** drinks per day (1 oz or 30 mL ethanol [e.g., 24 oz beer, 10 oz wine, or 3 oz 80-proof liquor]) in most men and no more than **one** drink per day in women and lighter-weight persons.	2–4 mmHg

Note.　DASH=Dietary Approaches to Stop Hypertension (U.S. Department of Health and Human Services 2004).

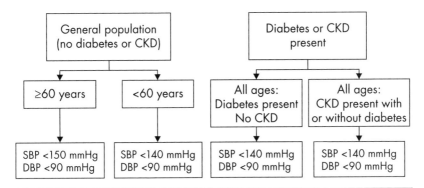

FIGURE 6–1. Treatment goals for hypertension.
Note. CKD = chronic kidney disease; DBP = diastolic blood pressure; SBP = systolic blood pressure.
Source. Adapted from James et al. 2014.

For patients over age 60, providers should treat with pharmacotherapy if the pressure is greater than 150/90 mmHg. Both of these targets to treatment are based on expert opinion and randomized controlled studies. These JNC 8 guidelines are more conservative than the JNC 7 guidelines, which suggested that normal blood pressure was less than 120/80 mmHg.

Patients between ages 18 and 69 who have chronic kidney disease (CKD), as defined by an estimated glomerular filtration rate of less than 60 mL/min per 1.73 m^2 for longer than 3 months, should be treated to a target of less than 140/90 mmHg. For patients over age 70 who have CKD, the JNC 8 report does not recommend a specific threshold for treatment. Although evidence is lacking, JNC 8 expert opinion recommends treatment for adults who have both diabetes and hypertension to less than 140/90 mmHg.

As shown in the JNC 8 guidelines in Figure 6–2, evidence supports use of thiazide-type diuretics (TDs), calcium channel blockers (CCBs), ACE inhibitors, or angiotensin receptor blockers (ARBs) in the general, nonblack population (with or without diabetes). TDs or CCBs should be first-line treatment for black patients, whether or not they have diabetes. In this population, ACE inhibitors and ARBs are less effective and may increase the risk for stroke. For black and nonblack adults who have CKD and hypertension, ACE inhibitors or ARBs should be first-line treatment for those with or without diabetes. For patients over age 75 with CKD, any of the four core treatments for hypertension may be used, as tolerated. Of note, β-blockers are no longer routinely used to treat hypertension but are often used for other reasons (e.g., heart failure, angina).

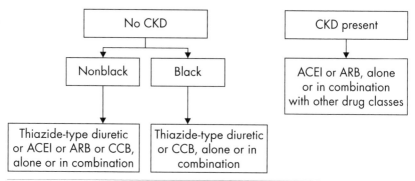

FIGURE 6–2.   Treatment of hypertension, based on age, diabetes, and chronic kidney disease.

Note.   ACEI = angiotensin-converting enzyme inhibitor; ARB = angiotensin receptor blocker; CCB = calcium channel blocker; CKD = chronic kidney disease.

Source.   Adapted from James et al. 2014.

There are three recommended approaches when initiating pharmacotherapy for hypertension:

1. Attempt to connect the patient with a primary care provider. If this is not possible, one medication should be started, with follow-up in 1 week. The initial medication should be a TD, CCB, ACE inhibitor, or ARB. If another type of medication is indicated (e.g., clonidine), we recommend referral to a primary care provider or cardiologist.
2. Start one medication, quickly followed by a second.
3. Start two medications at the same time if the patient has a blood pressure of greater than 160/100 mmHg.

When to Refer

Situations warranting referral to a primary care provider and/or cardiologist include the following:

- Complaint of a terrible headache by a patient with a diagnosis of hypertension
- Need for two or more medications for hypertension
- Secondary cause of hypertension
- Allergies or severe reactions to several blood pressure medications
- Metabolic issues, including low sodium, high potassium, and elevated creatinine
- Systolic blood pressure of greater than 180 mmHg or diastolic blood pressure greater than 120 mmHg

TABLE 6–4. Common drug class interactions

Antihypertensive medication class	Psychotropics	Caution
Diuretics	Lithium	Watch for dehydration and increased serum lithium level
Multiple taken at the same time	Venlafaxine	Potential for increased blood pressure
Multiple taken at the same time	Psychotropics with high α_1 blockade	Potential for hypotension
Any class	Monoamine oxidase inhibitors	1. Hypotension (α_1 blockade) 2. Hypertension (food with tyramine might cause a catecholamine surge and hypertensive crisis)
Any class	Stimulants	Potential for increased blood pressure

Special Treatment Considerations for the Psychiatric Patient Population

Close monitoring is especially important when working with patients who have hypertension and comorbid psychiatric illness. Because hypertension is generally considered a symptom-free disorder, mental health providers should be vigilant while checking vital signs and reconciling medications. Psychotropic medications can have an effect on blood pressure, in the form of either hypotension or hypertension. Providers should keep an accurate list of all medications and monitor for interactions (Table 6–4) and poor adherence. Patient education is paramount, because hypertension often has no immediate adverse consequences but can contribute to increased cardiovascular-related morbidity over time.

Case Discussion (*continued*)

Lithium is primarily metabolized by the kidney and should be used with caution in patients taking ACE inhibitors or ARBs. In Mrs. B's case, lithium is probably not the best initial treatment for bipolar depression because she has CKD. Lisinopril is renal protective; it should not be stopped. Mrs. B may benefit from another mood stabilizer or an atypical antipsychotic. Venlafaxine may increase blood pressure but is not absolutely contraindicated in this case.

The provider should closely monitor for elevations in blood pressure as the dose of venlafaxine is increased. The patient should be educated about all these clinical points and be an integral and active participant in the development of the treatment plan.

Clinical Highlights

- Identification and concurrent treatment of psychiatric comorbidities in patients with cardiovascular disease and hypertension are paramount. Patients with depressive, anxiety, psychotic, or other mental disorders are less likely to be adherent to the treatment plan.

- Patients with mental illness and comorbid hypertension are at significantly increased risk for adverse reactions from drug-drug interactions.

- It is best to treat to a target blood pressure goal, generally less than 140/90 mmHg.

- Thiazide-type diuretics, calcium channel blockers, ACE inhibitors, and angiotensin receptor blockers are the core medications used to treat hypertension. β-Blockers are no longer routinely used to treat hypertension.

- Mental health providers should routinely check the vital signs of all patients and closely monitor for hypertension. This should be standard practice.

Resources

For Patients

American Heart Association: http://www.heart.org
American Society of Hypertension: http://www.ash-us.org
UpToDate: http://www.uptodate.com

For Clinicians

Agency for Healthcare Research and Quality: http://www.ahrq.gov/ and
    http://www.guideline.gov
PsyResearch.org: http://psyresearch.org
PubMed: http://www.ncbi.nlm.nih.gov/pubmed

References

Bosworth HB, Bartash RM, Olsen MK, et al: The association of psychosocial factors and depression with hypertension among older adults. Int J Geriatr Psychiatry 18:1142–1148, 2003

Boulware LE, Daumit GL, Frick KD, et al: An evidence-based review of patient-centered behavioral interventions for hypertension. Am J Prev Med 21:221–232, 2001

Carroll D, Phillips AC, Gale CR, et al: Generalized anxiety and major depressive disorders, their comorbidity and hypertension in middle-aged men. Psychosom Med 72:16–19, 2010

Egan BM, Zhao Y, Axon RN: US trends in prevalence, awareness, treatment, and control of hypertension, 1988–2008. JAMA 303:2043–2050, 2010

Goff DC, Sullivan LM, McEvoy JP, et al: A comparison of ten-year cardiac risk estimates in schizophrenia patients from the CATIE study and matched controls. Schizophr Res 80:45–53, 2005

Goldstein BI, Fagiolini A, Houck P, et al: Cardiovascular disease and hypertension among adults with bipolar I disorder in the United States. Bipolar Disord 11:657–662, 2009

James PA, Oparil S, Carter BL, et al: 2014 evidence-based guideline for the management of high blood pressure in adults—report from the panel members appointed to the Eighth Joint National Committee (JNC 8). JAMA 311:507–520, 2014

Johannessen L, Strudsholm U, Foldager L, et al: Increased risk of hypertension in patients with bipolar disorder and patients with anxiety compared to background population and patients with schizophrenia. J Affect Disord 95:13–17, 2006

Lewington S, Clarke R, Qizilbash N, et al: Age-specific relevance of usual blood pressure to vascular mortality: a meta-analysis of individual data for one million adults in 61 prospective studies. Lancet 360:1903–1913, 2002

Nasrallah HA, Meyer JM, Goff DC, et al: Low rates of treatment for hypertension, dyslipidemia and diabetes in schizophrenia: data from the CATIE schizophrenia trial sample at baseline. Schizophr Res 86:15–22, 2006

U.S. Department of Health and Human Services: The Seventh Report of the Joint National Committee on Prevention, Detection, Evaluation, and Treatment of High Blood Pressure. Publ No 04-5230. Rockville, MD, National Institutes of Health, National Heart, Lung, and Blood Institute, National High Blood Pressure Education Program, August 2004. Available at: http://www.nhlbi.nih.gov/files/docs/guidelines/jnc7full.pdf. Accessed August 15, 2014.

U.S. Preventive Services Task Force: Screening for high blood pressure: U.S. Preventive Services Task Force reaffirmation recommendation statement. Ann Intern Med 147:783–786, 2007

Wolff T, Miller T: Evidence for the reaffirmation of the U.S. Preventive Services Task Force recommendation on screening for high blood pressure. Ann Intern Med 147:787–791, 2007

CHAPTER 7

Dyslipidemia

Erik R. Vanderlip, M.D.

Case Discussion

Mr. J is a 55-year-old black man with a history of hepatitis C, intermittent co-caine use, a 20 pack-year smoking history, chronic schizophrenia, hypertension, and poor dentition. He lives in a supported housing program near a community mental health clinic. His psychiatric medications include olanzapine 20 mg/day in addition to a risperidone long-acting injection every 2 weeks. He has been stable while out of the hospital and living somewhat independently for the past 4 years on this medication regimen. He does not routinely take his blood pressure medications and pays little attention to his diet. His body mass index is 31. He does not know if he has a significant family history of coronary artery disease and does not recall ever having a heart attack. He has been tested for diabetes and does not have it. His nonfasting total cholesterol (TC) is 260 mg/dL, high-density lipoprotein (HDL) cholesterol is 65 mg/dL, triglyceride level is 344 mg/dL, and low-density lipoprotein (LDL) (calculated) is 126 mg/dL.

Clinical Overview

Cholesterol is a waxy compound essential to the functioning of cell membranes in mammals. Cholesterol is acquired through direct ingestion of animal by-products (meats, eggs, lard) and through endogenous production in the liver. Although certain fats, such as trans fats, are more readily broken down and yield higher relative concentrations of cholesterol than others, most persons synthesize the majority of their cholesterol in the liver while fasting overnight. This process is dependent on 3-hydroxy-3-methylglutaryl-coenzyme A (HMG-CoA) reductase, the target of the famous statin class of cholesterol-lowering medications. After synthesis or ingestion, cholesterol is packaged in water-soluble lipoprotein molecules for transport to and from bodily tissues through the bloodstream. The relative quantity of cholesterol is accounted for by the mass of these circulating lipoproteins, identified by their relative density, and reported in a typical lipid panel. The fraction of cholesterol contained within LDL or non-HDL is most closely associated with risk for cardiovascular disease (CVD) biologically and epidemiologically (Di Angelantonio et al. 2009; Expert Panel on Detection, Evaluation, and Treatment of High Blood Cholesterol in Adults 2001; Stone et al. 2013).

CVD is the leading cause of death for adults in the United States. Dyslipidemia, defined as elevated TC, elevated LDL, or low HDL, is one of the leading independent risk factors for the development of CVD. Dyslipidemia is prevalent, affecting up to 25% of all U.S. adults (Expert Panel on Detection, Evaluation, and Treatment of High Blood Cholesterol in Adults 2001; Ford et al. 2003). As serum concentrations of LDL and TC increase, and HDL decreases, there is a significantly higher likelihood of myocardial infarction, stroke, and death (Kannel et al. 1971). Similarly, targeted lowering of TC and LDL levels in individuals with or without prior history of myocardial infarction significantly reduces the likelihood of morbidity and mortality resulting from subsequent cardiovascular events (Expert Panel on Detection, Evaluation, and Treatment of High Blood Cholesterol in Adults 2001; Stone et al. 2013; Taylor et al. 2013).

Numerous analyses have demonstrated excess mortality and morbidity due to CVD among individuals with severe and persistent mental illness (Colton and Manderscheid 2006; Druss et al. 2011; Miller et al. 2006; Saha et al. 2007; Sodhi et al. 2012). The prevalence of dyslipidemia among those with severe and persistent mental illness ranges from 25% to 70% (De Hert et al. 2011a; McEvoy et al. 2005) and is markedly higher than among age-matched population control subjects. This observation is likely the result of a confluence of multiple factors, which include, among others, sedentary lifestyle, poor diet, obesity, tobacco use, and treatment with antipsychotic or mood-stabilizing medications (Aliyazicioğlu et al. 2007; Compton et al. 2006; Daumit et al. 2005; Meltzer et al. 2011; Meyer and Koro 2004; Saari et al. 2005). In spite of this growing recognition, up to 88% of patients with schizophrenia diagnosed with dyslipidemia do not receive treatment, making it one of the most prevalent yet undertreated risk factors for CVD among those with severe mental illness (Nasrallah et al. 2006).

Practical Pointers

- Non–high-density lipoprotein (HDL) cholesterol (total cholesterol [TC] – HDL cholesterol) can be calculated without regard to fasting status. Nonfasting samples are more convenient for patients, especially in community-based mental health settings.
- Non-HDL cholesterol (TC – HDL cholesterol) may be a more reliable indicator of cardiovascular disease (CVD) risk than low-density lipoprotein, especially in persons with the metabolic syndrome phenotype common to those treated with second-generation antipsychotics (Blaha et al. 2008; Di Angelantonio et al. 2009).
- Screening and treating dyslipidemias in patients who have mental illness (particularly those taking an atypical antipsychotic) can significantly decrease risk for cardiac-related morbidity and mortality.

Diagnosis

Diagnosis and subsequent treatment of dyslipidemias are based on risk. Dyslipidemia occurs when cholesterol levels contribute excessively to an individual's CVD risk and the burden of pharmacotherapy or lifestyle modification is less than that risk. Because of the many trials utilizing statin therapy as the primary outcome demonstrating reductions in death or major cardiovascular events with significant reduction in cholesterol, treatment with statins to lower cholesterol remains the mainstay of cholesterol treatment (Expert Panel on Detection, Evaluation, and Treatment of High Blood Cholesterol in Adults 2001; Stone et al. 2013). Consequently, cholesterol is generally categorized as high and warranting intervention when the risk of treatment with a statin is offset by the potential for cardiovascular risk reduction over 10 years. Generally, individuals with greater than 7.5% risk of myocardial infarction or stroke in 10 years who are between ages 40 and 75 years and have an LDL cholesterol value greater than 70 mg/dL are eligible for statin therapy and therefore are classified as having dyslipidemia. Individuals with LDL values in excess of 190 mg/dL have such high lifetime risk that they may be candidates for lipid-lowering pharmacotherapy prior to age 40 (Table 7–1).

Until recent guidelines were released, individuals were given specific LDL targets (e.g., < 130 mg/dL, 100 mg/dL, or 70 mg/dL, depending on their cardiovascular risk). Many individuals failed to achieve these goals, requiring more intensive multidrug lipid-lowering regimens, which have not demonstrated effectiveness in reducing heart attacks or strokes (Stone et al. 2013). Current clinical evidence does not support any use of alternative lipid pharmacotherapies besides statins to achieve cholesterol reduction, and therefore a diagnosis of dyslipidemia depends primarily on an individual's candidacy for statin therapy.

TABLE 7–1. Four clinical classes of statin eligibility

Clinical characteristic	Type of prevention[a]	Applicable age range	Preferred statin intensity	Potential actions
Clinical presence of CVD[b]	Secondary	21–75	High	—
Serum LDL ≥190 mg/dL[c]	Primary	21–75	High	Work up potential secondary causes[d]
Type 2 diabetes[e]	Primary	40–75	Moderate to high	—
10-year risk >7.5%[e]	Primary	40–75	Moderate	—

Note. CVD = cardiovascular disease; LDL = low-density lipoprotein.

[a]Primary prevention takes place when there is no clinical evidence of disease. Secondary prevention applies to therapies in place after the clinical presence of disease.

[b]For list, refer to Tables 7–2 and 7–3.

[c]Individuals with non-high-density lipoprotein (HDL) cholesterol (total cholesterol – HDL cholesterol) greater than 220 mg/dL also fall into this category.

[d]Potential secondary causes (see Table 7–7).

[e]These recommendations apply to individuals with LDL cholesterol values of 70–189 mg/dL.

Source. Adapted from Stone et al. 2013.

TABLE 7–2. **Cardiovascular disease risk equivalents (10-year risk ~20%, risk-class high)**

Diabetes mellitus

Abdominal aortic aneurysm

Peripheral arterial disease

Symptomatic carotid artery stenosis

Source.   Adapted from Vanderlip et al. 2012.

Individuals with clinical atherosclerotic CVD—that is, acute coronary syndromes, history of myocardial infarction, stable or unstable angina, prior coronary or other arterial revascularization, stroke, transient ischemic attack, or atherosclerotic peripheral vascular disease—have a high (about 20%) risk of having another event in the subsequent 10 years. They should have cholesterol reduction for secondary prevention. They should be placed on the strongest form of statin therapy available and tolerable without regard to their LDL cholesterol values, unless such therapy is otherwise contraindicated (Table 7–1). Table 7–2 lists the set of conditions that are considered equal to this level of risk, known as CVD *risk equivalents.* Patients with existing severe congestive heart failure or end-stage renal disease requiring dialysis have not been shown to benefit from statin therapy and are an exception to this rule.

Candidates for primary prevention are classified based on the presence or absence of diabetes type 1 or 2 and the estimated 10-year risk of myocardial infarction or stroke. This risk estimate is derived from a risk prediction tool that is based on an individual's age, gender, race (white vs. nonwhite), smoking status, diabetes status, TC, HDL cholesterol, and most recent systolic blood pressure, as well as whether or not his or her blood pressure is currently being treated. The risk prediction tool can be accessed from the American Heart Association (AHA) CV [Cardiovascular] Risk Calculator (see "Resources" at the end of this chapter). The presence of one or two major risk factors for CVD (of which the majority of clients with severe and persistent mental illness have one) makes an individual a candidate for cholesterol screening (Table 7–3). Individuals who are in need of secondary prevention or who are at high risk and require primary prevention likely warrant the most intensive therapeutic regimens, whereas individuals at lower risk usually warrant more modest interventions.

Although the most current guidelines use LDL cholesterol as the primary value in determining risk, emerging evidence is pointing toward the use of non-HDL cholesterol as the primary criterion by which dyslipidemias may

TABLE 7–3. **Major risk factors for cardiovascular disease**

Family history of cardiovascular disease in first-degree relative (male < 55 years, female < 65 years)

Cigarette smoking

Hypertension, treated or untreated

Age (male ≥ 45 years, female ≥ 55 years)

High-density lipoprotein < 40 mg/dL

Source.   Adapted from Vanderlip et al. 2012.

be defined and managed (Sniderman and Kwiterovich 2013). This change may be particularly important to individuals with the constellation of metabolic abnormalities, which include obesity, impaired glucose tolerance, and high triglycerides—a pattern commonly encountered with antipsychotic therapy (Blaha et al. 2008; Newcomer 2005). Conveniently, non-HDL cholesterol can be calculated by subtracting HDL from the TC concentration and varies less than 2% between fasting and nonfasting states, making nonfasting samples reliable and valid (Sidhu et al. 2012). Cutoffs for non-HDL cholesterol are established as 30 mg/dL higher than LDL cutoffs, and non-HDL cholesterol can be lowered through the same therapies (Expert Panel on Detection, Evaluation, and Treatment of High Blood Cholesterol in Adults 2001) (see Table 7–1). For example, individuals with non-HDL cholesterol values greater than 220 mg/dL fall into the same class as those with LDL values greater than 190 mg/dL and warrant intervention and possible evaluation for secondary causes of abnormally high cholesterol (see Table 7–1). Clinicians may consider using non-HDL levels if they are unable to reliably get fasting LDL levels for a patient.

After cholesterol is measured and an individual's risk is determined, he or she can be appropriately categorized according to treatment intensity (Figure 7–1). Nonfasting TC, HDL, triglycerides, and hemoglobin A_{1c} encompass all the blood work necessary to determine risk category, especially if a clinician opts to use non-HDL cholesterol instead of LDL measurement.

Preventive Guidelines

The U.S. Preventive Services Task Force (2008) recommends screening males at average risk for dyslipidemias at age 35 and females at age 45. The primary guidelines for assessment and management of dyslipidemias in the United States are now governed by the American College of Cardiology (ACC) and the AHA. The most recent updates were made available in the fall of 2013 (Stone et al. 2013). For patients taking atypical antipsychotic medications, a consensus panel recommended obtaining cholesterol levels every 5 years in adults at average risk, although more recent experts have recommended yearly screening for patients who need ongoing antipsychotic treatment or for patients undergoing treatment who have gained in excess of 7% from their baseline weight (American Diabetes Association et al. 2004; De Hert et al. 2011b). Figure 7–1 presents a screening and treatment algorithm based on the AHA/ ACC guidelines from 2013, and Table 7–4 represents the recommended screening intervals for cardiovascular risk factors among patients taking second-generation antipsychotics.

Treatment Recommendations

Generally, individuals are candidates for low-, moderate-, or high-intensity cholesterol lowering. Individuals in need of high-intensity therapy need to have reductions in LDL or non-HDL cholesterol of around 50% or greater, whereas individuals in low-intensity regimens tend to need less than 30% reduction. Moderate-intensity therapies typically result in cholesterol reductions between 30% and 50%.

Treatment of dyslipidemias should begin with diet and lifestyle modifications. Table 7–5 lists common lifestyle interventions and their effect on cholesterol levels as well as any link toward improving CVD outcomes. Persons should be counseled to avoid trans and saturated fat consumption. Also, if it is clinically feasible, persons taking highly metabolically active antipsychotic medications (e.g., olanzapine, clozapine, thorazine), as well as somewhat less metabolically active medications (e.g., risperidone, quetiapine), should be given trials of less metabolically active therapies (e.g., aripiprazole, ziprasidone) (Stroup et al. 2011; Weiden 2007). Notably, most diet and lifestyle modifications result in low to moderate reduction of LDL cholesterol, usually less than 50%.

If, after 3 months, intensive diet and lifestyle modifications cannot be maintained or are insufficient to achieve lower cholesterol, or if the person is not a candidate for switching therapies to less metabolically active medications, pharmacotherapy for dyslipidemia should be considered. Because of their proven efficacy, ease of use, and relatively safe profiles, statin medications are the first choice and are well tolerated in patients (De Hert et al. 2006; Nelson et al. 2011; Taylor et al. 2013). Table 7–6 lists the statin therapies grouped by their treatment intensity. Simvastatin should be avoided if possible because of reported drug-drug interactions, and individuals taking dosages above 40 mg/day are more prone to myositis (U.S. Food and Drug Administration 2011). Statins are very rarely hepatotoxic and may be safely administered to patients with concurrent hepatitis C (provided that they are

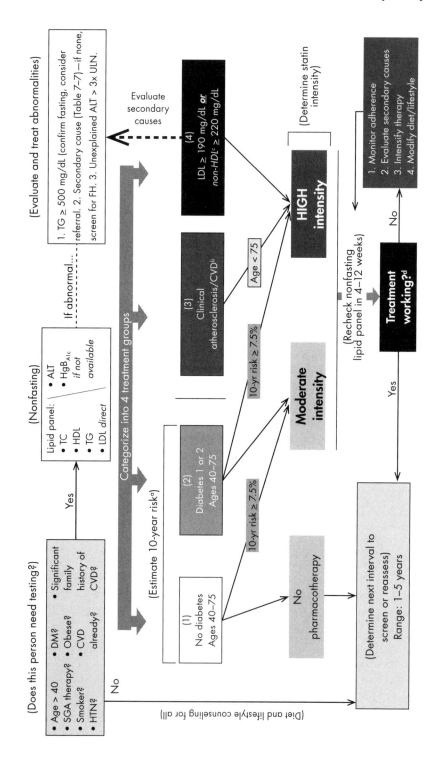

FIGURE 7–1. Screening, assessment, and treatment of dyslipidemias.

Note. ALT = alanine transaminase; CVD = cardiovascular disease; DM = diabetes mellitus; FH = familial hyperlipidemia; HDL = high-density lipoprotein cholesterol; HgB$_{A1c}$ = hemoglobin A$_{1c}$; HTN = hypertension; LDL = low-density lipoprotein cholesterol; SGA = second-generation antipsychotic; TC = total cholesterol; TG = triglycerides; ULN = upper limit of normal.

[a] Ten-year risk can be assessed through an online calculator available at: http://my.americanheart.org/professional/StatementsGuidelines/PreventionGuidelines/Prevention-Guidelines_UCM_457698_SubHomePage.jsp.

[b] See Table 7–1. Individuals older than age 75 on high-intensity statin therapy should discuss with their physicians lowering their treatment intensity to moderate, and discuss the risks and benefits of initiating statin therapy.

[c] Non-HDL cholesterol = total cholesterol – HDL cholesterol.

[d] Individuals undergoing high-intensity statin therapies generally have a 50% or greater reduction in LDL or non-HDL cholesterol, and it is generally under 100 mg/dL. Individuals undergoing moderate-intensity statin therapy should have a 30%–50% reduction in LDL or non-HDL. Although not the primary target with therapy, follow-up serum cholesterol levels can help monitor adherence and therapeutic efficacy.

Source. Adapted from Stone et al. 2013.

TABLE 7–4. Recommendations for metabolic monitoring of patients treated with second-generation antipsychotic medications

	Baseline	4 weeks	8 weeks	12 weeks	Quarterly	Annually
Personal/family history	X					X
Weight (BMI)	X	X	X	X	X	
Waist circumference	X					X
Blood pressure	X			X		X
Fasting plasma glucose	X			X		X
Fasting lipid profile	X			X		X

Note. BMI = body mass index.
Source. Adapted from American Diabetes Association et al. 2004.

TABLE 7–5. Selected lifestyle modifications and their effect on the lipid profile

Diet/intervention	Characteristic	Effect on cholesterol	Evidence for CVD reduction
Saturated fat	<7% saturated fat	Lowers LDL 9%–16%	Lowers
Cholesterol	<200 mg/day	Lowers LDL 9%–16%	Lowers
Total fat	25%–35% of total dietary caloric intake/day	Lowers LDL 9%–16%	Lowers
Fish	2 servings fatty fish/week	Lowers triglycerides	Lowers; likely not related to triglyceride lowering
Fiber, total + reduced saturated fat	>25 g/day	Lowers TC 2%–3%, LDL 7%	Lowers CVD risk
Plant stanols/sterols (e.g., Benecol spread)	2–3 g/day	Lowers TC 4%–11%, LDL 7%–15%	Not established
Soy proteins	26–50 g/day	Negligible	Not established
Tree nuts (i.e., almonds)	50–113 g/day (0.5–1 cup) isocaloric	Lowers TC 4%–21%, LDL 6%–29%	Lowers CVD
Alcohol	1–2 beverages/day	Raises HDL ~ 10%, lowers LDL ~ 6%	High consumption raises all-cause mortality
Red yeast rice extract; contains active statin compound	Various quantities, poor regulation	Raises HDL 5%, lowers LDL 30%–40%, lowers TC 40%–50%	Not established
Exercise, aerobic, moderate	30 min/day, 120 min/week	Raises HDL 9%, lowers LDL 5%, lowers TG 11%	Reduction in all-cause mortality
Portfolio diet	Combination of soy, nuts, fiber, and plant sterols	HDL negligible, TG negligible, lowers LDL 15%	Not established

Note. CVD=cardiovascular disease; HDL=high-density lipoprotein; LDL=low-density lipoprotein; TC=total cholesterol.
Source. Adapted from Kelly 2010; Van Horn et al. 2008.

TABLE 7–6.   Statin medications by dose and treatment intensity

Intensity class	LDL cholesterol effect	Drug/daily dosage	Notes
High	≥50% reduction	Atorvastatin 40–80 mg[a] Rosuvastatin 20–40 mg[b]	Higher potency is associated with higher rates of myalgias and side effects.
Moderate	30%–<50% reduction	Atorvastatin 10 mg[a] Rosuvastatin 5–10 mg[b] Simvastatin 20–40 mg[a] Pravastatin 40–80 mg[b] Lovastatin 40 mg[a] Fluvastatin 40 mg bid Pitavastatin 2–4 mg[b]	
Low	<30% reduction	Simvastatin 10 mg[a] Pravastatin 10–20 mg[b] Lovastatin 20 mg[a] Fluvastatin 20–40 mg Pitavastatin 1 mg[b]	Lower potency should be reserved for those intolerant of high- to moderate-intensity therapies.

Note.   LDL = low-density lipoprotein.
[a]Metabolized by cytochrome P450 (CYP) 3A4; grapefruit juice could raise drug levels; potential interactions with selected other therapies.
[b]No CYP metabolism; potentially fewer drug-drug interactions.

without liver failure) and to those with known liver disease. Baseline transaminase levels should be obtained before a patient begins taking a statin, but regular monitoring of liver function is no longer required (Andrus and East 2010). Nevertheless, it is reasonable to measure liver enzymes if symptoms suggesting hepatotoxicity arise (e.g., unusual fatigue or weakness, loss of appetite, abdominal pain, dark-colored urine, yellowing of the skin or sclera) (Stone et al. 2013). Individuals with greater than threefold elevations should have their statin use held until an underlying etiology can be found, and then periodic monitoring is indicated. Statins are contraindicated during pregnancy and breastfeeding.

Individuals with highly elevated initial cholesterol values (fasting calculated LDL or direct LDL > 190 mg/dL or fasting or nonfasting non-HDL cholesterol > 220 mg/dL) should be evaluated for secondary causes of dyslipidemias (see Figure 7–1 and Table 7–7). For this reason, as well as to classify initial 10-year risk and monitor therapeutic efficacy and adherence, periodic assessment of fasting LDL or nonfasting TC and HDL is necessary once treatment is initiated. Yearly assessment of the lipid profile is appropriate while a patient is undergoing therapy. Individuals should be placed on the highest-intensity regimen indicated and tolerated. Generally, higher-intensity statin regimens are associated with more side effects (e.g., myalgias, elevated liver enzymes) and less tolerance. Persons intolerant of higher-intensity regimens may opt for lower-intensity regimens. Those failing to meet approximate targets in cholesterol reduction after a trial of therapy should be evaluated for secondary causes of dyslipidemia, poor adherence to therapy, drug-drug interactions, and the potential to intensify their statin therapy as tolerated. Alternative drug therapies, such as niacin, fibrates, bile acid sequestrants, or ezetimibe, have not conclusively been shown to reduce the rate of stroke or myocardial infarction and are therefore not indicated.

Targeted treatment of elevated triglycerides and low HDL levels has not resulted in improvements in cardiovascular outcomes and is not recommended except in cases where the triglyceride concentration is above 500 mg/dL, at which point there is a heightened risk of pancreatitis (Keech et al. 2005).

When to Refer

Patients who should be referred to a primary care provider include the following:

- Patients with familial hyperlipidemias
- Patients in whom approximate cholesterol reduction goals are not achieved after adherence to a maximal dose of a high-potency statin medication (rosuvastatin, atorvastatin) for at least 1 month

TABLE 7–7. **Leading secondary causes of severely elevated blood cholesterol**

Secondary cause	Details
Disease/medical/genetic	Diabetes mellitus Hypothyroidism Chronic kidney disease Nephropathy, proteinuria Familial (genetic) hyperlipidemia Pregnancy[a]
Substance use	Excessive alcohol intake
Medications	Estrogen HIV antiretroviral therapy Antipsychotic medications Steroids, immunosuppressants Drug-drug interactions limiting statin efficacy
Diet	Extreme obesity High saturated and trans fat intake

[a]Pregnancy and lactation are contraindications to statin therapies.
Source.   Adapted from Stone et al. 2013; Vodnala et al. 2012.

- High-risk patients intolerant of statin medications
- Patients whose triglyceride concentrations are above 500 mg/dL, warranting independent treatment
- Patients with a history of myocardial infarction, bypass grafting, or percutaneous interventions such as stent placement
- Patients with very high serum cholesterol (non-HDL >220 mg/dL or LDL >190 mg/dL) warranting secondary workup

Special Treatment Considerations for the Psychiatric Patient Population

Because of myriad psychosocial issues plaguing patients with severe and persistent mental illness, achieving cholesterol reduction through diet and lifestyle modifications may be challenging. Nevertheless, emerging evidence supports the role of diet and lifestyle changes in managing obesity in those with severe mental illness (Chen et al. 2009; Daumit et al. 2013). Smoking cessation also may help to improve the lipid profile and should be pursued aggressively. Pravastatin may be considered for those in need of modest reduction in serum cholesterol because of its generic availability and relative paucity of drug-drug interactions with psychotropic medications. In the case that maximal doses of pravastatin fail to achieve needed therapeutic intensity, or when adherence to therapy during the evening is in question, atorvastatin (now generic) could be used because it is more potent and can be taken at any time during the day because of its long half-life (Cilla et al. 1996). Mental health clinicians engaging in pharmacotherapy for lipid disorders with patients are encouraged to be in contact with primary care clinicians in case referral is indicated and to obtain updated treatment recommendations.

Case Discussion (*continued*)

Mr. J has multiple risk factors for CVD, including his gender, age (55), smoking status, untreated hypertension (at this appointment, his systolic pressure is 154 mmHg), and TC of 265 mg/dL. His HDL level is above 60 mg/dL, which reduces his risk somewhat. Because Mr. J has no CVD risk equivalents (diabetes or known history of CVD [see Table 7–2]), his current 10-year risk of a major cardiovascular event or death is 15.8% (calculated using an online calculator). Because he is at greater than 7.5% risk, he would be a candidate for a moderate-intensity statin therapy. His LDL level, which was calculated in part on the triglyceride concentration, in this case is misleadingly low because his triglyceride concentration was high as a result of his not fasting. Therefore, his non-HDL value of 195 mg/dL is used to determine whether he needs an evaluation for a secondary cause (he does not because the non-HDL is less than 220 mg/dL) or to gauge his response to therapy. Because olanzapine is highly metabolically active, switching him to an equivalent dose of aripiprazole or ziprasidone (or another similarly weight-neutral first-generation antipsychotic such as perphenazine or haloperidol) should be considered, as should intensive diet and lifestyle modification and smoking cessation. If Mr. J has failed after 3 months to reduce his non-HDL value by around 30%–50% (100–140 mg/dL), he should try pravastatin at a moderate dose (40 mg) once in the evening, with the dose titrated every 1–3 months until his targets are obtained. If his basic goal of reduction by around 30% is not achieved after the maximum dose on a potent statin such as atorvastatin, he is intolerant of statins, or he is unable to consistently make diet and lifestyle modifications to reduce his cholesterol, he should be referred to primary care for further management.

Clinical Highlights

- Dyslipidemia is the most underrecognized and undertreated major cardiovascular risk factor present in individuals with severe mental illness.
- Nonfasting non–high-density lipoprotein (HDL) cholesterol (total cholesterol [TC] – HDL cholesterol) may be a more reliable indicator of cardiovascular risk than traditional low-density lipoprotein (LDL) cholesterol for those with severe mental illness.

Additionally, nonfasting non-HDL cholesterol is more convenient to measure and can be treated through similar therapies.

- Switching antipsychotic therapies to less metabolically active
drugs may help to improve the lipid profile.

- Intensive diet and lifestyle interventions for those with severe
mental illness have been shown to significantly reduce weight
and may improve cholesterol profiles, although they usually result in less than 50% reduction.

- Statin therapies are well tolerated, inexpensive, easy to use, and
highly effective at reducing cardiovascular risk for individuals at
moderate to high risk of subsequent events.

- Pravastatin, a relatively weak statin, has few drug-drug interactions, is generic, and is very well tolerated. It may be considered
as a first choice of the statins.

Resources

For Patients

American Heart Association: Cholesterol: Questions About the New
Guidelines? Available at: http://www.heart.org/HEARTORG/Condi-
tions/Cholesterol/Cholesterol_UCM_001089_SubHomePage.jsp
Mayo Clinic: Cholesterol: Top 5 Foods to Lower Your Numbers. Available at:
http://www.mayoclinic.com/health/cholesterol/CL00002

For Clinicians

American Heart Association: CV [Cardiovascular] Risk Calculator. Available at: http://my.americanheart.org/professional/StatementsGuide-
lines/PreventionGuidelines/
PreventionGuidelines_UCM_457698_SubHomePage.jsp
Eckel RH, Jakicic JM, Ard JD, et al: 2013 AHA/ACC Guideline on lifestyle management to reduce cardiovascular risk: a report of the American College
of Cardiology/American Heart Association Task Force on Practice Guidelines. Circulation Nov 12, 2013 [Epub ahead of print]. Available at: http://
circ.ahajournals.org/content/early/2013/11/11/01.cir.0000437740.48606.d1.
Stone NJ, Robinson JG, Lichtenstein AH, et al: 2013 ACC/AHA guideline on
the treatment of blood cholesterol to reduce atherosclerotic cardiovascular risk in adults: a report of the American College of Cardiology/Ameri-
can Heart Association Task Force on Practice Guidelines. J Am Coll
Cardiol 63(25, pt B):2889–2934, 2014

References

Aliyazicioğlu R, Kural B, Colak M, et al: Treatment with lithium, alone or in combination with olanzapine, relieves oxidative stress but increases atherogenic lipids in bipolar disorder. Tohoku J Exp Med 213:79–87, 2007

American Diabetes Association, American Psychiatric Association, American Association of Clinical Endocrinologists, et al: Consensus Development Conference on Antipsychotic Drugs and Obesity and Diabetes. Diabetes Care 27:596–601, 2004

Andrus MR, East J: Use of statins in patients with chronic hepatitis C. South Med J 103:1018–1022, 2010

Blaha MJ, Blumenthal RS, Brinton EA, et al: The importance of non-HDL cholesterol reporting in lipid management. J Clin Lipidol 2:267–273, 2008

Chen CK, Chen YC, Huang YS: Effects of a 10-week weight control program on obese patients with schizophrenia or schizoaffective disorder: a 12-month follow up. Psychiatry Clin Neurosci 63:17–22, 2009

Cilla DD Jr, Gibson DM, Whitfield LR, et al: Pharmacodynamic effects and pharmacokinetics of atorvastatin after administration to normocholesterolemic subjects in the morning and evening. J Clin Pharmacol 36:604–609, 1996

Colton CW, Manderscheid RW: Congruencies in increased mortality rates, years of potential life lost, and causes of death among public mental health clients in eight states. Prev Chronic Dis 3:A42, 2006

Compton MT, Daumit GL, Druss BG: Cigarette smoking and overweight/obesity among individuals with serious mental illnesses: a preventive perspective. Harv Rev Psychiatry 14:212–222, 2006

Daumit GL, Goldberg RW, Anthony C, et al: Physical activity patterns in adults with severe mental illness. J Nerv Ment Dis 193:641–646, 2005

Daumit GL, Dickerson FB, Wang NY, et al: A behavioral weight-loss intervention in persons with serious mental illness. N Engl J Med 368:1594–1602, 2013

De Hert M, Kalnicka D, Van Winkel R, et al: Treatment with rosuvastatin for severe dyslipidemia in patients with schizophrenia and schizoaffective disorder. J Clin Psychiatry 67:1889–1896, 2006

De Hert M, Correll CU, Bobes J, et al: Physical illness in patients with severe mental disorders, I: prevalence, impact of medications and disparities in health care. World Psychiatry 10:52–77, 2011a

De Hert M, Vancampfort D, Correll CU, et al: Guidelines for screening and monitoring of cardiometabolic risk in schizophrenia: systematic evaluation. Br J Psychiatry 199:99–105, 2011b

Di Angelantonio E, Sarwar N, Perry P, et al: Major lipids, apolipoproteins, and risk of vascular disease. JAMA 302:1993–2000, 2009

Druss BG, Zhao L, Von Esenwein S, et al: Understanding excess mortality in persons with mental illness: 17-year follow up of a nationally representative US survey. Med Care 49:599–604, 2011

Expert Panel on Detection, Evaluation, and Treatment of High Blood Cholesterol in Adults: Executive summary of the third report of the National Cholesterol Education Program (NCEP). JAMA 285:2486–2497, 2001

Ford ES, Mokdad AH, Giles WH, et al: Serum total cholesterol concentrations and awareness, treatment, and control of hypercholesterolemia among US adults: findings from the National Health and Nutrition Examination Survey, 1999 to 2000. Circulation 107:2185–2189, 2003

Kannel WB, Castelli WP, Gordon T, et al: Serum cholesterol, lipoproteins, and the risk of coronary heart disease. Ann Intern Med 74:1–12, 1971

Keech A, Simes RJ, Barter P, et al: Effects of long-term fenofibrate therapy on cardiovascular events in 9795 people with type 2 diabetes mellitus (the FIELD study): randomised controlled trial. Lancet 366:1849–1861, 2005

Kelly RB: Diet and exercise in the management of hyperlipidemia. Am Fam Physician 81:1097–1102, 2010

McEvoy JP, Meyer JM, Goff DC, et al: Prevalence of the metabolic syndrome in patients with schizophrenia: baseline results from the Clinical Antipsychotic Trials of Intervention Effectiveness (CATIE) schizophrenia trial and comparison with national estimates from NHANES III. Schizophr Res 80:19–32, 2005

Meltzer HY, Bonaccorso S, Bobo WV, et al: A 12-month randomized, open-label study of the metabolic effects of olanzapine and risperidone in psychotic patients: influence of valproic acid augmentation. J Clin Psychiatry 72:1602–1610, 2011

Meyer JM, Koro CE: The effects of antipsychotic therapy on serum lipids: a comprehensive review. Schizophr Res 70:1–17, 2004

Miller BJ, Paschall CB, Svendsen DP: Mortality and medical comorbidity among patients with serious mental illness. Psychiatr Serv 57:1482–1487, 2006

Nasrallah HA, Meyer JM, Goff DC, et al: Low rates of treatment for hypertension, dyslipidemia and diabetes in schizophrenia: data from the CATIE schizophrenia trial sample at baseline. Schizophr Res 86:15–22, 2006

Nelson LA, Graham MR, Lindsey CC, et al: Adherence to antihyperlipidemic medication and lipid control in diabetic Veterans Affairs patients with psychotic disorders. Psychosomatics 52:310–318, 2011

Newcomer JW: Second-generation (atypical) antipsychotics and metabolic effects: a comprehensive literature review. CNS Drugs 19:1–93, 2005

Saari KM, Lindeman SM, Viilo KM, et al: A 4-fold risk of metabolic syndrome: the Northern Finland 1966 Birth Cohort study. J Clin Psychiatry 66:559–563, 2005

Saha S, Chant D, McGrath J: A systematic review of mortality in schizophrenia: is the differential mortality gap worsening over time? Arch Gen Psychiatry 64:1123–1131, 2007

Sidhu D, Naugler C: Fasting time and lipid levels in a community-based population: a cross-sectional study. Arch Intern Med 172(22):1707–1710, 2012

Sniderman A, Kwiterovich PO: Update on the detection and treatment of atherogenic low-density lipoproteins. Curr Opin Endocrinol Diabetes Obes 20:140–147, 2013

Sodhi SK, Linder J, Chenard CA, et al: Evidence for accelerated vascular aging in bipolar disorder. J Psychosom Res 73:175–179, 2012

Stone NJ, Robinson JG, Lichtenstein AH, et al: 2013 ACC/AHA guideline on the treatment of blood cholesterol to reduce atherosclerotic cardiovascular risk in adults: a report of the American College of Cardiology/American Heart Association Task Force on Practice Guidelines. J Am Coll Cardiol 63(25, pt B):2889–2934, 2014

Stroup TS, McEvoy JP, Ring KD, et al: A randomized trial examining the effectiveness of switching from olanzapine, quetiapine, or risperidone to aripiprazole to reduce metabolic risk: Comparison of Antipsychotics for Metabolic Problems (CAMP). Am J Psychiatry 168:947–956, 2011

Taylor F, Huffman MD, Macedo AF, et al: Statins for the primary prevention of cardiovascular disease. Cochrane Database Syst Rev 1:CD004816, 2013

U.S. Food and Drug Administration: New Restrictions, Contraindications, and Dose Limitations for Zocor (Simvastatin) to Reduce the Risk of Muscle Injury. Rockville, MD, U.S. Food and Drug Administration, June 2011. Available at: http://www.fda.gov/Drugs/DrugSafety/ucm256581.htm. Accessed August 30, 2011.

U.S. Preventive Services Task Force: Screening for Lipid Disorders in Adults. Rockville, MD, U.S. Preventive Services Task Force, June 2008. Available at: http://www.uspreventiveservicestaskforce.org/uspstf/uspschol.htm. Accessed August 30, 2011.

Vanderlip ER, Fiedorowicz JG, Haynes WG: Screening, diagnosis, and treatment of dyslipidemia among persons with persistent mental illness: a literature review. Psychiatr Serv 63:693–701, 2012

Van Horn L, McCoin M, Kris-Etherton PM, et al: The evidence for dietary prevention and treatment of cardiovascular disease. J Am Diet Assoc 108:287–331, 2008

Vodnala D, Rubenfire M, Brook RD: Secondary causes of dyslipidemia. Am J Cardiol 110:823–825, 2012

Weiden PJ: Switching antipsychotics as a treatment strategy for antipsychotic-induced weight gain and dyslipidemia. J Clin Psychiatry 68(suppl):34–39, 2007

CHAPTER 8

Tobacco Dependence

Nicole M. Bekman, Ph.D.
Robert M. Anthenelli, M.D.

Case Discussion

Ms. A is a 56-year-old patient diagnosed with schizoaffective disorder who has been smoking one to two packs of cigarettes per day since she was 26 years old. She struggles with thought withdrawal and delusions of reference, as well as bouts of mania, but for several years clozapine has kept these symptoms well controlled. She expressed interest in quitting smoking after her general practitioner diagnosed hypertension and recently notified her that she is on the border of a diagnosis of chronic obstructive pulmonary disease. She also noted that smoking cigarettes has at times exacerbated symptoms of panic and anxiety.

Ms. A, like so many patients with similar backgrounds, has been smoking at a high rate for many years and is heavily dependent on nicotine. She has attempted to quit several times on her own but was not successful. Friends and health care providers have advised her that quitting smoking may worsen her psychiatric symptoms or, at best, be simply too difficult. Ms. A also has a previous history of methamphetamine dependence and, although she has been abstinent from methamphetamine for several years, has had lingering concerns that quitting smoking may trigger a relapse.

Clinical Overview

Despite a greater than 50% decline in smoking rates over the past 50 years (National Institute on Drug Abuse 2012), tobacco use continues to be the largest preventable cause of death and illness in the United States and accounts for more than 443,000 deaths annually in this country (Centers for Disease Control and Prevention 2008). Tobacco smoking is known to cause a host of illnesses, including cancer, cardiovascular disease, and respiratory disorders. Mortality rates are three times as high among smokers, who have an average life expectancy 10 years shorter that that of nonsmokers (Jha et al. 2013). Most importantly, quitting smoking prior to age 40 may reduce death related to continued smoking by approximately 90% (Jha et al. 2013). Prevention of smoking-related illness and deaths, and the costs incurred by smoking, is of critical concern to the nation's health.

Men and women struggling with mental illness smoke almost half (44%) of the cigarettes consumed in the United States and are twice as likely to smoke as adults without mental illness (Grant et al. 2004; Lasser et al. 2000). In addition, smokers with higher levels of psychological distress smoke more cigarettes daily than smokers experiencing lower levels of distress (Lawrence et al. 2009). Unlike in the general population, rates of smoking among individuals with mental illness have not declined over time. This may partially explain why individuals with severe mental illness die an average of 25 years earlier than individuals without mental illness (Prochaska 2011). A subset of this population, including individuals with serious mental illnesses such as schizophrenia, schizoaffective disorder, and bipolar disorder and individuals with substance use disorders, smoke at even higher rates. As a result, they are at increased risk for multiple smoking-related lung and cardiovascular diseases, including cancer (Colton and Manderscheid 2006).

In addition to having the same risk factors for smoking that the general population faces, individuals with mental illness are at increased risk for nicotine dependence as a result of genetic links between mental illness and abnormalities in cholinergic mechanisms and nicotinic receptors. For these individuals, nicotine may serve to ameliorate specific deficits in sensory processing, attention, cognition, and mood associated with these genetic precursors (George et al. 2003; Leonard et al. 2001). Some research has also indicated that tobacco smoke inhibits monoamine oxidase and may have other psychoactive properties that cause it to have an antidepressant effect (Newhouse et al. 2004). Additionally, individuals diagnosed with mental illness and substance use disorders have consistently been exposed to treatment environments, such as recovery homes and residential facilities, where smoking is common and even encouraged (i.e., by providing cigarettes as a behavioral reward). Despite these challenges, as in the general population, most smokers diagnosed with mental illness are interested in quitting smoking and, as difficult as it may be, a significant percentage of these individuals succeed at their efforts (Prochaska 2011).

Practical Pointers

- Patients are more successful at quitting smoking when they are *not* in crisis, are psychiatrically stable, and have no recent or planned changes in psychiatric medications.
- Patients should be encouraged to choose a target quit date (TQD) when they will have sufficient support (combined pharmacotherapy and psychosocial treatment is recommended).
- The clinician should closely monitor patients over the days and weeks immediately following their TQD to examine the following:
  - Successes and challenges
  - Nicotine withdrawal symptoms
  - Cravings to smoke
  - Psychiatric symptoms and medication side effects
  - Treatment adherence
  - Potential fluctuations in serum drug levels

Diagnosis

Tobacco smoke is highly addictive, and cigarettes have been uniquely designed to deliver nicotine to the brain in a manner that efficiently hijacks the meso-corticolimbic dopamine circuitry (Anthenelli 2005). Individuals who smoke a pack of cigarettes a day deliver nicotine to their reward system an average of 250 times per day (National Institute on Drug Abuse 2012). Table 8–1 lists the DSM-5 (American Psychiatric Association 2013) diagnostic criteria for tobacco use disorder.

To best help patients quit smoking, the clinician needs to recognize and help ameliorate (when possible) the common symptoms of nicotine withdrawal, which can begin within 2–3 hours of last tobacco use and peak within 2–3 days of quitting. These symptoms include the following:

- Nicotine cravings
- Anxiety
- Depression
- Drowsiness, difficulty sleeping, nightmares
- Irritability and agitation
- Headaches
- Increased appetite and weight gain
- Cognitive and attention deficits

Withdrawal symptoms are typically more severe within the first week of quitting smoking and decline steadily over the course of 1 month (Hughes

TABLE 8–1. **DSM-5 diagnostic criteria for tobacco use disorder**

A problematic pattern of tobacco use leading to clinically significant impairment or distress, as manifested by at least two of the following, occurring within a 12-month period:

1. Tobacco is often taken in larger amounts or over a longer period than was intended.
2. There is a persistent desire or unsuccessful efforts to cut down or control tobacco use.
3. A great deal of time is spent in activities necessary to obtain or use tobacco.
4. Craving, or a strong desire or urge to use tobacco.
5. Recurrent tobacco use resulting in a failure to fulfill major role obligations at work, school, or home (e.g., interference with work).
6. Continued tobacco use despite having persistent or recurrent social or interpersonal problems caused or exacerbated by the effects of tobacco (e.g., arguments with others about tobacco use).
7. Important social, occupational, or recreational activities are given up or reduced because of tobacco use.
8. Recurrent tobacco use in situations in which it is physically hazardous (e.g., smoking in bed).
9. Tobacco use is continued despite knowledge of having a persistent or recurrent physical or psychological problem that is likely to have been caused or exacerbated by tobacco.
10. Tolerance, as defined by either of the following:
    a. A need for markedly increased amounts of tobacco to achieve the desired effect.
    b. A markedly diminished effect with continued use of the same amount of tobacco.
11. Withdrawal, as manifested by either of the following:
    a. The characteristic withdrawal syndrome for tobacco (refer to Criteria A and B of the criteria set for tobacco withdrawal).
    b. Tobacco (or a closely related substance, such as nicotine) is taken to relieve or avoid withdrawal symptoms.

Source. Reprinted from American Psychiatric Association: *Diagnostic and Statistical Manual of Mental Disorders,* 5th Edition. Arlington, VA, American Psychiatric Association, 2013. Copyright 2013, American Psychiatric Association. Used with permission.

2007). For some individuals, however, withdrawal symptoms may persist for 3–4 months (Piasecki et al. 2002). In a meta-analysis, Aubin et al. (2012) found that there is considerable heterogeneity with regard to weight fluctuations experienced by individuals following smoking cessation, although people gained an average of 4.7 kg (10.4 lb) over 12 months, with most of the weight gain occurring within the first 3 months after cessation.

Preventive Guidelines

In 2009, the U.S. Preventive Services Task Force recommended that clinicians do the following:

- Ask all adults about tobacco use and provide tobacco cessation interventions for those who use tobacco products.
- Ask all pregnant women about tobacco use and provide augmented, pregnancy-tailored counseling for those who smoke.

Because of the severity of nicotine dependence among psychiatrically ill smokers, these recommendations are critical for all mental health professionals to implement in their routine clinical practice. Although many patients are motivated to quit smoking and some will seek the help of mental health professionals, many more individuals will not pursue such help. This ambivalence reflects fluctuations in their own motivational level, a desire to approach the problem on their own, or lack of knowledge about the effectiveness of tobacco cessation medications and counseling and/or about who might be able to assist them. Inquiring about a patient's tobacco use and offering to aid him or her in the process will not damage the rapport a provider has built with his or her patient but rather will let the patient know that the provider is able and willing to assist if and when the patient is ready to make a quit attempt. It is important that the clinician make these inquiries frequently and consistently and that patients are aware that quitting is a strong recommendation the provider is making for their health and well-being. Approaching patients about their tobacco use and options for smoking cessation can help break down barriers and move patients toward giving cessation a try.

Treatment Recommendations

Although all patients who are interested in quitting smoking should be offered smoking cessation medication, these medications work best when combined with either brief counseling (<5 minutes) or more intensive, evidence-based individual or group psychotherapy (>10 minutes) (Hughes 2000). Several approaches to counseling, including motivational interviewing, cognitive-behavioral therapy, and psychoeducation, have demonstrated effectiveness. Depending on the time frame available, several key topics are helpful to review with patients as the clinician proceeds with smoking cessation counseling (Table 8–2); some are more useful before the patient makes a quit attempt and others may be more helpful as the patient encounters difficulties along the way. Counseling may be particularly important for smokers diagnosed with a psychiatric condition because this would allow for more patient support and opportunities to develop alternative coping strategies for psychiatric symptoms or nicotine cravings. In fact, integrating smoking cessation into ongoing treatment of a patient's primary mental disorder may increase engagement, adherence, and success in quitting smoking (McFall et al. 2010).

As outlined in the U.S. Public Health Service's Clinical Practice Guideline "Treating Tobacco Use and Dependence" (Fiore et al. 2008), the "5 A's" is a mnemonic device that outlines intervention steps for health care providers to use with their nicotine-dependent patients (Figure 8–1). This and other similar mnemonics serve to remind providers to spend time discussing smoking cessation and providing advice, resources, and referrals for smoking-dependent patients. Additionally, providers can advise patients to take advantage of state and national quit lines (e.g., 800-QUIT-NOW), which provide self-help materials, brief telephone-based counseling, referral resources, and information on cessation medications (Schroeder and Morris 2010).

Combined use of first-line smoking cessation medications, approved by the U.S. Food and Drug Administration (FDA), and psychosocial treatments is the most effective treatment option available for nicotine-dependent individuals, whether or not they have been diagnosed with a psychiatric disorder (Fiore et al. 2008). Three types of medications have currently been approved by the FDA: nicotine replacement therapy (NRT), bupropion sustained release (SR), and varenicline (Table 8–3). All three of these medications improve smoking cessation rates and long-term abstinence rates (Fiore et al. 2008).

NRT is available in several formulations: transdermal patch, gum, lozenge, inhaler, and nasal spray. Each of these has a different pharmacokinetic profile. Nicotine nasal spray provides a bolus of nicotine that most closely mimics smoking a cigarette, whereas nicotine patches provide a slower, longer-acting delivery. Because quit rates associated with the use of NRT are relatively modest, with an overall risk ratio of abstinence for NRT of 1.58 (Stead et al. 2008), studies have examined the effectiveness of combining two deliveries of NRT. For example, combining a longer-acting NRT such as the patch with a shorter-acting form such as a lozenge or a spray may help to reduce withdrawal symptoms in general and also help to combat cravings experienced at a given moment (Stead et al. 2008). This treatment strategy may be especially helpful for patients with psychiatric illness, who are frequently heavier smokers and therefore more nicotine dependent than the general population. In a similar vein, some research has demonstrated that it may be

TABLE 8–2. Topics to discuss in smoking cessation counseling

Topic	Description
Motivation	Exploring reasons the patient would like to quit smoking, as well as changes in his or her motivation over time
Past quit attempts	Exploring what worked and what did not; reasons for relapse
Quit strategy	Setting a target quit date; strategies for cutting down, if the patient prefers that to quitting at once (e.g., reducing number of cigarettes per day, or targeting specific locations or activities where he or she smokes)
Withdrawal symptoms	Identifying, monitoring, and treating nicotine withdrawal symptoms, if they occur (e.g., discussing sleep hygiene for insomnia, or exercise and nutritional choices for weight gain, or ways to cope with irritability or mood fluctuations)
Smoking cessation medications	Education about medication options, potential side effects, and dosing schedule; medication compliance for cessation aids and other psychotropic medication (e.g., discussing where patient keeps his or her medication; recommending alarm clocks, automated phone reminders, or weekly pill boxes)
Monitoring	Careful monitoring of psychiatric symptoms and successes/failures of smoking cessation strategies
Triggers/cravings	Identifying triggers for smoking and ways to cope with cravings/urges (e.g., anticipating and avoiding temptation/trigger situations, strategies to reduce negative affect, changing routines or distracting attention to cope with urges)
Social support	Helping the patient to engage family, friends, associates, and other members of the treatment team in aiding patient's efforts toward smoking cessation
Rewards for not smoking	Helping patient identify benefits of not smoking and reward systems for recognizing successes (e.g., using money saved from not smoking to buy small, frequent rewards, such as movie tickets)
Lapse versus relapse	Discussing the possibility of lapses and troubleshooting how to manage those events should they occur (e.g., rereading a list of motivations to quit, refocusing on an enjoyable task, changing physical environment to remove tobacco availability or other smoking-related cues)

Ask	Identify and document tobacco use status for every patient at every visit.
Advise	In a clear, strong, and personalized manner, urge every tobacco user to quit.
Assess	Determine whether the tobacco user is willing to make a quit attempt at this time.
Assist	For the patient willing to make a quit attempt, use counseling and pharmacotherapy to help him or her quit.
Arrange	Schedule follow-up contact, in person or by telephone, preferably within the first week after the quit date.

FIGURE 8–1.   Five major steps toward intervention—the 5 A's.

Source.   Adapted from Agency for Healthcare Research and Quality 2012.

helpful to use NRTs in the week or two prior to the patient's TQD, to increase the likelihood of successful cessation and long-term abstinence (Wang et al. 2008).

Bupropion SR has been approved as a smoking cessation aid since 1997 and has been successful in improving rates of smoking cessation (odds ratio [OR] = 1.94; 95% confidence interval [CI], 1.72–2.19) (Hughes et al. 2007). Bupropion may help with smoking cessation by increasing catecholamine neurotransmitters in the synapse and reducing cravings and withdrawal symptoms. Additionally, bupropion may block nicotinic acetylcholine receptors, further reducing cravings and withdrawal (Mansvelder et al. 2007). The dosage of this medication should be titrated upward over a week or more in advance of the patient's TQD in order to reduce side effects and reach an effective dose before the quit attempt is made.

Varenicline was specifically designed as a smoking cessation medication and was approved for use as such in 2006. This medication acts as a partial agonist of a specific subtype of nicotinic receptor ($\alpha 4\beta 2$) involved in mediating nicotine's rewarding effects, easing withdrawal symptoms by partially stimulating dopaminergic neurons and blocking nicotine from binding to this

TABLE 8–3. Smoking cessation medications

Drug	Daily dosage	Treatment duration	Potential side effects
First-line treatments			
Nicotine replacement therapy			
Transdermal 24-hour patch (over the counter)	21 mg/day to start 7- and 14-mg patches for tapering dosage	8–12 weeks	Skin irritation, insomnia
Polacrilex (gum), 2- or 4-mg piece (over the counter)	1 piece/hour (<24 pieces/day)	8–12 weeks	Mouth irritation, sore jaw, dyspepsia, hiccups
Lozenge (over the counter)	2- or 4-mg dose (see dosage formula and titration schedule in package)	12 weeks	Hiccups, nausea, heartburn
Vapor inhaler (prescription only)	6–16 cartridges/day (delivers 4 mg/cartridge)	3–6 months	Mouth and throat irritation
Nasal spray (prescription only)	1–2 doses/hour; dose=1 mg (0.5 mg per nostril); maximum dosage 40 mg/day	3–6 months	Nasal irritation, sneezing, cough, tearing eyes
Approved non-nicotine medications			
Bupropion (sustained release)	150 mg/day for 3 days, then 150 mg bid; start 1 week before quit date	7–12 weeks; up to 6 months to maintain abstinence	Insomnia, dry mouth, neuropsychiatric symptoms including depression, suicidal thoughts, agitation *Contraindications:* seizures, eating disorders

TABLE 8–3. Smoking cessation medications (*continued*)

Drug	Daily dosage	Treatment duration	Potential side effects
First-line treatments (*continued*)			
Approved non-nicotine medications (continued)			
Varenicline	0.5 mg/day for 3 days, then 0.5 mg bid for 4 days, then 1 mg bid for 3 months; start 1 week before quit date	12–24 weeks	Nausea, headache, insomnia, vivid dreams, neuropsychiatric symptoms including depression, suicidal thoughts, agitation
Second-line treatments[a]			
Nortriptyline	75–100 mg/day; start 10–28 days prior to quit date at 25 mg/day and increase as tolerated	12 weeks	Dry mouth, sedation, dizziness, suicidal thoughts
Clonidine		3–10 weeks	Dry mouth, sedation, dizziness
Combination nicotine replacement therapy			

[a]Recommended in the Clinical Practice Guideline (Fiore et al. 2008) but not approved for this indication by the U.S. Food and Drug Administration.

receptor. This blockage may reduce the reinforcing effects of nicotine and make lapses to smoking less rewarding.

Nortriptyline and clonidine are recommended in the Clinical Practice Guideline as second-line medications (Fiore et al. 2008). Nortriptyline may be particularly useful for patients who have struggled with depression (Hall et al. 1998), whereas clonidine is an antihypertensive agent. Both are best used with patients who have not responded well to a first-line medication.

When to Refer

- If a patient experiences mild and transient psychiatric symptoms with significant interepisode recovery and has an ongoing relationship with a primary care provider (PCP), he or she may be better followed by that provider for tobacco cessation services.
- If a patient is experiencing significant medical complications related to tobacco use, his or her care may be best managed by a PCP in collaboration with the mental health practitioner as part of a comprehensive treatment plan.
- Mental health providers who do not have a medical license (e.g., psychologists, social workers) are recommended to work closely with the patient's PCP and/or psychiatrist to ensure that smoking cessation medications are readily available and that the effectiveness and toxicity of other psychotropic medications are closely monitored as the patient cuts down and/or quits use of tobacco products.

Special Treatment Considerations for the Psychiatric Patient Population

Treatments that work with the general population of smokers appear to be effective among patients with psychiatric illness, and several studies indicate that psychiatric symptoms do not worsen when patients participate in smoking cessation treatment (for a review, see Banham and Gilbody 2010). It is important to ensure that patients are not in an acute crisis, are psychiatrically stable, and have not had any recent or planned changes in medications prior to initiating smoking cessation treatment (Anthenelli 2005). Because rates of relapse for smoking are high in all populations, and particularly among individuals with mental illness, certain precautions can be taken to improve outcomes for these patients. As mentioned in the previous section, "Treatment Recommendations," combining medications with counseling increases rates of cessation and long-term abstinence. Additionally, incorporating smoking cessation treatment into ongoing psychiatric services may help to improve outcomes, particularly engagement and adherence (McFall et al. 2010). Given the importance of consistent use of medications, including aspects of medication compliance enhancement would also be valuable to ensure that patients regularly take their psychotropic and smoking cessation medications.

Other important considerations are the timing and duration of treatment. Given that patients with psychiatric illness are considerably more nicotine dependent than their non–psychiatrically ill counterparts, they may require longer treatment with more frequent follow-up visits. Treatment duration and frequency of follow-ups may vary, however, based on the patient's level of nicotine dependence, experiences during previous quit attempts, and history with treatment compliance. It is recommended that providers encourage patients to set their TQD within 2 weeks of initiating pharmacotherapy (or longer, depending on how well medications are tolerated); however, flexible TQDs may work in some individuals (Rennard et al. 2012). Given that relapses frequently occur within a few days of quitting, providers may schedule their first follow-up appointment for the day after the TQD to assess the patient's success in quitting, withdrawal symptoms, and side effects from smoking cessation and psychotropic medications. Weekly follow-ups may be recommended for the first 1–2 months following cessation to monitor psychiatric symptoms and changes in withdrawal symptoms and potential side effects.

Because cigarette smoking induces the cytochrome P450 1A2 isoenzyme system, patients are at some risk for heightened blood levels of certain psychotropic medications after quitting smoking (Table 8–4). It is important that providers assess the presence of side effects and adjust psychotropic medications accordingly to prevent toxicity.

Case Discussion (*continued*)

Ms. A meets with her provider to discuss treatment options for nicotine dependence. She has been stably treated for schizoaffective disorder with clozapine for several years and has not had any hospitalizations or suicidal ideation in the past year. On the basis of her history of several previous failed quit attempts, including some instances using NRT, and her intermittent bouts of mania that make the use of antidepressant smoking cessation aids (bupropion SR and nortriptyline) more risky, a trial of varenicline is initiated 1 week before her TQD (her upcoming birthday). Her doctor provides information about several behavioral smoking cessation programs in the area, one of which is held at the same community mental health agency where she attends weekly group therapy. She agrees to sign up for a group that will be starting the following week on the same day as her therapy group. Ms. A's provider checks plasma levels of clozapine prior to her TQD and monitors her closely over the following weeks.

TABLE 8–4.	Psychotropic drugs whose blood levels may be impacted by tobacco smoke or smoking cessation		
Antipsychotics	Antidepressants	Mood stabilizers	Anxiolytics
Haloperidol	Clomipramine	Carbamazepine	Desmethyldiazepam
Chlorpromazine	Desipramine		Oxazepam
Fluphenazine	Doxepin		
Olanzapine	Imipramine		
Clozapine	Nortriptyline		

Ms. A recruits the help of her family, her therapist, and friends in her group but finds it very difficult to quit smoking. Although she is able to quit smoking for 3 days, she has several lapses after that and finds it difficult to abstain completely. She meets with her provider weekly to monitor her nicotine withdrawal and psychological symptoms, and she continues to set goals, including a new TQD. On this second attempt, she is able to quit smoking successfully, and a minor adjustment is made to her clozapine dosage to minimize side effects. During her behavioral smoking cessation groups, she focuses on strategies to cope with cravings to smoke. Ms. A continues taking a regular dose of varenicline for the full 6 months to continue to assist in managing breakthrough cravings, and receives support and encouragement through monthly follow-up visits throughout the course of the medication.

Clinical Highlights

- Smokers with psychiatric illness are at significantly increased risk for dying from tobacco-related illnesses because they are more likely to smoke heavily and have more difficulty quitting smoking.
- Smokers with mental illness are usually more dependent on nicotine and may need longer courses of nicotine replacement therapy and other treatments.
- Patients who want to quit smoking are more likely to succeed when provided proven smoking cessation treatments that include smoking cessation medications in combination with supportive counseling.
- Smoking cessation is best attempted when patients are not in crisis, are psychiatrically stable, and have not had recent or planned changes in their medication.
- Smoking cessation may increase the blood levels of some psychotropic medications, thus increasing side effects. Patients should be closely monitored in the days and weeks following a quit attempt.

- Mental health professionals should become actively involved in smoking cessation treatment.

Resources

For Patients

Centers for Disease Control and Prevention: How to Quit. Atlanta, GA, Centers for Disease Control and Prevention, 2011. Available at: http://www.cdc.gov/tobacco/quit_smoking/how_to_quit/index.htm.

National Alliance on Mental Illness: Hearts & Minds: Smoking and Mental Illness. Arlington, VA, National Alliance on Mental Illness, 2010. Available at: http://www.nami.org/Content/NavigationMenu/Hearts_and_Minds/Smoking_Cessation/Smoking.pdf.

National Cancer Institute: Clearing the Air: Quit Smoking Today. NIH Publication No 08-1647. Bethesda, MD, National Cancer Institute, October 2008. Available at: http://smokefree.gov/sites/default/files/pdf/clearing-the-air-accessible.pdf.

U.S. Department of Health and Human Services Public Health Service: Help for Smokers and Other Tobacco Users. May 2008. Available at: http://www.ahrq.gov/patients-consumers/prevention/lifestyle/tobacco/helpsmokers.pdf.

For Clinicians

Hughes JR: Taking smoking cessation treatment seriously: the American Psychiatric Association's Practice Guideline for the Treatment of Patients With Nicotine Dependence. Addiction 93:469–470, 1998

University of California, San Francisco, Smoking Cessation Leadership Center: Behavioral Health Resources. San Francisco, University of California, 2010. Available at: http://smokingcessationleadership.ucsf.edu/MH_Resources.htm.

University of Colorado Denver Department of Psychiatry: Smoking Cessation for Persons With Mental Illnesses: A Toolkit for Mental Health. Denver, Colorado, 2009. Available at: http://smokingcessationleadership.ucsf.edu/Downloads/catolgue/MHtoolkitJan_2009.pdf.

U.S. Department of Health and Human Services Public Health Service: Treating Tobacco Use and Dependence. Rockville, MD, U.S. Department of Health and Human Services, May 2008. Available at: http://www.ncbi.nlm.nih.gov/books/NBK63952.

References

Agency for Healthcare Research and Quality: Five major steps to intervention (the "5 A's"). Rockville, MD, Agency for Healthcare Research and Quality, December 2012. Available at: http://www.ahrq.gov/professionals/clinicians-providers/guidelines-recommendations/tobacco/5steps.html. Accessed September 2013.

American Psychiatric Association: Diagnostic and Statistical Manual of Mental Disorders, 5th Edition. Washington, DC, American Psychiatric Association, 2013

Anthenelli RM: How—and why—to help psychiatric patients stop smoking. Curr Psychiatry 4:77–87, 2005

Aubin HJ, Farley A, Lycett D, et al: Weight gain in smokers after quitting cigarettes: meta-analysis. BMJ 345:e4439, 2012

Banham L, Gilbody S: Smoking cessation in severe mental illness: what works? Addiction 105:1176–1189, 2010

Centers for Disease Control and Prevention: Annual smoking-attributable mortality, years of potential life lost, and economic costs—United States, 2000–2004. MMWR Morb Mortal Wkly Rep 57:1226–1228, 2008

Colton CW, Manderscheid RW: Congruencies in increased mortality rates, years of potential life lost, and causes of death among public mental health clients in eight states. Prev Chronic Dis 3:A42, 2006

Fiore MC, Jaen CR, Baker TB, et al: Treating Tobacco Use and Dependence: 2008 Update. Clinical Practice Guideline. Rockville, MD, U.S. Department of Health and Human Services Public Health Service, 2008

George TP, Vessicchio JC, Termine A: Nicotine and tobacco use in schizophrenia, in Medical Illness and Schizophrenia. Edited by Meyer JM, Nasrallah HR. Washington, DC, American Psychiatric Publishing, 2003, pp 81–98

Grant BF, Hasin DS, Chou SP, et al: Nicotine dependence and psychiatric disorders in the United States: results from the National Epidemiologic Survey on Alcohol and Related Conditions. Arch Gen Psychiatry 61:1107–1115, 2004

Hall SM, Reus VI, Munoz RF, et al: Nortriptyline and cognitive-behavioral therapy in the treatment of cigarette smoking. Arch Gen Psychiatry 55:683–690, 1998

Hughes JR: New treatments for smoking cessation. CA Cancer J Clin 50:143–151, 2000

Hughes JR: Effects of abstinence from tobacco: valid symptoms and time course. Nicotine Tob Res 9:315–327, 2007

Hughes JR, Stead LF, Lancaster T: Antidepressants for smoking cessation. Cochrane Database Syst Rev 1:CD00031, 2007

Jha P, Ramasundarahettige C, Landsman V, et al: 21st-century hazards of smoking and benefits of cessation in the United States. N Engl J Med 368:341–350, 2013

Lasser K, Boyd JW, Woolhandler S, et al: Smoking and mental illness: a population-based prevalence study. JAMA 284:2606–2610, 2000

Lawrence D, Mitrou F, Zubrick SR: Smoking and mental illness: results from population surveys in Australia and the United States. BMC Public Health 9:1–14, 2009

Leonard S, Adler LE, Benhammou K, et al: Smoking and mental illness. Pharmacol Biochem Behav 70:561–570, 2001

Mansvelder HD, Fagen ZM, Chang B, et al: Bupropion inhibits the cellular effects of nicotine in the ventral tegmental area. Biochem Pharmacol 74:1283–1291, 2007

McFall M, Saxon AJ, Malte CA, et al: Integrating tobacco cessation into mental health care for posttraumatic stress disorder: a randomized controlled trial. JAMA 304:2485–2493, 2010

National Institute on Drug Abuse: Tobacco Addiction. Tobacco Addiction Research Report Series (NIH Publ No 12–4342). Bethesda, MD, National Institute on Drug Abuse, 2012

Newhouse P, Singh A, Potter A: Nicotine and nicotinic receptor involvement in neuropsychiatric disorders. Curr Top Med Chem 4:267–282, 2004

Piasecki TM, Fiore MC, McCarthy DE, et al: Have we lost our way? The need for dynamic formulations of smoking relapse proneness. Addiction 97:1093–1108, 2002

Prochaska JJ: Smoking and mental illness: breaking the link. N Engl J Med 365:196–198, 2011

Rennard S, Hughes J, Cinciripini PM, et al: A randomized placebo-controlled trial of varenicline for smoking cessation allowing flexible quit dates. Nicotine Tob Res 14:343–350, 2012

Schroeder SA, Morris CD: Confronting a neglected epidemic: tobacco cessation for persons with mental illnesses and substance abuse problems. Annu Rev Public Health 31:297–314, 2010

Stead LF, Perera R, Bullen C, et al: Nicotine replacement therapy for smoking cessation. Cochrane Database Syst Rev (1):CD000146, 2008

U.S. Preventive Services Task Force: Counseling and Interventions to Prevent Tobacco Use and Tobacco-Caused Disease in Adults and Pregnant Women: Reaffirmation Recommendation Statement (AHRQ Publ No 09-05131-EF-1), Rockville, MD, U.S. Preventive Services Task Force, 2009. Available at: http://www.uspreventiveservicestaskforce.org/uspstf09/tobacco/tobaccors2.htm. Accessed April 23, 2014.

Wang D, Connock M, Barton P, et al: 'Cut down to quit' with nicotine replacement therapies in smoking cessation: a systematic review of effectiveness and economic analysis. Health Technol Assess 12:iii–iv. ix–xi, 1–135, 2008

CHAPTER 9

Chronic Obstructive Pulmonary Disease

Abdulkader Alam, M.D.
Xixi Wong, M.D.
R. Michael Huijon, M.D.

Case Discussion

Mr. R is a 54-year-old man with a history of hypertension, gastroesophageal reflux disease, and schizophrenia, which is well controlled with clozapine. He has a 25-year history of smoking three packs of cigarettes per day. He presented with hemoptysis and required a hospital admission. He was diagnosed with acute bronchitis, as well as chronic obstructive pulmonary disease based on pulmonary function testing and chest X ray (see Figure 9–1).

Mr. R is obese, with a body mass index (BMI) of 41. He has symptoms of persistent dyspnea on exertion, intermittent productive cough, and frequent recurrent respiratory infections. He completed a course of antibiotics and was discharged home. He was subsequently referred to a smoking cessation program and started taking nicotine lozenges.

Clinical Overview

Chronic obstructive pulmonary disease (COPD) is called the "silent epidemic" and is a leading cause of death worldwide (Calverley and Walker 2003). The

111

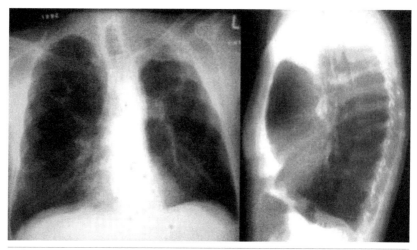

FIGURE 9–1.   Mr. R's chest X ray, showing hyperextended lung fields.

Global Initiative for Chronic Obstructive Lung Disease (2013) defines COPD as a disease state characterized by airflow limitation that is not fully reversible, is usually progressive, and is associated with an abnormal inflammatory response of the lungs to inhaled noxious particles or gases.

In addition to generating high health care costs, COPD imposes significant disability and impaired quality of life (Ferrer et al. 1997; Sullivan et al. 2000). Unlike many leading causes of death and disability, COPD is projected to rise in prevalence worldwide as the population ages and smoking becomes more commonplace (Feenstra et al. 2001). Although COPD is more common in individuals with mental illness, it often is underdiagnosed and unrecognized despite the high prevalence of smoking in this population.

Smoking prevention and smoking cessation are the keystone epidemiological measures necessary for counteracting the growing COPD epidemic.

Epidemiology, Risk Factors, and Impact of COPD

COPD affects more than 5% of the population and is a leading cause of morbidity and mortality worldwide (Centers for Disease Control and Prevention 2012). It is currently the third leading cause of death behind heart disease and cancer in the United States. In 2009, about 134,000 people died from COPD, and more than half (52.3%) were women (Miniño et al. 2011). A survey of patients with COPD found that their condition limits their ability to work (51%), to perform household chores (56%), to sleep (50%), and to participate in physical activities (70%), social activities (53%), and family activities (46%) (Schulman, Ronca, and Bucuvalas Inc 2001).

COPD represents a substantial socioeconomic burden for health care infrastructure. Current estimates suggest that COPD costs the United States alone almost $50 billion annually. It is also a significant cause of hospitalization in our aged population (National Center for Health Statistics, National Hospital Discharge Survey 1979–2006, unpublished data; Centers for Disease Control and Prevention 2011). Nonetheless, the data still greatly underestimate the total burden of COPD. This is because the disease usually is not diagnosed until it is clinically apparent and moderately advanced (Buist et al. 2007). Patients may not notice symptoms or may consider them normal (e.g., smoker's cough) and therefore delay presentation to their doctor.

Tobacco smoke is by far the most important risk factor for COPD. Approximately 85%–90% of COPD deaths are caused by smoking (Davis and Novotny 1989). Other important risk factors are occupational exposures, socioeconomic status, and genetic predisposition. Without major efforts in prevention, there will be an increasing number of end-stage COPD patients with an impaired quality of life.

COPD and Mental Illness

People with mental illness are much more likely to experience poor physical health than the general population. One study found that chronic pulmonary disease was the most prevalent comorbid condition in patients with severe mental illness (SMI) and was second in cost only to infectious diseases, with an average annual treatment cost of $8,277 per patient (Jones et al. 2004). In another study, individuals with SMI had over three times the odds of having chronic bronchitis and over five times the odds of having emphysema than a matched group of peers without SMI (Himelhoch et al. 2004). The prevalence of COPD is significantly higher among those with SMI than among those without SMI (Miller et al. 2006). Even when smoking was controlled for as a confounder, both people with schizophrenia and bipolar disorder were more likely to suffer from emphysema (Sokal et al. 2004). Although the association remains unclear, a higher incidence of COPD in the past two decades has been associated with the side effects of phenothiazine-related typical antipsychotics (Volkov 2009).

Individuals with mental illness, especially those with SMI, also have higher rates of premature death. Those with SMI are expected to lose an average of 25 years in life span. In about 60% of cases, this reduction is due to medical conditions such as cardiovascular, pulmonary, and infectious diseases. Chronic lower respiratory diseases were found to increase mortality risk three times in patients with SMI compared with those without SMI (Freeman and Yoe 2006).

Smoking and Mental Illness

Rates of cigarette smoking are very high among patients with psychotic and substance use disorders and fairly high among patients with depression, anxiety, and personality disorders. The prevalence of smoking is the highest among patients with schizophrenia, with an estimated range from 60% to 90% (Hahn et al. 2012). Furthermore, individuals with schizophrenia are more likely to be heavier smokers, smoke stronger cigarettes, start smoking at a younger age, and extract more nicotine from their cigarettes than smokers with other or without mental illnesses (George and Weinberger 2003; Kumari and Postma 2005; Ziedonis et al. 2003). Possible biological factors that lead to this high tobacco addiction with mental illness include an increased genetic vulnerability and cognitive-behavioral susceptibility (Hahn et al. 2012). Smoking may also be an attempt to self-medicate symptoms of depression, anxiety, loneliness, and other feelings common in this population (Kumari and Postma 2005). It has been shown to alleviate the side effects that are more common with the so-called typical antipsychotic medications. Studies suggest that individuals taking typical antipsychotics smoke significantly more than those taking atypical antipsychotics (Barnes et al. 2006).

Practical Pointers

- Tobacco smoke is the most important risk factor for chronic obstructive pulmonary disease (COPD). Approximately 85%–90% of COPD deaths are caused by smoking.
- The prevalence of COPD is higher in people with SMI, even after controlling for smoking.
- The prevalence of tobacco dependence is higher among individuals with schizophrenia than among individuals with other mental disorders.
- People with mental illness have three times the risk of chronic bronchitis, five times the risk of emphysema, and increased morbidity and mortality associated with COPD.

Diagnosis

COPD comprises both chronic bronchitis and emphysema. *Chronic bronchitis* is defined clinically as the presence of a chronic productive cough for 3 months during each of 2 consecutive years (after other causes of cough have been excluded). *Emphysema* is defined pathologically as an abnormal, permanent enlargement of the air spaces distal to the terminal bronchioles, accompanied by destruction of their walls and without obvious fibrosis.

Risk factors

- Smoking (number of pack-years smoked = packs of cigarettes per day × the number of years)
- Asthma
- Long-term exposure to aerosolized irritants (e.g., chemical dusts, fumes, vapors)
- Family history of lung disease

Symptoms

- Progressive and intermittent dyspnea
- Cough, usually worse in the mornings and productive of small amount of colorless sputum
- Wheezing, particularly during exertion and exacerbations
- Recurrent upper respiratory infections

Physical exam (findings are generally present only with severe disease)

- Pursed-lip breathing
- Cyanosis
- Barrel chest (hyperinflation)
- Hyperresonance on percussion
- Use of accessory respiratory muscles and/or intercostal retractions (Hoover's sign)
- Prolonged expiratory phase
- Decreased intensity of breath and heart sounds
- Wheezing during slow or forced breathing
- Mild dependent edema
- Digital clubbing

FIGURE 9–2. History and physical findings in chronic obstructive pulmonary disease.

Pathological changes in COPD occur in four different compartments of the lungs (central airways, peripheral airways, lung parenchyma, and pulmonary vasculature) and are variably present in individuals with the disease. History and physical findings in COPD are the same in people with and without mental illness (Figure 9–2).

Laboratory Tests

No laboratory test is diagnostic for COPD, but certain tests are sometimes performed to exclude other causes of dyspnea and comorbid diseases. Testing for α_1-antitrypsin deficiency should be done in COPD patients age 45 years or younger, in patients with emphysema without a history of smoking or with emphysema characterized by predominantly basilar changes on chest X ray, and in patients with a strong family history of emphysema.

Imaging

Chest X rays can be useful in supporting clinical suspicion for COPD. Radiographic features suggestive of COPD (usually seen in advanced disease) include the following:

• Increased bronchovascular markings and cardiomegaly (chronic bronchitis)
• Hyperinflation, flat hemidiaphragms, and possible bullous changes (emphysema)

Pulmonary Function Testing

Spirometry is the gold standard for confirming the diagnosis, determining the severity of the airflow limitation, assessing the response to medications, and following disease progression. COPD is confirmed when a patient with compatible symptoms is found to have irreversible airflow limitation. The clinical approach to COPD, which is the same in patients with or without mental illness, is summarized in Figure 9–3.

Preventive Guidelines

Given that COPD is strongly associated with cigarette smoking, smoking prevention and cessation are the most effective ways to prevent COPD (Godtfredsen et al. 2002). The U.S. Preventive Services Task Force (2008) strongly recommends screening adult patients for tobacco use and recommends that all current smokers receive cessation counseling and be offered pharmacological treatments. Key strategies for smokers who are not ready to quit include evoking and building motivation for change by focusing on the benefits of change and the risks associated with tobacco use, as well as addressing key barriers to cessation (e.g., stress, fear of weight gain, nicotine withdrawal). Key points for brief interventions on smoking, such as using the "5 A's," are noted in Table 9–1.

Screening

Early diagnosis and treatment can improve the quality of life of patients with COPD (Lacasse et al. 1996). The newest guidelines recommend evaluation for COPD in patients with respiratory symptoms and a history of COPD risk factors; physical examination is recommended, although it is rarely diagnostic for COPD because signs of airway limitations are generally not present until more advanced stages (Global Initiative for Chronic Obstructive Lung Disease 2013). Although spirometry is the gold standard for diagnosis of COPD, it should not be used for routine screening of otherwise healthy adults (U.S. Preventive Services Task Force 2008).

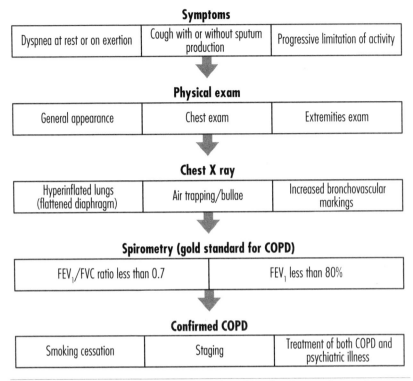

FIGURE 9–3.   Clinical assessment for chronic obstructive pulmonary disease (COPD).

Note. FEV_1 = forced expiratory volume after 1 second; FVC = forced vital capacity.

Patient Education

Education is critically important in patients with COPD and should address the following:

- Purpose and dosing of scheduled and as-needed medications
- Proper inhaler technique
- Importance of a well-balanced diet
- Need to seek medical care early during an exacerbation
- Need to avoid crowds during the cold and flu season
- Importance of washing hands often
- Value of recommended vaccinations (influenza and pneumococcal vaccines)
- Importance of physical activity, which may alleviate lung function decline
- Importance of optimizing treatment of existing psychiatric symptoms

TABLE 9–1. **Key points of treating tobacco use and dependence (the "5 A's")**

Ask: Systematically identify all tobacco users at every visit; implement an office-wide system that ensures that tobacco use is queried and documented.

Advise: Strongly urge all tobacco users to quit.

Assess: Determine the patient's willingness to make a quit attempt.

Assist: Help the patient with a quit plan; provide practical counseling, treatment, and social support; and recommend the use of approved pharmacotherapy.

Arrange: Schedule follow-up contact, either in person or via telephone.

Five first-line pharmacotherapies: Sustained-release bupropion, nicotine gum, nicotine inhaler, nicotine nasal spray, and nicotine patch.

- At least one of these medications should be prescribed in the absence of contraindications.

Source. "5 A's": Agency for Healthcare Research and Quality 2012.

Treatment Recommendations

Both nonpharmacological and pharmacological interventions are important in the management of patients with COPD. Smoking cessation is a crucial step in the management of COPD in all stages and continues to be the most important therapeutic intervention for COPD. The long-term benefits of smoking cessation in COPD patients are well documented; quitting smoking has been found to be rapidly followed by a substantial improvement in cough, expectoration, breathlessness, and wheezing (Anthonisen et al. 1994; Pisinger and Godtfredsen 2007). Risk factor reduction (e.g., an annual influenza vaccine) is important for all patients with COPD to improve mortality rates in patients with chronic hypoxemia. Pulmonary rehabilitation improves symptoms, exercise capacity, and quality of life (Reardon et al. 1994).

Generally, pharmacotherapy is added in a stepwise fashion; however, for patients who present with severe disease, a stepwise approach may not always be the best choice. The mainstays of drug therapy for stable symptomatic COPD are inhaled bronchodilators (β_2 agonists and anticholinergics) and inhaled corticosteroids. A simplified algorithm for COPD pharmacotherapy in ambulatory care is shown in Figure 9–4.

When to Refer

COPD is a complex disease that requires health care providers to work together to produce an optimal outcome. Patients should always be followed

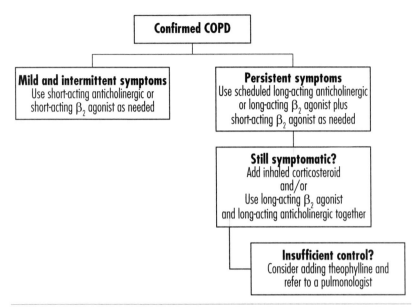

FIGURE 9–4.   Algorithm for pharmacological management of chronic obstructive pulmonary disease (COPD) in an ambulatory setting.
Source.   Adapted from Global Initiative for Chronic Obstructive Lung Disease 2013.

by a primary care provider. A pulmonary specialist should be involved for any of the following situations:

- Uncertain diagnosis
- Disease onset before age 40 years
- Frequent exacerbations (two or more per year)
- Severe COPD
- Rapidly progressive disease course
- Comorbid illness (osteoporosis, heart failure, bronchiectasis, lung cancer)
- Evaluation for surgery
- Presence of fever or weight loss

Ethical and Palliative Care Issues in COPD

Many patients have an interest in discussing advance care plans, but their wishes tend to be passive and unspoken. Clinicians are encouraged to initiate and facilitate conversations about advance care planning with all patients with COPD at routine outpatient visits. The goal is to give patients control over their health care decisions and to reassure patients that their wishes will be carried out at the end of their lives.

Special Treatment Considerations for the Psychiatric Patient Population

Many patients with severe mental disorders go years without preventive medical treatment, and it is not uncommon to observe high rates of under-diagnosed and undertreated medical problems in these patients (Miller et al. 2006). First, diagnosis can be more challenging because patients with mental illness and a sedentary lifestyle are unlikely to report symptoms. Hence, clinicians are encouraged to ask patients, especially those who smoke, about symptoms of COPD. Second, patients with significant cognitive or functional impairment may be unable to effectively participate in their own care (e.g., patients with dementia may have difficulty with self-administering inhaled therapy) (Zarowitz and O'Shea 2012).

Psychiatric comorbidities, including depression, anxiety, and psychosis, have been well documented in patients with COPD. Estimates of depression among patients with COPD range from 37% to 71% (Solano et al. 2006). Up to 55% of patients with COPD complain of anxiety symptoms (Vögele and von Leupoldt 2008).

Pharmacological Considerations in People With Mental Illness and COPD

*   Switching from typical to atypical antipsychotic medications often reduces smoking frequency (Kumari and Postma 2005).
*   Neuroleptic side effects, such as acute laryngeal dystonia or tardive dyskinesia, can worsen dyspnea in patients with COPD.
*   Opioids and most hypnotics, sedatives, and anxiolytics have a respiratory-depressing effect and need to be used with caution in patients with COPD, or avoided if possible.
*   The co-occurrence of anxiety and COPD is common and can be difficult to manage. Selective serotonin reuptake inhibitors, buspirone, cognitive-behavioral therapy, and pulmonary rehabilitation can be helpful in treating anxiety.
*   The effect of antidepressants on breathing is controversial. Nortriptyline was shown to be effective at treating both anxiety and depressive symptoms in patients with COPD (Borson et al. 1992)
*   Monitoring the blood levels of medications in people with mental illness both before and during smoking cessation is advised. Metabolism of tricyclic antidepressants and some antipsychotics (e.g., clozapine, olanzapine, haloperidol, asenapine) is increased when a person is smoking (tobacco induces cytochrome P450 1A2).

- Management of sleep problems in patients with COPD should focus particularly on minimizing sleep disturbance (limiting cough and dyspnea) and avoiding use of hypnotics.

Case Discussion (*continued*)

At presentation, Mr. R's 25-year history of heavy smoking, symptoms of dyspnea and chronic cough, and chest X ray were all suggestive of a diagnosis of COPD, which was confirmed with spirometry. Although acute bronchitis is the most likely cause of his hemoptysis, his smoking history of 75 pack-years also puts him at risk for lung cancer. He should be evaluated for lung cancer and followed by a pulmonologist, in addition to getting routine care by his primary care provider.

Mr. R should be carefully counseled on smoking cessation and offered pharmacotherapy. He has begun to quit smoking, so his clozapine level needs to be monitored for potential toxicity. Nutritional screening and weight loss education should be performed due to his elevated BMI. His elevated BMI also increases his risk for obstructive sleep apnea, which could complicate his COPD and hypertension. Also, he needs to be provided with education about appropriate medication use, infection risk reduction, diet, exercise, hygiene, and sleep. Finally, a discussion on advance medical planning should be started in case of subsequent COPD exacerbations.

Clinical Highlights

- Chronic obstructive pulmonary disease (COPD) is a common condition with high mortality.
- COPD prevalence seems to be highest in people with mental illness, contributing to the high morbidity seen in individuals with SMI.
- There is evidence of a disparity in clinical attention to COPD in individuals with mental illness despite a very high prevalence of smoking.
- COPD should be considered and confirmed with spirometry in all patients who report any combination of the following: dyspnea, chronic cough, chronic sputum production, and history of exposure to triggers of COPD.
- Correct diagnosis of COPD is important because appropriate management can decrease symptoms (especially dyspnea), reduce the frequency and severity of exacerbations, improve health status, improve exercise capacity, and prolong survival.
- All patients with COPD should be advised to quit smoking, educated about COPD, vaccinated for influenza and pneumococcal illnesses, and counseled on nutrition, physical activity, functional ability, exacerbations, and end-of-life decision making.

- Interventions that improve COPD outcomes by decreasing symptoms and preventing acute exacerbations could substantially decrease the costs associated with this disease.

Resources

For Patients

Agency for Healthcare Research and Quality: Help for Smokers and Other Tobacco Users: Quit Smoking. Rockville, MD, Agency for Healthcare Research and Quality, May 2008. Available at: http://www.ahrq.gov.

Mayo Clinic: Diseases and Conditions: COPD. Available at: http://www.mayoclinic.com/health/copd/DS00916.

For Clinicians

American College of Chest Clinicians: Evidence-based clinical practice guidelines. Available at: http://www.chestnet.org.

Global Initiative for Chronic Obstructive Lung Disease: Guidelines for professionals in the diagnosis and treatment of COPD. Available at: http://www.goldcopd.com.

References

Anthonisen NR, Connett JE, Kiley JP, et al: Effects of smoking intervention and the use of an inhaled anticholinergic bronchodilator on the rate of decline of FEV1. The Lung Health Study. JAMA 272:1497–1505, 1994

Barnes M, Lawford BR, Burton SC, et al: Smoking and schizophrenia: is symptom profile related to smoking and which antipsychotic medication is of benefit in reducing cigarette use? Aust Z J Psychiatry 40:575–580, 2006

Borson S, McDonald GJ, Gayle T, et al: Improvement in mood, physical symptoms, and function with nortriptyline for depression in patients with chronic obstructive pulmonary disease. Psychosomatics 33:190–201, 1992

Buist AS, McBurnie MA, Vollmer WM, et al: International variation in the prevalence of COPD (the BOLD Study): a population-based prevalence study. Lancet 370:741–750, 2007

Calverley PM, Walker P: Chronic obstructive pulmonary disease. Lancet 362:1053–1061, 2003

Centers for Disease Control and Prevention: Chronic obstructive pulmonary disease among adults—United States, 2011. MMWR Morb Mortal Wkly Rep 61:938–943, 2012

Davis RM, Novotny TE: The epidemiology of cigarette smoking and its impact on chronic obstructive pulmonary disease. Am Rev Respir Dis 140(3 Pt 2):S82–84, 1989

Feenstra TL, van Genugten ML, Hoogenveen RT, et al: The impact of aging and smoking on the future burden of chronic obstructive pulmonary disease: a model analysis in the Netherlands. Am J Respir Crit Care Med 164:590–596, 2001

Ferrer M, Alonso J, Morera J, et al: Chronic obstructive pulmonary disease stage and health-related quality of life. Ann Intern Med 127:1072–1079, 1997

Freeman E, Yoe JT: The poor health status of consumers of mental healthcare: behavioral disorders and chronic disease. Presentation to the National Association of State Mental Health Program Directors Medical Directors Work Group, May 2006

George TP, Weinberger AH: Nicotine and tobacco use in schizophrenia, in Medical Illness and Schizophrenia. Edited by Meyer JM, Nasrallah HA. Washington, DC, American Psychiatric Publishing, 2003, pp 223–245

Global Initiative for Chronic Obstructive Lung Disease: Global Strategy for the Diagnosis, Management, and Prevention of Chronic Obstructive Pulmonary Disease. Vancouver, WA, Global Initiative for Chronic Obstructive Lung Disease, 2013

Godtfredsen NS, Vestbo J, Osler M, et al: Risk of hospital admission for COPD following smoking cessation and reduction: a Danish population study. Thorax 57:967–972, 2002

Hahn C, Hahn E, Dettling M, et al: Effects of smoking history on selective attention in schizophrenia. Neuropharmacology 62:1897–1902, 2012

Himelhoch S, Lehman A, Kreyenbuhl J, et al: Prevalence of chronic obstructive pulmonary disease among those with serious mental illness. Am J Psychiatry 161:2317–2319, 2004

Jones DR, Macias C, Barreira PJ, et al: Prevalence, severity, and co-occurrence of chronic physical health problems of persons with serious mental illness. Psychiatr Serv 55:1250–1257, 2004

Kumari V, Postma P: Nicotine use in schizophrenia: the self medication hypotheses. Neurosci Biobehav Rev 29:1021–1034, 2005

Lacasse Y, Wong E, Guyatt GH, et al: Meta-analysis of respiratory rehabilitation in chronic obstructive pulmonary disease. Lancet 348:1115–1119, 1996

Miller B, Paschall CB, Svendsen D: Mortality and medical comorbidity in patients with serious mental illness. Psychiatr Serv 57:1482–1487, 2006

Miniño AM, Murphy SL, Xu J, et al: Deaths: final data for 2008. Natl Vital Stat Rep 59:1–126, 2011

Pisinger C, Godtfredsen NS: Is there a health benefit of reduced tobacco consumption? A systematic review. Nicotine Tob Res 9:631–646, 2007

Reardon J, Awad E, Normandin E, et al: The effect of comprehensive outpatient pulmonary rehabilitation on dyspnea. Chest 105:1046–1052, 1994

Schulman, Ronca, and Bucuvalas Inc: Confronting COPD in America: Executive Summary. New York, Schulman, Ronca, and Bucuvalas Inc, 2001

Sokal J, Messias E, Dickerson FB: Comorbidity of medical illnesses among adults with serious mental illness who are receiving community psychiatric services. J Nerv Ment Dis 192:421–427, 2004

Solano JP, Gomes B, Higginson IJ: A comparison of symptom prevalence in far advanced cancer, AIDS, heart disease, chronic obstructive pulmonary disease and renal disease. J Pain Symptom Manage 31:58–69, 2006

Sullivan SD, Ramsey SD, Lee TA: The economic burden of COPD. Chest 117:5S–9S, 2000

Vögele C, von Leupoldt A: Mental disorders in chronic obstructive pulmonary disease (COPD). Respir Med 102:764–773, 2008

Volkov VP: Respiratory diseases as a cause of death in schizophrenia [in Russian]. Probl Tuberk Bolezn Legk 6:24–27, 2009

U.S. Preventive Services Task Force: Screening for chronic obstructive pulmonary disease using spirometry: U.S. Preventive Services Task Force recommendation statement. Ann Intern Med 148:529–534, 2008

Zarowitz BJ, O'Shea T: Chronic obstructive pulmonary disease: prevalence, characteristics, and pharmacologic treatment in nursing home residents with cognitive impairment. J Manag Care Pharm 18:598–606, 2012

Ziedonis D, Williams JM, Smelson D: Serious mental illness and tobacco addiction: a model program to address this common but neglected issue. Am J Med Sci 326:223–230, 2003

SECTION III

Endocrine and Metabolic Disorders in the Psychiatric Patient Population

CHAPTER 10

Diabetes

Sarah K. Rivelli, M.D., F.A.C.P.
Virginia O'Brien, M.D.

Case Discussion

Ms. F, a 30-year-old woman with obesity and hypertension, is seeking help for management of her depression. She says she does not feel motivated to do anything and has been forgetting to take her medications. She reports feeling too tired to prepare meals and she craves carbohydrates and sweets. As a result, she often purchases cake or fast food when going home from work. This has caused her to gain 3.6 kg (8 lb) in the last 2 months. She feels tired, cannot concentrate, and is not sleeping well. She feels unmotivated and tends to stay at home and watch TV. Although she knows she is depressed, she is reluctant to take any additional medications because the last medication she tried caused sedation and weight gain.

Clinical Overview

Diabetes is a disease in which the body does not produce or effectively respond to insulin, leading to hyperglycemia. It affects an estimated 8.3% of the U.S. population and is the seventh leading cause of death in the United States (Centers for Disease Control and Prevention, Division of Diabetes Translation 2011). Approximately 20.9 million people have been diagnosed with diabetes, and another 7 million are currently undiagnosed. The burden of illness falls more heavily on people over age 65 years, who make up 26.9% of those with diabetes. If the prevalence of diabetes continues to grow at a steady rate, it is estimated that about 25% of Americans will have diabetes by 2030 (Boyle et al. 2010). Diabetes is the leading cause of new blindness, kidney failure, and non-traumatic limb amputations. Patients with diabetes have a two- to fourfold increased risk of mortality, stroke, and cardiovascular disease.

There are two main types of diabetes: type 1 and type 2. In type 1 diabetes, the body makes insufficient insulin due to dysfunction of β-cells of the pancreas. Onset tends to occur prior to age 30 years, and exogenous insulin is required indefinitely. Symptom onset may be sudden and be characterized by weight loss, fatigue, frequent urination, thirst, and diabetic ketoacidosis.

Type 2 diabetes is much more common and makes up about 90% of all diabetes cases. Onset tends to occur after age 40 years, and the disease frequently goes undiagnosed. In fact, 25% of people with type 2 diabetes are not aware they have it. The pathophysiology of type 2 diabetes includes impaired sensitivity to insulin and lack of control over hepatic glucose production, which leads to excessive liver gluconeogenesis. Insulin levels may actually be high when type 2 diabetes is first diagnosed. Over time, pancreatic β-cell dysfunction ensues and patients become dependent on insulin. Risk factors for type 2 diabetes include age, obesity, sedentary lifestyle, family history, and a history of gestational diabetes. (Modifiable risk factors for type 2 diabetes are listed in Table 10–1.) Higher rates of diabetes are also seen in those of certain racial or ethnic backgrounds, such as non-Hispanic blacks (approximately 13%) and Hispanics/Latinos (approximately 12%). Insulin resistance occurs for 5–10 years prior to the development of type 2 diabetes. During this "at-risk" period, glucose levels slowly rise and impaired fasting glucose may be detected. This condition is called "prediabetes" and impacts almost one in every three Americans.

Depression and Diabetes

Depression is a risk factor for the development of type 2 diabetes. In one prospective study of older adults, participants who reported high levels of depressive symptoms were more likely to develop diabetes, with a hazard ratio of 1.6 (Carnethon et al. 2007). A prospective study of adults over age 55 that diagnosed depression by psychiatric interview also showed a 65% increased risk for incident diabetes among those with depression, even after controlling for confounders such as body mass index (BMI), family history, and hypertension (Campayo et al. 2010). Similarly, a meta-analysis of 13 studies that used mostly self-reported symptoms to measure depression found that baseline depression predicted diabetes with a pooled relative risk of 1.60 (95% confidence interval [CI], 1.37–1.88) (Mezuk et al. 2008).

Of note, common risk factors exist between depression and diabetes. Even after adjustment for lifestyle factors such as physical activity, depres-

TABLE 10–1. **Modifiable risk factors for type 2 diabetes among patients with mental illness**

Sedentary lifestyle

Lack of exercise

Poor diet

Obesity

Medications causing weight gain

Poor access to routine medical screening

Poor adherence to medical regimen

Depression

sive symptoms increase the risk of developing diabetes by about 40% (Lustman et al. 2006).

Patients with diabetes also appear to be at increased risk for developing depression. A meta-analysis of large-scale prospective studies revealed significantly elevated rates of depression among people with type 2 diabetes compared with control subjects (17.6% vs. 9%, odds ratio [OR] = 1.6 [95% CI, 1.2–2.0]) (Ali et al. 2006). Finally, there is a clear positive association between hyperglycemia in diabetes and depression, with a larger effect size noted for hyperglycemia and elevated risk of major depressive disorder (Lustman et al. 2000). Thus, the relationship between diabetes and depression appears bidirectional, with each being a significant risk factor for the development of the other.

Patients with comorbid depression and diabetes fare worse than those with diabetes who are not depressed. Depressed patients with diabetes are less adherent to self-care regimens. Moreover, depression is associated with poorer glycemic control (Katon et al. 2012; Lustman et al. 2000) and increased cardiovascular risk factors (Katon et al. 2004a). Depression is also associated with increased complications from diabetes, such as retinopathy and nephropathy, and with higher rates of disability, dementia, and mortality (see Rustad et al. 2011 for review).

Schizophrenia and Diabetes

Patients with schizophrenia are at higher risk than individuals in the general population for development of diabetes, even prior to treatment with antipsychotics. Studies of antipsychotic-naïve individuals with schizophrenia have shown the presence of insulin resistance (Dasgupta et al. 2010; Venkatasubramanian et al. 2007). Moreover, insulin resistance among patients with schizophrenia appears to be independent of lipid abnormalities and weight in some studies (Dasgupta et al. 2010).

Dementia and Diabetes

Diabetes is a risk factor for the development of both Alzheimer's dementia and vascular dementia. A meta-analysis of prospective studies revealed increased relative risks of 1.5 (95% CI, 1.20–1.77) for Alzheimer's dementia and 2.48 (95% CI, 2.08–2.96) for vascular dementia (Cheng et al. 2012). Microvascular lesions, atherosclerosis, and recurrent hypoglycemia are associated with cognitive deficits in elderly patients with diabetes and likely explain the relationship between diabetes and dementia. Some limited evidence suggests that treatment of vascular risk factors, including diabetes, leads to the delay and attenuation of cognitive decline. Thus, diabetes should be treated in patients with mild cognitive impairment and dementia to improve cognitive outcomes.

Practical Pointers

- The relationship between diabetes and depression is bidirectional, each being a risk for the development of the other.
- Obesogenic medications should be used with caution in patients with type 2 diabetes in order to limit weight gain.
- Lifestyle modification is first-line treatment for patients with prediabetes and psychiatric illness.
- Metformin is generally safe and can be prescribed to at-risk individuals with prediabetes to attenuate weight gain and prevent progression to diabetes.
- First-line treatment of type 2 diabetes in patients with mental illness does not differ from treatment in the general population.
- Cognitive-behavioral therapy, motivational interviewing, and collaborative care models have shown positive results for improving health in patients with comorbid diabetes and depression.

Diagnosis

The diagnosis of diabetes requires one of the following:

- Fasting blood glucose of >126 mg/dL on 2 separate days
- Symptoms of hyperglycemia plus a random plasma glucose of ≥200 mg/dL
- Two-hour plasma glucose of ≥200 mg/dL during an oral glucose tolerance test (OGTT), with results duplicated on a separate day
- Hemoglobin A_{1c} (HbA_{1c}) of ≥6.5%

Prediabetes can be identified with the same tests used to diagnose diabetes and is defined as follows:

- Fasting blood glucose of 100–125 mg/dL
- Two-hour plasma glucose of 140–199 mg/dL during an OGTT
- HbA_{1c} of 5.7%–6.4%

Symptoms of prediabetes may include thirst, frequent urination, increased appetite, fatigue, frequent infections, slow healing of cuts or wounds, blurry vision, and numbness or tingling in extremities. Patients whose testing is consistent with prediabetes should be monitored yearly.

A simple screening and diagnostic test for diabetes is the HbA_{1c} test. The use of HbA_{1c} values for diagnosis was recently updated (American Diabetes Association 2014) to improve the diagnostic rate for diabetes. The fact that neither fasting nor the OGTT is required for the HbA_{1c} test is especially relevant for patients with mental illness, because it is often challenging to obtain fasting test results or to perform the OGTT. The HbA_{1c} value gives a sense of average blood glucose levels in the past 120 days.

Screening for diabetes should be considered in all adults over age 45 or those who are overweight (BMI$\geq$25) with one or more of the following risk factors:

- Physical inactivity
- First-degree relative with diabetes
- High-risk race/ethnicity (e.g., African American, Latino, Native American, Asian American, Pacific Islander)
- Having delivered a baby weighing more than 4 kg (9 lb), or having been diagnosed with gestational diabetes mellitus
- Hypertension (having blood pressure of $\geq$140/90 mmHg, or taking an antihypertensive)
- A high-density lipoprotein cholesterol level of <35 mg/dL and/or a triglyceride level of >250 mg/dL
- Polycystic ovary syndrome (in women)
- HbA_{1c} of $\geq$5.7%, impaired glucose tolerance, or impaired fasting glucose on previous testing
- Other clinical conditions associated with insulin resistance (e.g., severe obesity, acanthosis nigricans)
- History of cardiovascular disease

Preventive Guidelines

Identifying individuals at risk for type 2 diabetes and managing these risks can help in prevention. In addition to considering the guidelines listed below, clinicians should consider patients with depression and schizophrenia to be particularly at risk, especially if they are also taking a medication associated with weight gain and/or metabolic syndrome.

Guidelines for diabetes prevention include lifestyle modifications such as exercise and low-fat, low-caloric, or low-glycemic diets that promote weight loss. Overweight patients should aim to lose 7% of their body weight by using low-fat or calorie-restricted diets. Three large follow-up studies of lifestyle intervention in the general population yielded sustained reductions of 34%–58% in the rate of conversion to type 2 diabetes (Diabetes Prevention Program Research Group et al. 2009; Knowler et al. 2002; Lindstrom et al. 2003).

Lifestyle interventions should include patient-led, specific objectives that can be recalled using the acronym FIRM: **F**ew in number, **I**ndividualized, **R**ealistic, and **M**easurable. Mental illness should not necessarily be a barrier to these interventions, although studies show limited efficacy in inpatient settings and greater improvement among outpatients.

Evidence-based specific targets for exercise include moderate-intensity aerobic physical activity for 150 minutes per week over 3–4 days of the week (Diabetes Prevention Program Research Group et al. 2009).

Pharmacological interventions for prevention of progression to diabetes are also available. Metformin therapy can be considered for those with impaired glucose tolerance, impaired fasting glucose, or an HbA_{1c} of 5.7%–6.4%, especially for patients with a BMI greater than 35, individuals older than age 60 years, and women with prior gestational diabetes. Metformin does not cause hypoglycemia but decreases hepatic glucose output, increases sensitivity to insulin, and promotes mild weight loss. Metformin is generally well tolerated, aside from transient gastrointestinal side effects such as dyspepsia. However, it should not be used in patients with a creatinine level greater than 1.4 mg/dL (corresponding to a glomerular filtration rate [GFR] < 30) or in pregnant patients. The risk of lactic acidosis is thought to be very low (1 per 100,000) (Nathan et al. 2009). Long-term use is associated with vitamin B_{12} deficiency, which should be monitored for periodically.

Agents such as α-glucosidase inhibitors, orlistat, and thiazolidinediones have been shown to have varying degrees of success in decreasing incident diabetes. Screening for diabetes should occur at least annually for patients who have prediabetes, to ensure they have not progressed to diabetes.

Treatment Recommendations

The treatment of diabetes is based on self-management, including self-monitoring of glucose, lifestyle modifications such as improving diet and exercise, and medications. Self-management includes exploration of attitudes toward illness, discussion of barriers to adherence and concerns about treat-

TABLE 10–2. **Glycemic goals in the treatment of diabetes**

Glycemic test	Goal
Hemoglobin A_{1c}	<7%
Preprandial capillary plasma glucose	70–130 mg/dL
Peak postprandial capillary plasma glucose	<180 mg/dL

ment, and motivation enhancement; for these areas of management, the psychiatrist may be particularly well equipped to handle such issues.

Glycemic treatment goals are shown in Table 10–2. HbA_{1c} is monitored every 3 months if treatment is being titrated; once goals are reached, it can be monitored every 6–12 months. Home capillary plasma glucose self-monitoring should occur at least three times daily for patients taking insulin; once-daily monitoring may be sufficient for patients taking oral agents.

Initial treatment of type 2 diabetes includes lifestyle modifications to promote weight loss and metformin. Both metformin and a combination of exercise and dietary changes can lower HbA_{1c} by 1%–2%. For weight loss, either low-carbohydrate, low-fat, calorie-restricted or Mediterranean diets appear to be effective. Aerobic physical activity is recommended for a total of at least 150 minutes per week and can lead to benefits even in the absence of weight loss. If HbA_{1c} is near goal (<7.5%), a 3- to 6-month period of lifestyle change only, without medication, may be tried. Bariatric surgery should be considered for all patients with a BMI greater than 35 and diabetes.

Metformin can be started at 500 mg/day and titrated upward every 5–7 days as tolerated to a dosage of 1,000 mg bid (Nathan et al. 2009). Although metformin is contraindicated in patients with a GFR under 30, psychiatrists should refer patients to a primary care provider (PCP) if the GFR falls below 60 so closer monitoring of renal function can be implemented.

Additional oral agents exist for type 2 diabetes (Table 10–3). If after initiating lifestyle modifications and metformin, a patient's blood glucose remains above goal, addition of a sulfonylurea or thiazolidinedione is generally recommended (Nathan et al. 2009).

Management of diabetes requires regular follow-up and close monitoring of associated conditions to prevent complications. Table 10–4 lists blood pressure and lipid goals that a patient should maintain, and Table 10–5 lists tests that should be done annually to monitor for potential complications of diabetes.

The most potent strategies to prevent nephropathy and retinopathy are glycemic and blood pressure control. Blood pressure should be measured at every visit until goals are reached and then every few months thereafter. For

TABLE 10–3. Oral diabetic agents

Class	Agent	Comments
Biguanides	Metformin (Glucophage, Riomet cherry-flavored liquid) Metformin ER (Fortamet, Glumetza, Glucophage XR)	No hypoglycemia GI side effects Rare lactic acidosis Contraindicated in renal insufficiency (GFR <30) Vitamin B_{12} deficiency
Sulfonylureas	Glipizide (Glucotrol, Glucotrol XL) Glimepiride (Amaryl) Glyburide (DiaBeta, Micronase)	Hypoglycemia Weight gain
Thiazolidinediones/glitazones	Pioglitazone (Actos)	Weight gain Heart failure Rare hepatotoxicity
Dipeptidyl peptidase–4 inhibitors	Sitagliptin (Januvia) Saxagliptin (Onglyza)	Modest effect on HbA_{1c} levels No hypoglycemia, urticaria, angioedema Small risk of pancreatitis
α-Glucosidase inhibitors	Acarbose (Precose) Miglitol (Glyset)	Modest effect on HbA_{1c} levels GI side effects
Oral β-cell stimulators	Repaglinide (Prandin) Nateglinide (Starlix)	Hypoglycemia Weight gain Short half-life

Note. ER = extended release; GFR = glomerular filtration rate; GI = gastrointestinal; HbA_{1c} = hemoglobin A_{1c}; XL = extended release; XR = extended release.

TABLE 10–4. Blood pressure and lipid goals

Measure	Goal
Blood pressure	
Systolic	<140 mmHg
Diastolic	<90 mmHg
Fasting lipid panel	
Total	<200 mg/dL
Triglycerides	<150 mg/dL
Low-density lipoprotein	<100 mg/dL[a]
High-density lipoprotein	>40 mg/dL (men); >50 mg/dL (women)

[a]Low-density lipoprotein goal is <70 mg/dL among patients with cardiovascular disease.

a patient with blood pressure that is not at goal or with albuminuria and/or elevated creatinine levels, an angiotensin-converting enzyme inhibitor or angiotensin II receptor blocker should be initiated and the patient should be referred to a PCP. Blood pressure control generally requires multiple agents, however. Dosing at least one agent at bedtime appears to improve the chance of achieving blood pressure control.

Lipids should be monitored annually, with more frequent testing if a lifestyle intervention or medication has been started. Hyperlipidemia treatment in patients with diabetes is no different from that used for isolated hyperlip-

TABLE 10–5. Recommended monitoring for potential complications of diabetes

Complication	Test	Frequency
Renal failure and end-stage renal disease due to nephropathy	Urine albumin Serum creatinine or calculated glomerular filtration rate	Annually
Blindness due to retinopathy	Dilated comprehensive eye examination	Annually
Nonhealing ulcers and lower extremity amputation from neuropathy	Foot examination, including inspection, pulses, monofilament test, vibration, and pinprick sensation	Annually

TABLE 10–6. **Specialist referrals for patients with recently diagnosed diabetes**

Purpose	Referral
Comprehensive eye examination	Ophthalmologist or optometrist
Female reproductive health	Obstetrician/gynecologist or family practitioner
Medical nutrition management	Registered dietitian
Self-management education	Diabetes educator
Periodontal examination	Dentist

idemia. A statin can be initiated if lipid levels exceed the targets and lifestyle intervention is unsuccessful.

Patients with type 1 or 2 diabetes and elevated cardiovascular risk should be offered daily low-dose aspirin (75–162 mg) for primary prevention of cardiovascular disease. Elevated cardiovascular risk is defined as risk greater than 10% in the next 10 years and applies to most men older than 50 years or women older than 60 years who have at least one additional major risk factor, such as hypertension, hyperlipidemia, albuminuria, smoking, or family history of premature cardiovascular disease (see Chapter 5, "Coronary Artery Disease"). Patients should be counseled not to smoke and be offered smoking cessation therapies. Patients with newly diagnosed diabetes require multidisciplinary care and should be referred to the providers listed in Table 10–6.

When to Refer

Situations warranting referral to a PCP include the following:

- Severe symptoms such as polyuria, polydipsia, confusion, blurry vision, or sudden weight loss
- $HbA_{1c} > 9\%$
- Initiating insulin
- Untreated diabetes and existing complications (e.g., neuropathy, proteinuria, retinopathy, cardiovascular disease)
- Patient is pregnant or becomes pregnant
- Patient cannot tolerate metformin and HbA_{1c} is not at goal
- $GFR < 60$

Special Treatment Considerations for the Psychiatric Patient Population

Medications that can cause weight gain are risk factors for the development of type 2 diabetes. Such medications exist in all classes of psychotropic drugs: antidepressants, mood stabilizers, and antipsychotics. Mirtazapine, paroxetine, lithium, valproic acid, tricyclic antidepressants (TCAs), and second-generation antipsychotics (SGAs) all cause weight gain to varying degrees. Of note, valproic acid can lead to polycystic ovary syndrome, which is associated with insulin resistance and type 2 diabetes.

Previous research suggested a link between antidepressant use and diabetes, but this relationship is explained by antidepressants being a marker for depression, which is associated with diabetes. Antidepressants that are associated with sedation and weight gain do confer risk for diabetes. For example, TCAs are associated with weight gain and hyperglycemia, whereas serotonin reuptake inhibitors such as fluoxetine have been shown to reduce hyperglycemia, normalize glucose homeostasis, and increase insulin sensitivity (Goodnick 2001). Dual-mechanism antidepressants (e.g., duloxetine and venlafaxine) do not appear to disrupt glucose homeostatic dynamics significantly (McIntyre et al. 2006). Sertraline was found to be an effective treatment for depression in diabetes and reduced recurrent depression in a follow-up study (Lustman et al. 2000). Glycemic control improved equally for patients with depression recovery whether they had been taking sertraline or placebo (Lustman et al. 2000). In contrast, nortriptyline has been shown to be an effective treatment for depression in patients with diabetes but at the cost of hyperglycemia (Lustman et al. 1997).

Among the first-generation antipsychotics (FGAs), chlorpromazine carries the highest risk of increasing weight and risk for type 2 diabetes (Werneke et al. 2013). Weight gain is relatively low with the high-potency FGAs perphenazine, fluphenazine, and haloperidol. SGAs not only cause weight gain but worsen glycemic control in patients with diabetes and lead to hyperglycemia in patients without a preexisting diagnosis of diabetes. Clozapine and olanzapine are the most likely to increase weight and appetite, stimulate overeating, and increase risk of type 2 diabetes. Quetiapine, risperidone, paliperidone, asenapine, and iloperidone confer more moderate risk for weight gain, whereas ziprasidone, aripiprazole, and lurasidone are not associated with weight gain. Mechanisms by which SGAs cause weight gain are complex; antihistaminergic and anticholinergic properties appear to be relevant. Sedation and dry mouth lead to decreased activity and increased oral intake, respectively. Weight gain occurs early after initiation of antipsychotic treatment. Prevention of weight gain through early intervention with lifestyle modification appears more effective than intervening once weight loss has occurred (Werneke et al. 2013).

Metformin prevents and attenuates SGA-induced weight gain, leading to weight loss of 2.5–3.0 kg (5.5–6.6 lb) across trials (Maayan et al. 2010). Topiramate also has shown a consistent though less potent impact on weight gain in a smaller number of trials. Topiramate leads to a reduction of about 2.5 kg (5.5 lb) over an 8- to 12-week period (Maayan et al. 2010). Additional options for therapy with less evidence include orlistat for weight loss, and α-glucosidase inhibitors or thiazolidinediones for antipsychotic-associated prediabetes. Nonpharmacological interventions, such as cognitive-behavioral therapy (CBT) and nutritional counseling, also lead to about 3 kg (6.6 lb) of weight loss (Caemmerer et al. 2012). Moreover, nonpharmacological interventions have also been shown to decrease waist circumference, total and low-density lipoprotein cholesterol levels, and triglyceride levels. Interestingly, both individual and group interventions appear effective. Evidence shows that patients with schizophrenia can successfully participate in lifestyle interventions (Daumit et al. 2013). In fact, dropout rates are significantly lower in nonpharmacological than in pharmacological intervention studies. A combination pharmacological and behavioral intervention is likely the most effective strategy, although head-to-head comparisons of a combination strategy versus single strategies are limited (Wu et al. 2012).

In the interest of diabetes prevention, psychiatrists should consider changing therapies if the patient is already obese or has gained significant weight—typically defined as 7% or more of the baseline weight—while taking an agent. This is even more important if the patient already has one or more risk factors for diabetes, such as physical inactivity or family history of diabetes. A patient's baseline weight should be considered when starting pharmacotherapy so that agents with high weight gain liability can be avoided.

Psychiatrists might use some pharmacological therapies to the patient's advantage by targeting multiple problems with a single medication. For example, in a patient with diabetes, depression, and nicotine dependence, bupropion might be a good option for treating depression and can aid in smoking cessation and has no propensity to cause weight gain.

CBT has been shown to effectively treat depression among patients with type 2 diabetes. In combination with diabetes education, CBT significantly improved HbA_{1c} at 6-month follow-up (Lustman et al. 1998). Motivational interviewing has shown promise in improving glycemic control, blood pressure, and lipids in patients with type 2 diabetes (Chen et al. 2012; Gabbay et al. 2013).

Treatment of depression alone does not appear to be sufficient to lead to improved diabetes outcomes. A collaborative care intervention for depression in primary care patients with diabetes was effective in treating depression, but

HbA$_{1c}$ levels were unchanged (Katon et al. 2004b). However, another collaborative care intervention designed to address depression, poorly controlled diabetes, and cardiovascular risk factors led to significantly improved HbA$_{1c}$, blood pressure, lipid profile, and depression (Katon et al. 2013). This intervention included a nurse care manager who followed patients and assisted the PCP in prescribing medications for depression, hypertension, and diabetes, as indicated. It included routine measurement, systematic follow-up, and treat-to-target guidelines based on evidence-based therapies. Not surprisingly, the improved outcomes were associated with greater success in achieving guideline-recommended treatment in the intervention group. Finally, patients in the intervention group were more satisfied with both their behavioral and medical care than the usual care group. Thus, coordinated comprehensive interventions that address both medical and behavioral health problems can have significant impact in improving overall health.

Case Discussion (*continued*)

Ms. F's clinical presentation meets the criteria for diabetic screening. She has obesity, hypertension, fatigue, and uncontrolled depression, all of which place her at risk for diabetes. Her HbA$_{1c}$ is 6.3%, which places her in the prediabetic range. Her renal function is normal. The psychiatrist's approach is to aggressively treat both her depression and her prediabetes to prevent progression to type 2 diabetes. For depression, the clinician prescribes bupropion, an antidepressant that limits weight gain, after learning that Ms. F has not tried and failed this medication in the past. The clinician also prescribes metformin 500 mg/day with breakfast, with the intent to titrate the dose in about 1 week.

The clinician also counsels Ms. F about how to set specific goals for diet and exercise. The patient agrees to try walking three times a week for 15–20 minutes to start. The clinician plans to check Ms. F's weight every few months and to recheck her HbA$_{1c}$ in 1 year. In the interim, the patient is being referred to a PCP for coordinated care.

Clinical Highlights

- Diabetes is common in the psychiatric population, possibly due to biological interplay between mental illness and diabetes, but also due to use of psychiatric medications that increase risk of obesity and diabetes.
- Screening for diabetes in psychiatric patients requires a simple lab test, such as hemoglobin A$_{1c}$, fasting blood glucose, or oral glucose tolerance test.
- Management of uncomplicated type 2 diabetes is founded on principles of self-management and behavior change.

- Lifestyle intervention counseling should be provided to all patients with prediabetes and diabetes.
- Metformin is well tolerated and can help prevent progression to diabetes in patients with prediabetes.

Resources

For Patients

American Diabetes Association: http://www.diabetes.org
Behavioral Diabetes Institute: http://www.behavioraldiabetesinstitute.org
Stop Diabetes: http://www.stopdiabetes.com

For Clinicians

American Association of Clinical Endocrinologists: https://www.aace.com
American Diabetes Association: http://www.diabetes.org

References

Ali S, Stone MA, Peters JL, et al: The prevalence of depression in adults with type II diabetes: a systematic review and meta-analysis. Diabet Med 23:1165–1173, 2006

Boyle JP, Thompson TJ, Gregg EW, et al: Projection of the year 2050 burden of diabetes in the US adult population: dynamic modeling of incidence, mortality, and prediabetes prevalence. Popul Health Metr 8:1–12, 2010

Caemmerer J, Correll CU, Maayan L: Acute and maintenance effects of non-pharmacologic interventions for antipsychotic associated weight gain and metabolic abnormalities: a meta-analytic comparison of randomized controlled trials. Schizophr Res 140:159–168, 2012

Campayo A, de Jonge P, Roy JF, et al: Depressive disorder and incident diabetes mellitus: the effect of characteristics of depression. Am J Psychiatry 167:580–588, 2010

Carnethon MR, Biggs ML, Barzilay JI, et al: Longitudinal association between depressive symptoms and incident type 2 diabetes mellitus in older adults. Arch Intern Med 167:802–807, 2007

Centers for Disease Control and Prevention, Division of Diabetes Translation: Long-Term Trends in Diagnosed Diabetes. Atlanta, GA, Centers for Disease Control and Prevention, October 2011. Available at: http://www.cdc.gov/diabetes/statistics/slides/long_term_trends.pdf. Accessed May 2013.

Chen SM, Creedy D, Lin HS, et al: Effects of motivational interviewing intervention on self-management, psychological and glycemic outcomes in type 2 diabetes: a randomized controlled trial. Int J Nurs Stud 49:637–644, 2012

Cheng G, Huang C, Deng H, et al: Diabetes as a risk factor for dementia and mild cognitive impairment: a meta-analysis of longitudinal studies. Intern Med J 42:484–491, 2012

Dasgupta A, Singh OP, Rout JK, et al: Insulin resistance and metabolic profile in antipsychotic naïve schizophrenia patients. Prog Neuropsychopharmacol Biol Psychiatry 34:1202–1207, 2010

Daumit GL, Dickerson FB, Wang NY, et al: A behavioral weight-loss intervention in persons with serious mental illness. N Engl J Med 368:1594–1602, 2013

Diabetes Prevention Program Research Group, Knowler WC, Fowler SE, et al: 10-year follow-up of diabetes incidence and weight loss in the Diabetes Prevention Program Outcomes Study. Lancet 374:1677–1686, 2009

Gabbay RA, Anel-Tiangco RM, Dellasega C, et al: Diabetes nurse case management and motivational interviewing for change (DYNAMIC): results of a 2-year randomized controlled pragmatic trial. J Diabetes 5:349–357, 2013

Goodnick PJ: Use of antidepressants in treatment of comorbid diabetes mellitus and depression as well as in diabetic neuropathy. Ann Clin Psychiatry 13:31–34, 2001

Katon WJ, Lin EH, Russo J, et al: Cardiac risk factors in patients with diabetes mellitus and major depression. J Gen Intern Med 19:1192–1199, 2004a

Katon WJ, Von Korff M, Lin EH, et al: The Pathways Study: a randomized trial of collaborative care in patients with diabetes and depression. Arch Gen Psychiatry 61:1042–1049, 2004b

Katon W, Lyles CR, Parker MM, et al: Association of depression with increased risk of dementia in patients with type 2 diabetes: the Diabetes and Aging Study. Arch Gen Psychiatry 69:410–417, 2012

Katon WJ, Young BA, Russo J, et al: Association of depression with increased risk of severe hypoglycemic episodes in patients with diabetes. Ann Fam Med 11:245–250, 2013

Knowler W, Barrett-Conner E, Fowler S, et al: Reduction in the incidence of type 2 diabetes with lifestyle intervention or metformin. N Engl J Med 346(6):393–403, 2002

Lindstrom J, Eriksson J, Louheranta A, et al: The Finnish Diabetes Prevention Study (DPS): lifestyle intervention and 3-year results on diet and physical activity. Diabetes Care 26:3230–3236, 2003

Lustman PJ, Griffith LS, Clouse RE, et al: Effects of nortriptyline on depression and glycemic control in diabetes: results of a double-blind, placebo-controlled trial. Psychosom Med 59:241–250, 1997

Lustman PJ, Griffith LS, Freedland KE, et al: Cognitive behavior therapy for depression in type 2 diabetes mellitus. Ann Intern Med 129:613–621, 1998

Lustman PJ, Anderson RJ, Freedland KE, et al: Depression and poor glycemic control: a meta-analytic review of the literature. Diabetes Care 23:934–942, 2000

Lustman PJ, Clouse RE, Nix BD, et al: Sertraline for prevention of depression recurrence in diabetes mellitus: a randomized, double-blind, placebo-controlled trial. Arch Gen Psychiatry 63:521–529, 2006

Maayan L, Vakhrusheva J, Correll CU, et al: Effectiveness of medications used to attenuate antipsychotic-related weight gain and metabolic abnormalities: a systematic review and meta-analysis. Neuropsychopharmacology 35:1520–1530, 2010

McIntyre RS, Soczynska JK, Konarski JA, et al: The effect of antidepressants on glucose homeostasis and insulin sensitivity: synthesis and mechanisms. Expert Opin Drug Saf 5(1):157–168, 2006

Mezuk B, Eaton W, Albrecht S, et al: Depression and type 2 diabetes over the lifespan. Diabetes Care 31:2383–2390, 2008

Nathan D, Buse JB, Davidson MB, et al: Medical management of hyperglycemia in type 2 diabetes: a consensus algorithm for the initiation and adjustment of therapy. Diabetes Care 32:193–203, 2009

Rustad JK, Musselman DL, Nemeroff CB: The relationship of depression and diabetes: pathophysiological and treatment implications. Psychoneuroendocrinology 36:1276–1286, 2011

Venkatasubramanian G, Chittiprol S, Neelakantachar N, et al: Insulin and insulin-like growth factor-1 abnormalities in antipsychotic-naïve schizophrenia. Am J Psychiatry 164:1557–1560, 2007

Werneke U, Taylor D, Sanders TA: Behavioral interventions for antipsychotic induced appetite changes. Curr Psychiatry Rep 15:347, 2013

Wu R, Jin H, Gao K, et al: Metformin for treatment of antipsychotic-induced amenorrhea and weight gain in women with first episode schizophrenia: a double-blind, randomized, placebo-controlled trial. Am J Psychiatry 168:813–821, 2012

CHAPTER 11

Obesity

Matthew Reed, M.D., M.S.P.H.

Case Discussion

Mr. I, a 54-year-old white man with chronic paranoid schizophrenia, pre-diabetes (hemoglobin A_{1c} of 6.0), hypertension, and hyperlipidemia, returns to the clinic after starting olanzapine 3 months earlier. Mr. I, who is 5′8″, has gained 9 kg (20 lb) since his last visit and now weighs 113 kg (250 lb). He has been stable on olanzapine and volunteers regularly at the local animal shelter. He lives in a local board-and-care home and has a limited social support network but is accompanied to this visit by his sister.

Clinical Overview

Epidemiology of Obesity Among the General Population

It is estimated that 36% of adults and 17% of children in the United States are obese (Ogden et al. 2012). The prevalence of obesity among adults (ages 20–74) has more than doubled from 1976 to 2008 (Ogden and Carroll 2010). Obesity affects most major organ systems and is associated with various significant health conditions, including diabetes, cardiovascular disease, dyslipidemia, and cancer (see Table 11–1 for a more complete list). The American Medical Association (2013) recently designated obesity a distinct disease, citing its connection with cardiovascular disease and type 2 diabetes. Obesity

TABLE 11–1. Health conditions associated with obesity

Endocrine	Diabetes
	Dyslipidemia
Cardiovascular	Hypertension
	Coronary artery disease
	Stroke
Cancer	Colorectal
	Breast
	Endometrial
Gastrointestinal	Gastroesophageal reflux disease
	Cholelithiasis
	Fatty liver disease
Renal	Nephrolithiasis
Reproductive	Infertility, pregnancy complications
	Polycystic ovary syndrome
	Erectile dysfunction
Pulmonary	Obstructive sleep apnea
Musculoskeletal	Osteoarthritis
	Low back pain

Source. Adapted from Tsai and Wadden 2013.

is also associated with an overall increase in mortality at body mass index (BMI) levels greater than 30–35 (Berrington de Gonzalez et al. 2010; Flegal et al. 2013; Tsai and Wadden 2013).

Epidemiology of Obesity Among Those With Serious Mental Illness

Adults with serious mental illness (SMI) are defined as persons age 18 and older who have a mental illness (based on the *Diagnostic and Statistical Manual of Mental Disorders*) that has substantially interfered with one or more major life activities in the past year (Insel 2013). Individuals with SMI die on average 13–30 years earlier than the general population (Colton and Manderscheid 2006). Much of the excess mortality can be attributed to cardiovascular disease, for which obesity is a major risk factor (Osby et al. 2000, 2001). Obesity's effect on the development of cardiovascular disease appears to be largely mediated through worsening blood pressure, cholesterol, and diabetes (Emerging Risk Factors Collaboration et al. 2011). The majority of research on obesity and mental health has involved individuals with schizophrenia and affective disorders. The prevalence of obesity in this population is 1.5–2.0 times greater than in the general population (American Diabetes Association et al. 2004). The underlying etiology for the increased prevalence is not completely understood; however, there is some evidence that mental illness itself and the medications used to treat it are contributors to obesity.

The extent to which SMI itself may contribute to weight gain is not clear. Some studies have shown the prevalence of obesity to be increased among drug-naïve individuals with bipolar disorder or schizophrenia. More recent research has not corroborated this (Padmavati et al. 2010; Sengupta et al. 2008; Thakore 2004; Thakore et al. 2002). There is, however, strong evidence that antipsychotics, mood stabilizers, and some antidepressants have contributed to the increased prevalence of obesity among individuals with psychiatric illness. Antipsychotics, as a class, have been associated with the greatest weight gain; however, there is considerable variation among individual agents. Generally, the second-generation (or atypical) antipsychotics (SGAs) have been shown the lead to the greatest weight gain (Correll et al. 2009; Kahn et al. 2008; Lieberman et al. 2005; Patel et al. 2009; Sikich et al. 2008). Olanzapine, for example, has been associated with up to 13.9 kg (30.6 lb) of weight gain in the first 12 months of use (Kahn et al. 2008). Three newer agents (iloperidone, asenapine, and particularly lurasidone) are purported to have less associated weight gain, but comparative studies are lacking (Citrome 2011). Among mood stabilizers, valproate and to a lesser extent lithium have been associated with significant weight gain (Bowden et al. 2010; Sachs et al. 2006). Among antidepressants, mirtazapine, paroxetine, and the tricyclic antidepressants are most often associated with weight gain, whereas bupropion has been associated with modest weight loss (Aronne and Segal 2003). Table 11–2 provides a ranking of the weight gain potential of the various psychotropic agents.

Practical Pointers

- Mental health providers are uniquely qualified to diagnose and initiate treatments for obesity among adults with serious mental illness.
- Mental health providers
  - Are more familiar with psychotropic agents.
  - Have a better understanding of effective treatment modalities less likely to contribute to obesity.
  - Understand the psychosocial contributors to weight gain.
  - May be the only medical professional their patients see regularly.

TABLE 11–2.　**Ranking of weight gain propensity among psychotropic agents**

Most weight gain	Clozapine
	Olanzapine
Moderate weight gain	Quetiapine
	Risperidone
	Perphenazine
	Valproate
	Lithium
	Mirtazapine
	Tricyclic antidepressants (amitriptyline, imipramine, doxepin)
Least weight gain	Haloperidol
	Fluphenazine
	Ziprasidone
	Asenapine
	Aripiprazole
	Lurasidone
	Lamotrigine
	Most selective serotonin reuptake inhibitors

Source.　Based on data from Aronne and Segal 2003; Bowden et al. 2010; Citrome 2011; Lieberman et al. 2005; Sachs et al. 2006; Sikich et al. 2008.

Diagnosis

According to the National Heart, Lung, and Blood Institute (1998), individuals with BMI of 30 or greater are considered obese. Table 11–3 lists the weight classifications for adults, ranging from underweight through three levels of obesity. There is some controversy as to whether increased mortality begins at a BMI of 25 or 35. Earlier studies showed an increased mortality beginning with a BMI greater than 25, but a more recent systematic review and meta-analysis showed increased mortality beginning with a BMI of 35 kg/m^2. Being overweight (BMI 25–30) was actually associated with *lower* all-cause mortality (Berrington de Gonzalez et al. 2010; Flegal et al. 2013). Although it is unclear whether being overweight conveys increased mortality risk, being overweight is correlated with the development of type II diabetes, hypertension, sleep apnea, and cardiovascular disease (Tsai and Wadden 2013).

TABLE 11–3. **Weight classifications for adults**

	Body mass index
Underweight	<18.5
Normal weight	18.5–24.9
Overweight	25.0–29.9
Grade I obesity	30.0–34.9
Grade II obesity	35.0–39.9
Grade III obesity	≥40

Source. Adapted from National Heart, Lung, and Blood Institute 1998.

An initial evaluation for obesity should include measurement of a patient's BMI and waist circumference. Waist circumference measurements should be limited to individuals who are overweight or have Grade I obesity (BMI = 25.0–34.9). Little additional risk information is obtained from measuring the waist circumference of those weighing more or less than this. Waist circumference measurements provide an estimate of visceral adiposity. Increased visceral adiposity is associated with an elevated risk for diabetes, hypertension, and nonalcoholic fatty liver disease (National Heart, Lung, and Blood Institute 1998). Waist circumference should be measured in a horizontal plane over the iliac crests after exhalation. A circumference of 35 inches or greater for women and 40 inches or greater for men is considered elevated (National Heart, Lung, and Blood Institute 1998).

At the time of initial evaluation, a complete personal weight history and family history for obesity should be obtained. The personal weight history should include instances of successful weight loss, with a focus on how the weight loss was achieved. Reasons for returned weight gain should also be explored. Recommended laboratory evaluations include fasting glucose or hemoglobin A1c, thyroid-stimulating hormone, liver-associated enzymes, and fasting lipids.

Preventive Guidelines

Prevention of obesity among patients with SMI involves careful patient assessment, promotion of obesity-preventing behaviors, and frequent monitoring. Many components of the assessment are already routinely obtained during the intake evaluation of patients in a behavioral health clinic. Seven key assessment domains are detailed in Table 11–4. Factors related to any one of these domains may increase or decrease the likelihood of developing obe-

TABLE 11–4. **Individual patient assessment domains for the prevention and treatment of obesity**

Weight history	Including personal history of weight gain (and loss), as well as family history
Medication profile	Thorough evaluation for obesity-related medications
Dietary habits	A detailed understanding of what a patient eats day to day
Physical activity	Formal exercise program as well as general activity level
Social support	Network of family and friends
Economic status	Source of patient's funds (e.g., public assistance, earned wages)
Living arrangements	Place of residence (e.g., apartment, board-and-care facility, family home)

sity. For example, a patient with limited means is more likely to purchase cheaper, highly processed foods, which are associated with weight gain. The same patient, living alone in an apartment, may have more difficulty preparing healthy meals than someone living in a board-and-care facility that provides meals. Individualized assessment increases the likelihood that any intervention to prevent or treat obesity will be effective.

A patient's medication profile should be thoroughly evaluated for obesity-related medications. In addition to psychotropic medications, the following medications have been associated with weight gain: glucocorticoids, diabetes medications (not including metformin), antihistamines (especially cyprohep-tadine), hormonal agents (progestins), β-blockers (especially propranolol), and α-blockers (especially terazosin) (Tsai and Wadden 2013). The glucocorticoids and SGAs are associated with the greatest weight gain. Patients who are going to be taking a medication associated with weight gain may benefit from initiation of a behavioral program at the time the medication is prescribed rather than waiting for obesity to develop (Gabriele et al. 2009).

Following individualized assessment, patients should be encouraged to engage in well-established obesity-preventing behaviors. Such behaviors include reading food labels, eating smaller portions, eating adequate fiber (25 g/day), eating five servings of fruits and vegetables per day, and exercising 45–60 minutes per day (Tsai and Wadden 2013). Getting adequate sleep (6–9 hours per night) has also been associated with less weight gain (Patel and Hu 2008).

Prevention of obesity among patients with SMI who are taking psychotropic medications requires frequent monitoring. The American Diabetes Association, American Psychiatric Association, American Association of Clinical Endocrinologists, and North American Association for the Study of Obesity developed a consensus statement on obesity monitoring with antipsychotic use (American Diabetes Association et al. 2004). The consensus recommendation is for baseline BMI measurements before the individual starts taking an antipsychotic medication, followed by repeat measurements at 4, 8, and 12 weeks (Table 11–5). Thereafter, measurements should be made quarterly. Waist circumference should also be measured at baseline and annually. If at any time during therapy the patient gains 5%–7% or more of his or her baseline weight, consideration should be given for switching to another medication with less associated weight gain. When switching any psychotropic agent, gradual cross-titration is recommended.

Treatment Recommendations

The treatment of obesity among patients with SMI is similar in many respects to treatment of obesity among the general population. Comprehensive lifestyle modification remains a cornerstone of treatment. The goal of treatment for overweight and obese individuals with SMI should be a 10% reduction in baseline body weight (National Heart, Lung, and Blood Institute 1998). Among those individuals with SMI, greater emphasis should be given to identifying obesity-related medications they may be taking. Measures to mitigate the effects of these medications should be a top priority. Once the diagnosis of obesity has been established, the clinician can undertake the treatment strategy summarized by the mnemonic A-SCAR, as detailed in Table 11–6.

Assessment was discussed in the previous section, with a summary of the seven domains listed in Table 11–4. Switching psychotropic medications is the initial recommendation for patients who have gained 5%–7% or more of their body weight while taking a medication known to cause weight gain. As shown earlier in Table 11–2, olanzapine is among the SGAs most likely to cause weight gain. If a patient is psychiatrically stable but gaining weight while taking olanzapine, switching to an agent with less associated weight gain, such as aripiprazole or ziprasidone, may be an appropriate intervention. When changing medications, gradual cross-titration is recommended. Titration off clozapine should be given careful consideration due to the potential for serious psychiatric sequelae (American Diabetes Association et al. 2004).

Comprehensive lifestyle modifications include dietary changes, physical activity, and cognitive-behavioral components. Lifestyle modification has been shown to decrease the amount of weight gain associated with atypical

TABLE 11–5. Monitoring protocol for patients taking second-generation antipsychotics

	Baseline	4 weeks	8 weeks	12 weeks	Quarterly	Annually
Personal/family history	X					X
Body mass index	X	X	X	X	X	
Waist circumference	X					X

Source. Adapted from American Diabetes Association et al. 2004.

TABLE 11–6.	A-SCAR: treatment of obesity among individuals with serious mental illness
Assess	Assess patient's weight history, medication profile, dietary habits, level of physical activity, social supports, economic status, and living arrangements.
Switch	Switch patient to a medication less likely to contribute to obesity.
Change	Change lifestyle to include dietary, exercise, and cognitive-behavioral modifications.
Add	Add another medication to assist with weight loss or minimize ongoing weight gain.
Refer	Refer for bariatric surgery as a last resort in carefully selected patients.

antipsychotic medications (Gabriele et al. 2009). When lifestyle modification is initiated before medication treatment begins, subsequent weight gain is decreased. When the modification is initiated after medication treatment has started, weight loss occurs. The length of the intervention program correlates with the amount of weight loss. One systematic literature review found that patients lost an average of 2.63 kg (5.80 lb) with 12- to 16-week interventions, 4.24 kg (9.35 lb) with 6-month interventions, and 3.05 kg (6.72 lb) with 12- to 18-month interventions (Gabriele et al. 2009). The U.S. Preventive Services Task Force (USPSTF) recommends only high-intensity interventions, defined as 12–26 sessions in a year (Moyer and U.S. Preventive Services Task Force 2012). The composition of high-intensity interventions, while not formally defined, has included diet, exercise, and CBT components administered by dietitians, psychologists, fitness trainers, and nurses.

Many weight loss diets have proven to be effective. The key feature of a successful diet is calorie restriction. Macronutrient composition is less important than patients' adherence to a low-calorie diet they can tolerate (Wadden et al. 2012). A diet of 1,200–1,500 kcal/day is recommended for a person weighing less than 113 kg (250 lb) to achieve a calorie deficit of 500–1,000 kcal/day. This calorie deficit will result in approximately a 10% reduction in baseline weight over 6 months (National Heart, Lung, and Blood Institute 1998; Tsai and Wadden 2013). A diet of 1,500–1,800 kcal/day is indicated if the person weighs 113 kg (250 lb) or more. Federal guidelines suggest macronutrient composition of 15% protein, less than 30% fat (less than 7% saturated fat), and the remainder carbohydrates (predominantly complex carbohydrates) (National Heart, Lung, and Blood Institute 1998). Meal replacement diets, in which two meals per day are replaced with nutritional shakes, have shown good weight loss results, and patients with SMI may have an easier time adhering to these diets (Heymsfield et al. 2003). Web-based resources for structuring a diet can be found at the end of this chapter in the "Resources" section.

A significant amount of research has been done on the effectiveness of exercise on weight loss. Randomized controlled trials have shown that walking about 4 miles/hour for 30 minutes/day 5 days per week is associated with about a 1%–3% loss of baseline body weight, which is roughly equivalent to maintenance of body weight (Physical Activity Guidelines Advisory Committee 2009). Significantly more exercise is required to actually lose weight. Exercise programs have been shown to be most effective for maintenance of weight loss. One encouraging meta-analysis by Bravata et al. (2007) found that use of the simple pedometer with a focus on goal setting to reach particular step counts each day was associated with a small but significant reduction in BMI. On average, study participants who used pedometers walked 1 mile more each day compared with control subjects. Use of pedometers among those with SMI may present a cost-effective way to encourage increased physical activity and maintenance of weight loss obtained through dietary means.

Cognitive-behavioral interventions are essential for any successful weight loss program. As listed in Table 11–7, key components of these interventions include self-monitoring, goal setting, stimulus control, behavior replacement, problem solving, and cognitive restructuring (Fabricatore 2007). Self-monitoring typically involves keeping a food record, maintaining an exercise log (or automated log such as with a pedometer), and frequent (weekly) weight checks. These are well-established behavioral mechanisms to promote weight loss and maintenance of weight loss (Dalle Grave et al. 2003). All patients should be taught to self-monitor. Goal setting provides motivation for continued adherence to any program. Stimulus control can be as simple as removing access to unhealthy foods and avoiding situations that typically trigger the desire to eat. Behavior replacement aims to provide alternative healthy behaviors to counter internal cues to eat (such as depressed mood). An example would be a patient who typically reaches for a snack when depressed but instead goes on a walk. The alternative behavior should be pleasurable to the patient. Learning to problem-solve is key for a person to adapt to changing circumstances and maintain a weight loss program. Patients are trained to identify the problem, brainstorm solutions, weigh the pros and cons of each solution, and finally select a solution (Fabricatore 2007). Cognitive restructuring involves identifying dysfunctional thoughts and replacing them with more rational or accurate ones. Dysfunctional thoughts are typically identified through the use of "thought records." Cognitive-behavioral interventions focused on restructuring maladaptive cognitions regarding diet and weight have demonstrated greater weight reduction than diet and physical activity counseling (Das et al. 2012).

TABLE 11–7. **Key components of cognitive-behavioral interventions**

Self-monitoring

Goal setting

Stimulus control

Behavior replacement

Problem solving

Cognitive restructuring

Numerous medications have been investigated to treat antipsychotic-induced weight gain and obesity in general. Medications with the most evidence supporting their use include metformin, topiramate, phentermine, lorcaserin, and orlistat. Metformin is the most studied agent. It inhibits hepatic gluconeogenesis and improves skeletal muscle insulin sensitivity. Its effects on weight are thought to be secondary to a reduction in appetite (Lee and Morley 1998). A meta-analysis indicated that metformin led to a mean weight loss of 2.93 kg (6.46 lb) over the 12–16 weeks of the studies included (Fiedorowicz et al. 2012). Although metformin may potentially play a role in weight management among patients with SMI, its empirical use among patients without diabetes or prediabetes is premature and has not been approved by the U.S. Food and Drug Administration (FDA). Of all the weight loss agents, the combination pill phentermine-topiramate produces the most weight loss (8%–11% of initial weight) (Tsai and Wadden 2013). However, use of phentermine, a sympathomimetic, among patients with SMI is usually avoided because of its potential for psychosis, dysphoria, and abuse. Use of topiramate is also limited given its poor tolerability (psychomotor retardation, drooling, dizziness, headache, and mild cognitive impairment). Lorcaserin, a serotonin 5-HT$_{2c}$ receptor agonist, was recently approved by the FDA for weight loss. However, it is not recommended among patients with SMI given its potential for serotonin syndrome, depression, and suicidality. Orlistat, a lipase inhibitor, has been disappointing in reversing psychotropic-induced weight gain. It is also poorly tolerated due to gastrointestinal upset.

Bariatric surgery is the most efficacious treatment for severe obesity. The three most common bariatric surgeries done in the United States are adjustable gastric banding, Roux-en-Y gastric bypass, and sleeve gastrectomy (with reported BMI reductions of 2.4, 9.0, and 10.1, respectively) (Padwal et al. 2011). Bariatric surgery is indicated for patients either with a BMI of 40 or greater or with a BMI of 35–39.9 and comorbid conditions (type 2 diabetes, sleep apnea, or disabling arthritis) who have failed lifestyle and medication interventions. Laparoscopic gastric banding has FDA approval for patients with a BMI of 30 or greater and type 2 diabetes (Tsai and Wadden 2013). Although efficacious, bariatric surgery is associated with significant complications, including band slippage, erosion of anastomosis, and micronutrient deficiencies. Furthermore, the perioperative complications are not insignificant. Thirty-day mortality rates have been estimated at 0.2% for laparoscopic gastric bypass and 2.1% for open gastric bypass (Longitudinal Assessment of Bariatric Surgery Consortium 2009). Typically, patients must undergo psychiatric evaluation to ensure their appropriateness for surgery. A diagnosis of SMI is generally felt to be an exclusionary criterion; however, there have been published reports of patients with stable schizophrenia undergoing bariatric surgery with good outcomes (Das et al. 2012). Any consideration of bariatric surgery in a patient with SMI would require close collaboration between mental health providers, primary medical doctors, and bariatric surgery specialists to ensure appropriate candidate selection and adequate follow-up and support.

Treatment selection parameters based on BMI for patients with SMI are summarized in Table 11–8.

When to Refer

Table 11–9 lists specific indications about when to refer a patient for further medical evaluation. Mental health providers are well trained to understand the psychosocial aspects contributing to an individual patient's development of obesity and the factors that may impede successful weight loss. As with any intervention requiring behavioral change, a patient's motivation to change is key. Miller and Rollnick's clinical principles of motivational interviewing, which include expression of empathy, development of discrepancy, avoidance of argument, rolling with resistance, and supporting self-efficacy, can be applied to individuals with obesity and mental illness (Miller and Rollnick 2002). When physicians express empathy and support self-efficacy, patients *feel* valued. In turn, they will often be more open about their goals and difficulties. With this basic trust, the physician can assist the patient to become cognizant of discrepancies between current behaviors and desired outcomes. Resistance in the process should be viewed not as failure but rather as an opportunity to reaffirm the patient's own autonomy and explore the resistance together.

Special Treatment Considerations for the Psychiatric Patient Population

The treatment of obesity among patients with SMI requires a collaborative approach among mental health and primary care providers. Mental health

TABLE 11–8. Treatment selection based on body mass index for patients with severe mental illness

Treatment	Body mass index (BMI)				
	25.0–26.9	27.0–29.9	30.0–34.9	35.0–39.9	≥40
Switch medication	If patient has gained >5% of his or her baseline body weight since initiating treatment				
Make lifestyle modification (diet, exercise, and cognitive-behavioral therapy)	If patient has comorbid type 2 diabetes, obstructive sleep apnea, or disabling osteoarthritis		Indicated	Indicated	Indicated
Add metformin	If patient is prediabetic or diabetic and does not have any contraindications (e.g., hepatic, renal, or cardiac disease)				
Add sympathomimetic or lorcaserin (5-HT$_{2C}$ agonist)	Usually contraindicated given the potential for exacerbating mental illness				
Refer for bariatric surgery	Not indicated	Not indicated	Not indicated	Unclear	Unclear

Source. Adapted from Tsai and Wadden 2013.

TABLE 11–9. **When to refer a patient to a primary care doctor or bariatric specialist**

If the patient develops any of the following:

Prediabetes/diabetes

Hypertension

Hyperlipidemia

Sleep apnea

If the patient is stable from a psychiatric standpoint, has a body mass index of ≥40, and wishes to pursue bariatric surgery

If the patient has been unable to maintain a healthy weight by using caloric restriction, exercise, and cognitive-behavioral therapy

If the patient has chronic and severe myofascial or joint pain due to obesity

providers play a key role in treating obesity because many of the psychotropic medications prescribed are associated with increased weight gain and subsequent development of diabetes, hypertension, hyperlipidemia, and coronary artery disease. Should these adverse outcomes develop, primary care providers can assist in proper treatment of these conditions while obesity continues to be addressed collaboratively between mental health and primary care providers.

Case Discussion (*continued*)

The treatment of obesity in Mr. I, who has chronic paranoid schizophrenia, could proceed in a stepwise fashion using the mnemonic A-SCAR as follows:

Assess the patient. Mr. I now has a BMI of 38, which falls in the Grade III obesity range (see Table 11–3), increasing his mortality risk. Further assessment would include a weight history (including prior success in losing weight) and discussion of his dietary and exercise habits. It is helpful if Mr. I has at least some support from his sister, who brought him to the appointment, as well as staff at the board and care.

Switch medications. Mr. I has gained more than 5% of his baseline body weight since starting olanzapine. He appears stable from a psychiatric point of view, as demonstrated by the fact that he has been volunteering regularly at the animal shelter. Therefore, switching to an antipsychotic that has less association with weight gain would be the next step.

Change lifestyle. The patient should begin a high-intensity lifestyle modification program (12–26 visits in the first year) focused on diet, exercise, and cognitive-behavioral interventions. The clearly defined goal should be for a 10% decrease in body weight within the first 6 months, followed by maintenance of the weight loss for at least 1 year. His sister and board-and-care operator may be able to assist with dietary modifications. Use of a pedometer (with regular goal setting) may be a simple method for increasing exercise.

Add a medication. The addition of metformin is likely indicated for this patient with prediabetes. Metformin could be started in collaboration with his primary care physician.

Refer for surgery. Bariatric surgery is not currently indicated. It may become a consideration if Mr. I fails to lose weight with the above interventions. The case for bariatric surgery would be strengthened should he develop full type II diabetes, disabling osteoarthritis, or obstructive sleep apnea. With a BMI of 38 kg/m^2, he would need one or more of these additional comorbidities before surgery would be indicated. Prior to any consideration for bariatric surgery, there would need to be careful consultation with his primary medical doctor and bariatric surgery specialists. He would also have to be stable from a mental health standpoint.

Clinical Highlights

- Thirty-six percent of adults and 17% of children in the United States are obese. The prevalence of obesity among adults (ages 20–74) has more than doubled from 1976 to 2008.

- The prevalence of obesity among those with serious mental illness (SMI) is 1.5–2.0 times greater than among the general population.

- Individuals with SMI die on average 13–30 years earlier than the general population. Much of the excess mortality can be attributed to cardiovascular disease, for which obesity is a major risk factor.

- There is strong evidence that antipsychotics, mood stabilizers, and some antidepressants have contributed to the increased prevalence of obesity among individuals with psychiatric illness.

- Treatment of obesity among individuals with SMI is possible. Key components can be remembered using the mnemonic A-SCAR (see Table 11–6).

- Patient motivation is important to achieving change. Motivational interviewing, with a focus on expression of empathy, development of discrepancy, avoidance of argument, rolling with resistance, and supporting self-efficacy, is beneficial.

- Referral to primary care physicians for assistance in treating associated medical conditions while maintaining a collaborative focus on the primary issue of obesity management is likely to yield the best patient outcomes.

Resources

For Patients

Let's Move: http://www.letsmove.gov
Obesity Action Coalition: http://www.obesityaction.org

For Clinicians

American College of Physicians: Physicians' Information and Education Resource (PIER) Module on Obesity: Available at: http://smartmedicine.acponline.org

Clinical Guidelines on the Identification, Evaluation, and Treatment of Overweight and Obesity in Adults: The Evidence Report. 1998. Available at: http://www.ncbi.nlm.nih.gov/books/NBK2003/. Updated guide referred to as "Obesity 2" should be released in 2014.

U.S. Department of Health and Human Services, National Institutes of Health, National Heart, Lung, and Blood Institute: Managing overweight and obesity in adults: systematic evidence review from the Obesity Expert Panel, 2013. Available at: http://www.nhlbi.nih.gov/health-pro/guidelines/in-develop/obesity-evidence-review/obesity-evidence-review.pdf. Accessed August 18, 2014.

References

American Diabetes Association, American Psychiatric Association, American Association of Clinical Endocrinologists, et al: Consensus development conference on antipsychotic drugs and obesity and diabetes. Diabetes Care 27:596–601, 2004

American Medical Association: AMA adopts new policies on second day of voting at annual meeting [press release]. Available at: http://www.ama-assn.org/ama/pub/news/news/2013/2013-06-18-new-ama-policies-annual-meeting.page.

Aronne LJ, Segal KR: Weight gain in the treatment of mood disorders. J Clin Psychiatry 64(suppl):22–29, 2003

Berrington de Gonzalez A, Hartge P, Cerhan JR, et al: Body-mass index and mortality among 1.46 million white adults. N Engl J Med 363:2211–2219, 2010

Bowden CL, Mosolov S, Hranov L, et al: Efficacy of valproate versus lithium in mania or mixed mania: a randomized, open 12-week trial. Int Clin Psychopharmacol 25:60–67, 2010

Bravata DM, Smith-Spangler C, Sundaram V, et al: Using pedometers to increase physical activity and improve health: a systematic review. JAMA 298:2296–2304, 2007

Citrome L: Iloperidone, asenapine, and lurasidone: a brief overview of 3 new second-generation antipsychotics. Postgrad Med 123:153–162, 2011

Colton CW, Manderscheid RW: Congruencies in increased mortality rates, years of potential life lost, and causes of death among public mental health clients in eight states. Prev Chronic Dis 3:A42, 2006

Correll CU, Manu P, Olshanskiy V, et al: Cardiometabolic risk of second-generation antipsychotic medications during first-time use in children and adolescents. JAMA 302:1765–1773, 2009

Dalle Grave R, Centis E, Marzocchi R, et al: Major factors for facilitating change in behavioral strategies to reduce obesity. Psychol Res Behav Manag 6:101–110, 2003

Das C, Mendez G, Jagasia S, et al: Second-generation antipsychotic use in schizophrenia and associated weight gain: a critical review and meta-analysis of behavioral and pharmacologic treatments. Ann Clin Psychiatry 24:225–239, 2012

Emerging Risk Factors Collaboration, Wormser D, Kaptoge S, et al: Separate and combined associations of body-mass index and abdominal adiposity with cardiovascular disease: collaborative analysis of 58 prospective studies. Lancet 377:1085–1095, 2011

Fabricatore AN: Behavior therapy and cognitive-behavioral therapy of obesity: is there a difference? J Am Diet Assoc 107:92–99, 2007

Fiedorowicz JG, Miller DD, Bishop JR, et al: Systematic review and meta-analysis of pharmacological interventions for weight gain from antipsychotics and mood stabilizers. Curr Psychiatry Rev 8:25–36, 2012

Flegal KM, Kit BK, Orpana H, et al: Association of all-cause mortality with overweight and obesity using standard body mass index categories: a systematic review and meta-analysis. JAMA 309:71–82, 2013

Gabriele JM, Dubbert PM, Reeves RR: Efficacy of behavioural interventions in managing atypical antipsychotic weight gain. Obes Rev 10:442–455, 2009

Heymsfield SB, van Mierlo CA, van der Knaap HC, et al: Weight management using a meal replacement strategy: meta and pooling analysis from six studies. Int J Obes Relat Metab Disord 27:537–549, 2003

Insel T: Director's Blog: Getting Serious About Mental Illnesses. Bethesda, MD, National Institute of Mental Health, July 2013. Available at: http://www.nimh.nih.gov/about/director/2013/getting-serious-about-mental-illnesses.shtml. Accessed January 20, 2014.

Kahn RS, Fleischhacker WW, Boter H, et al: Effectiveness of antipsychotic drugs in first-episode schizophrenia and schizophreniform disorder: an open randomised clinical trial. Lancet 371:1085–1097, 2008

Lee A, Morley JE: Metformin decreases food consumption and induces weight loss in subjects with obesity with type II non-insulin-dependent diabetes. Obes Res 6:47–53, 1998

Lieberman JA, Stroup TS, McEvoy JP, et al: Effectiveness of antipsychotic drugs in patients with chronic schizophrenia. N Engl J Med 353:1209–1223, 2005

Longitudinal Assessment of Bariatric Surgery Consortium: Perioperative safety in the longitudinal assessment of bariatric surgery. N Engl J Med 361:445–454, 2009

Miller WR, Rollnick S: Motivational Interviewing: Preparing People for Change, 2nd Edition. New York, Guilford, 2002

Moyer VA, U.S. Preventive Services Task Force: Screening for and management of obesity in adults: U.S. Preventive Services Task Force recommendation statement. Ann Intern Med 157:373–378, 2012

National Heart, Lung, and Blood Institute: Obesity Education Initiative Expert Panel on the Identification, Evaluation, and Treatment of Obesity in Adults: Clinical Guidelines on the Identification, Evaluation, and Treatment of Overweight and

Obesity in Adults. Bethesda, MD, National Heart, Lung, and Blood Institute, 1998

Ogden CL, Carroll MD: Prevalence of Overweight, Obesity, and Extreme Obesity Among Adults—United States, Trends 1960–1962 through 2007–2008. NCHS Health E-Stat, June 2010. Available from: http://www.cdc.gov/nchs/data/hestat/obesity_adult_07_08/obesity_adult_07_08.pdf. Accessed February 18, 2014.

Ogden CL, Carroll MD, Kit BK, et al: Prevalence of obesity in the United States, 2009–2010. NCHS Data Brief, No 82. Hyattsville, MD, National Center for Health Statistics, 2012

Osby U, Correia N, Brandt L, et al: Time trends in schizophrenia mortality in Stockholm county, Sweden: cohort study. BMJ 321:483–484, 2000

Osby U, Brandt L, Correia N, et al: Excess mortality in bipolar and unipolar disorder in Sweden. Arch Gen Psychiatry 58:844–850, 2001

Padmavati R, McCreadie RG, Tirupati S: Low prevalence of obesity and metabolic syndrome in never-treated chronic schizophrenia. Schizophr Res 121:199–202, 2010

Padwal R, Klarenbach S, Wiebe N, et al: Bariatric surgery: a systematic review and network meta-analysis of randomized trials. Obes Rev 12:602–621, 2011

Patel JK, Buckley PF, Woolson S, et al: Metabolic profiles of second-generation antipsychotics in early psychosis: findings from the CAFE study. Schizophr Res 111:9–16, 2009

Patel SR, Hu FB: Short sleep duration and weight gain: a systematic review. Obesity (Silver Spring) 16:643–653, 2008

Physical Activity Guidelines Advisory Committee: Physical Activity Guidelines Advisory Committee report, 2008. To the Secretary of Health and Human Services. Part A: executive summary. Nutr Rev 67:114–120, 2009

Sachs G, Bowden C, Calabrese JR, et al: Effects of lamotrigine and lithium on body weight during maintenance treatment of bipolar I disorder. Bipolar Disord 8:175–181, 2006

Sengupta S, Parilla-Escobar MA, Klink R, et al: Are metabolic indices different between drug-naive first-episode psychosis patients and healthy controls? Schizophr Res 102:329–336, 2008

Sikich L, Frazier JA, McClellan J, et al: Double-blind comparison of first- and second-generation antipsychotics in early-onset schizophrenia and schizoaffective disorder: findings from the Treatment of Early Onset Schizophrenia Spectrum Disorders (TEOSS) study. Am J Psychiatry 165:1420–1431, 2008

Thakore JH: Metabolic disturbance in first-episode schizophrenia. Br J Psychiatry Suppl 47:S76–S79, 2004

Thakore JH, Mann JN, Vlahos I, et al: Increased visceral fat distribution in drug-naive and drug-free patients with schizophrenia. Int J Obes Relat Metab Disord 26:137–141, 2002

Tsai AG, Wadden TA: In the clinic: obesity. Ann Intern Med 159:ITC3-1–ITC3-15; quiz ITC3-16, 2013

Wadden TA, Webb VL, Moran CH, et al: Lifestyle modification for obesity: new developments in diet, physical activity, and behavior therapy. Circulation 125:1157–1170, 2012

CHAPTER 12

Metabolic Syndrome

Natasha Cunningham, M.D.
Sarah K. Rivelli, M.D., F.A.C.P.

Case Discussion

Mr. M is a 42-year-old man with schizophrenia. He was hospitalized psychiatrically for an exacerbation of his psychotic symptoms 6 months ago. At that time, his antipsychotic was switched from haloperidol to olanzapine. Since his discharge, he has gained 8 kg (18 lb) and been diagnosed with type 2 diabetes; his last hemoglobin A_{1c} (HbA$_{1c}$) level was 7%. Routine labs are checked by his psychiatrist, and Mr. M is found to have a total cholesterol level of 210 mg/dL, a high-density lipoprotein (HDL) level of 35 mg/dL, a low-density lipoprotein (LDL) level of 155 mg/dL, and triglycerides of 140 mg/dL. His current weight is 111 kg (245 lb), and his body mass index (BMI) is 33.2. His current blood pressure (BP) in the clinic is 135/85 mmHg.

Clinical Overview

Metabolic syndrome is a constellation of findings associated with increased risk of cardiovascular disease (CVD). This syndrome is also known as *syndrome X* or *hyperglycemia-dyslipidemia syndrome*. Metabolic syndrome results from abdominal obesity, which leads to insulin resistance, dyslipidemia, hypertension, endothelial dysfunction, and vascular inflammation. The National Cholesterol Education Program Adult Treatment Panel III (ATP III) (Expert Panel on Detection, Evaluation, and Treatment of High Blood Cholesterol in Adults 2001; Grundy et al. 2005) and the International Diabetes Federation (IDF) (Alberti et al. 2006) have developed similar guidelines for diagnosis of metabolic syndrome (see Table 12–2 in the section "Diagnosis" later in this chapter). Compared with the ATP III guidelines, the IDF guidelines have slightly lower, ethnicity-specific waist circumference cutoffs, which have been shown to translate into a 15%–20% higher prevalence of metabolic syndrome in U.S. urban populations (Adams et al. 2005). However, the associated increase in cardiovascular risk in metabolic syndrome is between 32% and 45% regardless of which guidelines are used for diagnosis (Lawlor et al. 2006).

The prevalence of metabolic syndrome in the United States has been increasing over the last several decades, from 22% in a survey from 1988–1994 (Ford et al. 2002) to 34.5% in a survey from 1999–2002 (Ford 2005). There has been a consistently higher prevalence among older adults, women, and Mexican Americans. Weight gain is the single greatest risk factor for the development of metabolic syndrome. An increase in weight of 2.25 kg (4.96 lb) over 16 years is associated with a 21%–45% increased risk of developing metabolic syndrome, and the prevalence is 60% among obese individuals versus 5% among those with normal weight.

The prevalence of metabolic syndrome among individuals with schizophrenia in the United States has been estimated to be 60%, almost double the prevalence in the general population (Papanastasiou 2012). In parallel, the risk of death due to CVD in patients with schizophrenia has been shown to be 2–3 times higher than in the general population (Osborn et al. 2007). The most common cause of death among individuals with serious mental illness is CVD, and the predicted survival for this population is about 20–25 years shorter than that of age-matched peers (Tiihonen et al. 2009).

Henry Maudsley noted an association between schizophrenia and diabetes as early as 1979, long before the development of the second-generation antipsychotics (SGAs). Antipsychotic-naïve patients with schizophrenia have been shown to have impaired glucose tolerance, increased insulin resistance, and increased visceral fat compared with control subjects (Thakore et al. 2002; Venkatasubramanian et al. 2007). Nonaffected relatives of individuals with schizophrenia have been found to have glucose intolerance and increased prevalence of type 2 diabetes (Fernandez-Egea et al. 2008). Interestingly, a genetic association between schizophrenia and an allele that confers risk for diabetes has been found, suggesting shared genetic vulnerability (Hansen et al. 2011). Overall, there is an approximately threefold increased risk for diabetes among those with schizophrenia (Papanastasiou 2012). Moreover, patients with severe mental illness are less likely to eat fruits and vegetables, are less likely to exercise, and tend to smoke cigarettes, all of which confer increased cardiovascular risk.

In addition to this elevated baseline risk, SGAs cause weight gain, dyslipidemia, and insulin resistance. Sedation from medications leads to decreased physical activity and thus weight gain and decreased cardiovascular health. For example, clinically significant weight gain, which is defined as a gain greater than 7% of baseline body weight, has been reported in up to 68% of patients taking olanzapine (Simpson et al. 2005). Younger, treatment-naïve patients appear to be most vulnerable to weight gain. In fact, olanzapine has been associated with an average weight gain of 15.5 kg (34.1 lb) after 1 year of treatment in treatment-naïve patients (Zipursky et al. 2005).

The American Diabetic Association, American Psychiatric Association, American Association of Clinical Endocrinologists, and North American Association for the Study of Obesity developed consensus guidelines (American Diabetes Association et al. 2004) recommending baseline evaluation and monitoring for metabolic syndrome in patients prescribed SGAs (Table 12–1).

Practical Pointers

- Metabolic syndrome confers an increased risk of cardiovascular disease (CVD).
- The association of CVD risk factors is synergistic, leading to substantially more risk than each of the risk factors individually.
- Both a diagnosis of schizophrenia and use of second-generation antipsychotics (SGAs) are associated with an increased risk of developing metabolic syndrome.
- Patients taking SGAs should be routinely monitored and treated for metabolic side effects of these medications.
- Switching to a different antipsychotic and lifestyle modification are first-line interventions for SGA-related metabolic syndrome.
- Medications are available to mediate antipsychotic-associated weight gain.

Diagnosis

The diagnosis of metabolic syndrome was developed by expert consensus groups based on clinical and epidemiological studies. It includes the presence of various health factors that tend to occur together and confer elevated cardiovascular morbidity and mortality risk. The diagnostic criteria for metabolic syndrome are summarized in Table 12–2.

Preventive Guidelines

No specific guidelines are targeted at the prevention of metabolic syndrome; however, close monitoring and early detection by psychiatrists are impor-

TABLE 12–1. Monitoring protocol for patients taking second-generation antipsychotics

	Baseline	4 weeks	8 weeks	12 weeks	Quarterly	Annually	Every 5 years
Personal/family history	X					X	
Weight (BMI)	X	X	X	X	X	X	
Waist circumference	X					X	
Blood pressure	X			X		X	
Fasting plasma glucose	X			X		X	
Fasting lipid profile	X			X			X

Note.   BMI = body mass index.
Source.   Adapted from American Diabetes Association et al. 2004.

TABLE 12–2. Metabolic syndrome: diagnostic criteria

Three of the following criteria:

Abdominal obesity	Men: waist circumference≥40 in. (102 cm) Women: waist circumference≥35 in. (88 cm)
Hypertriglyceridemia	Serum TG≥150 mg/dL
Low HDL cholesterol	Men: serum HDL<40 mg/dL Women: serum HDL<50 mg/dL
Elevated blood pressure	BP≥130/85 mmHg Or medication for HTN
Impaired fasting glucose	Fasting BG≥100[a] Or medication for diabetes

Note. BG=blood glucose; BP=blood pressure; HDL=high-density lipoprotein; HTN=hypertension; TG=triglycerides.
[a]Hemoglobin A_{1c} (HbA$_{1c}$)≥6.5% is now used for the diagnosis of diabetes. HbA$_{1c}$≥ 5.7% has a 91% specificity for impaired fasting glucose (BG≥100 mg/dL) (American Diabetes Association 2010).
Source. Adapted from Alberti et al. 2006; Expert Panel on Detection, Evaluation, and Treatment of High Blood Cholesterol in Adults 2001.

tant in mitigating its development and negative effects. Implementation of guidelines for monitoring for metabolic syndrome has been suboptimal, with compliance rates reaching only 40% in some studies (Barnes et al. 2008). Effective implementation requires practice change at the clinic level in terms of culture, work flow, leveraging informatics via the use of reminders, routine order sets, and feedback to providers on their practice.

Several approaches have been explored for the prevention of the driving factors of metabolic syndrome: abdominal obesity and insulin resistance (Adams et al. 2005). Dietary changes with a goal of decreasing weight and increasing insulin sensitivity include the Mediterranean diet, DASH (Dietary Approaches to Stop Hypertension) diet, and low glycemic index diet. All three emphasize increasing fruits and vegetables, decreasing refined carbohydrates and sugar, and eliminating sugared beverages, and all have shown efficacy in general populations (Azadbakht et al. 2005; Brand-Miller et al. 2003; Kastorini et al. 2011). Exercise is also an important component of weight loss or maintenance. The Council on Clinical Cardiology and the Council on Nutrition, Physical Activity, and Metabolism recommend 30 minutes daily of vigorous physical activity such as brisk walking (Thompson et al. 2003). Finally, treatment with metformin was shown to decrease the risk of developing metabolic syndrome or type 2 diabetes in a study of 3,234 obese individuals; however, metformin was less effective than intensive lifestyle change in this study (Knowler et al. 2002).

Avoidance of agents with high metabolic risk, particularly in treatment-naïve and younger patients, who are most at risk for such adverse effects, is an effective prevention strategy. The importance of preventing weight gain early in treatment cannot be emphasized enough, because it is very difficult for patients to lose weight and maintain weight loss once weight gain has occurred. Meta-analytic results show a three- to fourfold increase in the amount of weight gain among antipsychotic-naïve and young patients randomized to olanzapine or risperidone compared with older patients, whereas haloperidol does not have this effect (Alvarez-Jiménez et al. 2008a).

Treatment Recommendations

We recommend maintaining close contact with primary care providers (PCPs) and notifying them of any new diagnosis made or any new medications initiated. However, many patients under the care of a psychiatrist do not have a PCP. We recommend that any patient who develops metabolic syndrome be offered referral to a PCP if he or she does not already have one. However, if there are barriers to connecting with a PCP, the psychiatrist should feel empowered to start first-line medications to treat the components of metabolic syndrome. There are several circumstances when a treating psychiatrist should seek expert consultation. A patient should be referred to a PCP or endocrinologist if his or her blood sugar is persistently above 200 mg/dL despite treatment, if symptomatic hypoglycemia exists, or if diabetic ketoacidosis occurs. A patient whose BP is persistently above 180/100 mmHg should be referred to a PCP. A patient should be referred for emergent evaluation if he or she has symptomatic hypertension characterized by blurred vision, headache, or chest pain in the setting of significantly elevated BP. Another indication for referral to a PCP is if a patient does not tolerate or does not respond to first-line medications. Details of treatment of the cardiovascular risk factors present in metabolic syndrome can be found in Table 12–3.

Treatment With Metformin

Metformin appears to have a variety of beneficial effects in patients with obesity, prediabetes, diabetes, and metabolic syndrome. Metformin improves peripheral insulin sensitivity, decreases hepatic insulin resistance, decreases hepatic neoglucogenesis, protects pancreatic β-cells from glucotoxicity, decreases lipid levels, decreases appetite and carbohydrate absorption, and promotes modest weight loss (Cicero et al. 2012). Metformin leads to an average decrease of 1.5% in HbA_{1c}. Metformin can safely and efficaciously be combined with all oral antidiabetic agents and insulin and is generally the initial agent prescribed for type 2 diabetes. It is an important agent for the prevention of type 2 diabetes and is recommended for patients with docu-

TABLE 12–3. Treatment of cardiovascular risk factors associated with metabolic syndrome

Risk factor	Treatment	Treatment considerations	When to refer
Diabetes mellitus or prediabetes	Metformin	Contraindicated in renal dysfunction (Cr>1.4 mg/dL), severe congestive heart failure, or cirrhosis with ascites Common side effects: GI upset (nausea, vomiting, abdominal pain) Rare side effect: lactic acidosis	Persistent fasting blood sugar above 200 mg/dL despite treatment Signs or symptoms of diabetic ketoacidosis: nausea, vomiting, abdominal pain, ketonuria, and anion gap metabolic acidosis Signs or symptoms of hypoglycemia: tremor, palpitations, anxiety, diaphoresis, hunger, and resolution with eating Intolerance of or contraindication to metformin
Obesity	Metformin or topiramate	Consider switching to psychiatric medication with lower metabolic risk	Concern for obesity-associated complications such as obstructive sleep apnea, obesity hypoventilation syndrome, or severe osteoarthritis
	Metformin	Contraindicated in renal dysfunction (Cr>1.4 mg/dL), severe congestive heart failure, or cirrhosis with ascites Common side effects: GI upset (nausea, vomiting, abdominal pain) Rare side effect: lactic acidosis	

TABLE 12–3. **Treatment of cardiovascular risk factors associated with metabolic syndrome** *(continued)*

Risk factor	Treatment	Treatment considerations	When to refer
Obesity *(continued)*	Topiramate	Contraindicated in chronic metabolic acidosis or history of renal calculi Use with caution in renal or hepatic dysfunction Common side effects: anorexia, somnolence, dizziness, nervousness, ataxia Rare hyperammonemia or metabolic acidosis; stop topiramate and check ammonia and bicarbonate in case of fatigue, anorexia, or altered mental status	
Dyslipidemia	Statin (HMG-CoA reductase inhibitor)	Contraindicated in cirrhosis; check liver function prior to initiation Common side effects: myalgias, headache, GI upset (abdominal pain, nausea, constipation) Rare rhabdomyolysis; stop statin and check creatine kinase if significant muscle pain or weakness Initiate therapy in any patient with clinical atherosclerotic cardiovascular disease with high-intensity statin	History of myocardial infarction Intolerance of or contraindication to statin

TABLE 12–3. Treatment of cardiovascular risk factors associated with metabolic syndrome (*continued*)

Risk factor	Treatment	Treatment considerations	When to refer
Hypertension	ACE-I	Contraindicated in patients with renal failure (Cr>2 mg/dL) or hyperkalemia (K>4.5 mEq/L), bilateral renal artery stenosis, severe aortic stenosis, hereditary angioedema, or anaphylaxis without a known trigger Common side effect: cough Monitor basic metabolic profile prior to initiation and 1–2 weeks after initiation	Persistent BP above 180/110 mmHg despite treatment Symptomatic hypertension: chest pain, headache, or blurred vision associated with very high BP Renal failure: Cr>2 mg/dL Intolerance of or contraindication to ACE-I Increase of Cr greater than 50% or to a level greater than 3 with initiation of ACE-I Increase of potassium to >5 mEq/L associated with initiation of ACE-I

Note.   ACE-I=angiotensin-converting enzyme inhibitor; BP=blood pressure; Cr=creatinine; GI=gastrointestinal; HMG-CoA=3-hydroxy-3-methylglutaryl–coenzyme A; K=potassium mented prediabetes. It is particularly effective for patients with a BMI of 35 or greater and those ages 25–44 years. Metformin should be considered for individuals with risk factors for type 2 diabetes, such as family history of diabetes in first-degree relatives, elevated triglycerides, reduced HDL cholesterol, and hypertension.

The most common side effects from metformin include nausea, diarrhea, abdominal pain, and metallic taste (Cicero et al. 2012). The starting dosage is 500 mg bid, with the dosage titrated gradually to 1,000 mg bid, as tolerated and to effect. Rarely, metformin can cause lactic acidosis; this risk is increased in patients with poor renal clearance. For this reason, metformin should be used with caution in patients with an estimated glomerular filtration rate of less than 45 mL/min and is contraindicated in patients with an estimated glomerular filtration rate of less than 30 mL/min (Rocha et al. 2013), severe heart failure, or cirrhosis with ascites. We recommend that psychiatrists initiate metformin only in patients with creatinine levels that are less than 1.5 mg/dL. Metformin should also be avoided 24–78 hours before surgery and before intravenous injection of iodinated contrast media, because its use may increase the risk of nephropathy. Long-term use of metformin is associated with a risk of vitamin B_{12} deficiency, with studies reporting an approximately threefold risk per gram/day of use and an absolute risk of about 7% over 4 years (Sando et al. 2011).

Diabetes

For the treatment of type 2 diabetes or impaired fasting glucose, we recommend initiation of metformin. We recommend PCP referral for patients who cannot tolerate metformin or who have contraindications to this medication. Referral is also indicated for patients with signs and symptoms of hypoglycemia, such as tremor, palpitations, diaphoresis, hunger, and resolution with eating, or diabetic ketoacidosis, characterized by nausea, vomiting, abdominal pain, ketonuria, and anion gap metabolic acidosis.

Obesity

Many studies have evaluated pharmacological and nonpharmacological strategies for attenuating antipsychotic-associated weight gain. A review and meta-analysis of 17 studies of behavioral interventions for antipsychotic-associated weight gain and metabolic changes found a cumulative average of 3.12 kg (6.88 lb) less weight gain in the intervention group, with associated improvements in waist circumference, body fat percentage, and other metabolic parameters (Alvarez-Jiménez et al. 2008b). The number needed to treat to prevent weight gain greater than 7% was 4 across these interventions. There was no significant difference in outcomes across interventions, with similar results for group and individual interventions, nutritional counseling, and cognitive-behavioral therapy (CBT), as well as across various study durations. However, other reviews have indicated an advantage for behavioral techniques such as CBT compared with education on diet and nutrition alone (Papanastasiou 2012). We recommend referral to behavioral interventions for weight loss or nutritional counseling when these are available for any patient experiencing weight gain associated with psychiatric medication.

A large meta-analysis of 32 studies evaluating pharmacological interventions for antipsychotic-associated weight gain identified five medications whose effect differed from that of placebo (Maayan et al. 2010). Of these medications, the two that are available in the United States are topiramate and metformin. Because of metformin's favorable effect on insulin sensitivity, this medication should be the first pharmacological intervention for antipsychotic-associated weight gain. In this review, metformin had the most studies supporting its efficacy, was associated with a weight gain that was 2.94 kg (6.48 lb) lower than that with placebo, and had a number needed to treat of 3 to prevent clinically significant (>7%) weight gain. Metformin has been effective in treating antipsychotic-associated weight gain at dosages as low as 750 mg/day, which are generally well tolerated (Wu et al. 2008). Maintaining patients on metformin 500–1,000 mg/day is a reasonable strategy for the prevention or treatment of weight gain. Of note, studies suggest that metformin appears to have more impact in aiding weight loss after it has occurred than in preventing weight gain (Papanastasiou 2012), but we recommend prevention of weight loss as the primary goal.

For patients who cannot tolerate metformin, topiramate is an effective alternative. When taken in conjunction with SGAs, topiramate has been associated with weight gain that is about 2.5 kg (5.5 lb) less than weight gain with placebo across studies. One positive study found that a dose of 200 mg/day was significantly more effective than 100 mg/day (Ko et al. 2005). Topiramate should be started at 25 mg/day and the dose increased by 25 mg weekly and as tolerated until a dose of 200 mg/day is reached. The most common side effects of topiramate include anorexia, somnolence, dizziness, nervousness, cognitive blunting, and ataxia; adverse effects can be exacerbated by rapid titration. Topiramate should be used with caution even in cases of mild renal impairment (such as creatinine clearance of <70%) or hepatic impairment, and the target dose should be decreased by 50% (to 100 mg/day) and the drug titrated more slowly (increased by 25 mg every 2 weeks). Rarely, topiramate has been associated with closed-angle glaucoma, and the medication should be stopped immediately if the patient experiences acute visual changes or eye pain. Topiramate is a carbonic anhydrase inhibitor and causes a decrease in serum bicarbonate; it should be avoided in patients with chronic metabolic acidosis or a history of renal calculi (Mirza et al. 2009).

Metabolic acidosis is associated with fatigue and hyperventilation. If any of these symptoms develop, topiramate should be discontinued and electrolyte, bicarbonate, and ammonia levels should be checked. There are no specific guidelines for monitoring ammonia or bicarbonate levels in patients taking topiramate, but the clinician should consider monitoring these within 2–4 weeks of initiating this medication.

We recommend PCP referral for all patients with obesity, but especially for patients with obesity-related health issues such as obstructive sleep apnea, obesity hypoventilation syndrome, or severe osteoarthritis. Such patients may also be eligible for weight loss surgery such as gastric banding which is highly effective for weight loss and decreases the impact of these comorbidities, although its availability may be rather limited as a function of health insurance and because programs select patients who have only relatively low psychiatric comorbidity.

Dyslipidemia

Fasting plasma lipids should be obtained at baseline when initiating a new treatment and, if an SGA is being prescribed, at 3 months. If lipids are normal at 3-month follow-up, then monitoring every 5 years is appropriate, although some groups have recommended more frequent monitoring. If lipids are abnormally high, more frequent monitoring is warranted. Patients with clinical atherosclerotic CVD (history of myocardial infarction, angina, coronary revascularization, stroke, transient ischemic attack, and peripheral arterial disease) do not necessarily need lipid testing. New guidelines recommend that such patients should simply be offered high-intensity statin therapy (Keaney et al. 2014).

All patients older than 21 years with an LDL cholesterol level greater than 190 mg/dL should be treated for hyperlipidemia. For patients with diabetes ages 40–75 years, treatment is recommended for anyone with an LDL level greater than 70 mg/dL. For patients without diabetes who have an LDL level of 70–189 mg/dL, treatment is recommended if the 10-year risk of atherosclerotic CVD is more than 7.5% using the American Heart Association's CV (Cardiovascular) Risk Calculator (http://my.americanheart.org/cvrisk-calculator).

The mainstay of treatment for dyslipidemia is a 3-hydroxy-3-methylglutaryl–coenzyme A (HMG-CoA) reductase inhibitor, also called a statin. Statins have been shown to have a mortality benefit independent of their lipid-lowering effect and are thus considered first-line treatments of dyslipidemia. It may be useful for a psychiatrist to become comfortable with using a statin of his or her choosing. Simvastatin is inexpensive, has moderate lipid-lowering effect, is relatively well tolerated, and is frequently used first line for the treatment of dyslipidemia. Patients who do not achieve goal cholesterol levels on simvastatin 40 mg/day should be switched to a more potent statin. Rosuvastatin and atorvastatin have more potent lipid-lowering effects than other statin medications (Jones et al. 2003) and are recommended for any patient with clinical atherosclerotic CVD.

The most common side effects from statins include gastrointestinal symptoms such as nausea, abdominal pain, constipation, headache, and myalgias. In rare, more serious cases, patients can develop rhabdomyolysis, which, when severe, may result in kidney injury. Caution should be taken not to use statins in combination with inhibitors of cytochrome P450 (CYP) 3A4, because doing so may increase the risk of adverse effects. Statins should be discontinued and a creatine kinase (CK) level checked if patients develop significant muscle pain or weakness. Experts recommend against the routine monitoring of CK levels in asymptomatic patients, however (Thompson et al. 2006). Statins are contraindicated in patients with cirrhosis, and a baseline hepatic panel should be checked prior to initiation.

Hypertension

Normal BP consists of a systolic pressure of less than 140 mmHg and diastolic pressure of less than 80 mmHg. There are different approaches to hypertension treatment targets, but we recommend that patients with severe mental illness be followed closely and often, with a lower threshold for recommending lifestyle modification or antihypertensive medications. Stage 1 hypertension is defined as an average systolic BP greater than 139 mmHg or average diastolic BP greater than 89 mmHg on two or more separate readings occurring on two different visits after an initial screening. Patients with readings falling between normal and stage 1 are classified as having prehypertension and should be monitored at least yearly for the development of hypertension.

Lifestyle interventions for hypertension share similar features to those for weight gain, metabolic syndrome, and type 2 diabetes. The DASH diet has been shown to lower SBP by about 10 mmHg (Appel et al. 1997), whereas salt restriction alone has less impact. For every 10 kg of weight lost, BP tends to decrease by 10–15 mmHg on average. Smoking cessation, exercise, and limiting alcohol intake also improve BP control.

For the treatment of elevated BP in patients with metabolic syndrome, we recommend use of an angiotensin-converting enzyme (ACE) inhibitor (e.g., lisinopril, captopril, enalapril, ramipril). Additionally, diazide-type diuretics may be used as first-line treatment. We recommend that psychiatrists become comfortable with a single ACE inhibitor of their choice because all have similar efficacy and side-effect profiles. ACE inhibitors should be used with caution, however, in patients with renal failure or in patients taking lithium. ACE inhibitors raise lithium levels on average 35% and increase the risk for lithium-related toxicity (Meyer et al. 2005). The most common side effect is dry cough (Dicpinigaitis 2006). Rarely, ACE inhibitors can cause acute kidney injury or hyperkalemia shortly after initiation. For this reason, ACE inhibitors are contraindicated in patients with significant chronic kidney disease, known bilateral renal artery stenosis, or borderline hyperkalemia. We recommend that ACE inhibitors be initiated only in patients with creatinine levels less than 2 mg/dL and potassium levels less than 4.5 mEq/L. The European Society of Cardiology recommends checking renal function and electrolytes prior to initiation and 1–2 weeks after initiation of an ACE inhibitor. A mild to moderate increase in creatinine is expected after the initiation of an ACE inhibitor, but an increase of greater than 50% or to a creatinine level greater than 3 mg/dL should prompt discontinuation of the medication and referral to a PCP for further evaluation (Dickstein et al. 2008). Even more rarely, ACE inhibitors can cause angioedema due to dysregulation of the renin-angiotensin-aldosterone system, leading to increased bradykinin, nitric oxide release, vasodilatation, and hypotension (Nussberger et al. 2002). ACE inhibitors are contraindicated in patients with hereditary angioedema and should be used with caution in patients with a history of anaphylaxis without a clearly identified trigger. These medications are also contraindicated in patients with severe aortic stenosis (Dickstein et al. 2008). β-Blockers should not routinely be considered as first-line treatment for hypertension.

In summary, we recommend consistent screening and monitoring for the components of metabolic syndrome by all psychiatrists. This is even more essential if the patient is particularly prone to metabolic syndrome because of personal or family history, being overweight, having a diagnosis of schizophrenia, and/or taking medications, such as the SGAs, that have a high propensity to cause metabolic syndrome.

When to Refer

Diabetes Mellitus

- Persistent fasting blood sugar above 200 mg/dL despite treatment
- Signs or symptoms of diabetic ketoacidosis: nausea, vomiting, abdominal pain, ketonuria, and anion gap metabolic acidosis
- Signs of symptoms of hypoglycemia: tremor, palpitations, anxiety, diaphoresis, hunger, and resolution with eating
- Intolerance or contraindication to metformin

Obesity

- Concern for obesity-associated complications such as obstructive sleep apnea, obesity hypoventilation syndrome, or severe osteoarthritis

Dyslipidemia

- History of myocardial infarction
- Intolerance of or contraindication to statin

Hypertension

- Persistent BP above 180/110 despite treatment
- Symptomatic hypertension: chest pain, headache, or blurred vision associated with very high BP
- Renal failure: Cr > 2 mg/dL
- Intolerance of or contraindication to ACE inhibitor
- Increase of Cr greater than 50% or to a level greater than 3 with initiation of ACE inhibitor
- Increase of potassium to >5 mEq/L associated with initiation of ACE inhibitor

Special Treatment Considerations for the Psychiatric Patient Population

In individuals with psychiatric illness, especially those taking SGAs, weight reduction (or prevention of weight gain) and improved insulin sensitivity remain the primary preventive interventions. Behavioral interventions have been shown to be effective in preventing weight gain, with a meta-analysis of 17 randomized controlled trials showing that patients receiving behavioral interventions gained 3.12 kg (6.88 lb) less than control subjects (Caemmerer et al. 2012). The interventions included CBT, nutritional counseling and support, and exercise interventions, all of which were found to be effective among patients with schizophrenia.

SGAs significantly contribute to increased metabolic risk factors for CVD, and these risk factors have been shown to be undertreated in populations with psychiatric illness. Metabolic syndrome is alarmingly frequent among patients with mental illness. Forty-one percent of patients with schizophrenia enrolled in the CATIE trial had metabolic syndrome (McEvoy et al. 2005). Compared with the general population, males in the CATIE trial were 138% more likely to have metabolic syndrome, while women were 251% more likely to meet such criteria (McEvoy et al. 2005). Moreover, risk factors for metabolic syndrome where also found to be untreated, despite patients being in psychiatric care and sufficiently stable to be enrolled in a research trial: the rate of untreated diabetes was 30%, untreated hypertension was 62% and untreated hyperlipidemia was 88% (McEvoy et al. 2005). In many circumstances, patients with severe mental illness have barriers to accessing

TABLE 12–4. **Metabolic effects of atypical antipsychotics, from low to high metabolic risk**

Drug	Weight gain	Risk for diabetes	Risk for dyslipidemia
Lurasidone	–	–	–
Ziprasidone	+/–	+/–	–
Aripiprazole	+	+/–	–
Asenapine	++	+	–
Iloperidone	++	++	++
Paliperidone	+++	++	+
Risperidone	+++	++	+
Quetiapine	+++/++++	+++	+++
Clozapine	++++	++++	+++
Olanzapine	++++	++++	+++

Source.   Adapted from American Diabetes Association et al. 2004 and "Drugs for Psychotic Disorders" 2010.

primary care, including challenges with insurance and transportation and difficulty in navigating the health system. For these reasons, we recommend that psychiatrists screen and monitor for metabolic syndrome and then initiate first-line therapies accordingly. Carefully chosen antipsychotic therapy, lifestyle interventions, and the use of a limited number of medications to offset metabolic syndrome could significantly improve the cardiovascular health of patients (Knowler et al. 2002).

Antipsychotic medications have differing metabolic effects. Generally, first-generation antipsychotics have lower rates of metabolic side effects and should be used as first-line agents in individuals with symptoms of metabolic syndrome or who have high cardiovascular risk. Among the SGAs, there is a range of metabolic effects, with clozapine and olanzapine having the most impact and aripiprazole having a significantly lower metabolic effect (Table 12–4). Additionally, some of the newer SGAs (lurasidone, asenapine) are reported to have low rates of metabolic effects. Paliperidone and iloperidone appear to confer moderate metabolic risk, similar to that of risperidone. Consideration of switching to a lower-risk agent is the first recommended intervention for patients who develop metabolic syndrome (Zipursky et al. 2005).

Additionally, psychiatric medications other than antipsychotics can be associated with weight gain and thus increased risk for metabolic syndrome. Among antidepressants, amitriptyline, mirtazapine, and paroxetine are associated with the highest levels of weight gain and related histaminic (H_1) blockade. Bupropion is considered weight neutral, and has even been associated with mild potential weight loss in some studies (Serretti and Mandelli 2010). Among mood stabilizers, both valproic acid and lithium have been associated with significant weight gain (Biton et al. 2001; Chengappa et al. 2002). Valproic acid also increases risk for polycystic ovary syndrome in women, which is associated with insulin resistance and metabolic syndrome. Lamotrigine is associated with less weight gain than other mood stabilizers (Biton et al. 2001). The antiepileptic topiramate is used off label for mood stabilization and is associated with weight loss (Chengappa et al. 2002); however, there is minimal evidence to support the use of topiramate monotherapy for the treatment of bipolar disorder or acute mania (Rosa et al. 2011).

Case Discussion (*continued*)

Mr. M's clinical presentation currently meets criteria for metabolic syndrome: low HDL cholesterol, impaired fasting glucose (type 2 diabetes), and elevated BP. His waist circumference is not reported, but he is at high risk of abdominal obesity with a BMI of 33. These metabolic changes were likely triggered by the weight gain he experienced after switching from a first-generation antipsychotic to olanzapine. First, his psychiatrist should review his psychiatric history to assess if switching from olanzapine to an antipsychotic with lower metabolic risk is appropriate. Mr. M should also be offered referral to a PCP if he does not already have one. If it is decided that Mr. M should continue to take olanzapine or another SGA, his psychiatrist should ensure that the patient is being monitored appropriately. His weight, BP, and lipid panel have all been assessed. His glucose has likely been checked with his recent diabetes diagnosis. His psychiatrist should make sure that Mr. M's personal and family medical history, especially concerning CVD, are up to date and should check a waist circumference if this has not been obtained.

If Mr. M has not started taking metformin for his type 2 diabetes, this would be an appropriate medication for his psychiatrist to prescribe at this time. Prior to starting this medication, Mr. M will need to be screened for heart failure or cirrhosis with ascites (by history) and renal function (by creatinine level). Metformin would serve the dual function of treating his diabetes and potentially decreasing further weight gain associated with SGAs. Mr. M's psychiatrist could also consider starting medications for dyslipidemia and hypertension. A liver function panel should be checked prior to starting a statin for his dyslipidemia. If his renal function is normal and he is not taking lithium, an ACE inhibitor is first-line treatment for BP in a patient with diabetes. Mr. M should also be referred for behavioral interventions to assist with weight loss and, if he is a smoker, smoking cessation.

Clinical Highlights

- Patients with serious mental illness and those taking psychotropic medications are at increased risk for metabolic syndrome. Those taking second-generation antipsychotics (SGAs) should be monitored on a regular basis for the development of metabolic syndrome.

- Metabolic syndrome is diagnosed when a patient has three of the following: abdominal obesity, elevated triglycerides, low high-density lipoprotein cholesterol, elevated blood pressure (BP), and impaired fasting glucose.

- Many patients in psychiatric care are not seen by primary care providers (PCPs). First-line treatments for the components of metabolic syndrome provided by psychiatrists could significantly improve cardiovascular health in patients with psychiatric illness.

- Interventions to prevent the development of metabolic syndrome in patients taking SGAs include switching to a lower-risk agent, evidence-based behavioral interventions for weight loss, and starting a medication, such as metformin, that has been shown to minimize weight gain.

- We recommend the following as first-line treatments for metabolic syndrome: metformin for diabetes or significant weight gain; an HMG-CoA reductase inhibitor (statin) for any patient with clinical atherosclerotic cardiovascular disease or dyslipidemia; and an ACE inhibitor for elevated BP.

- All patients who develop metabolic syndrome should be offered referral to a PCP. More urgent referral should be offered for patients with persistently elevated blood sugars, hypoglycemia, diabetic ketoacidosis, persistently elevated BP (hypertensive urgency), or symptomatic hypertension (hypertensive emergency).

Resources

For Patients

American Diabetes Association: http://www.diabetes.org

American Heart Association: Getting Healthy. Available at: http://www.heart.org/HEARTORG/GettingHealthy/GettingHealthy_UCM_001078_SubHomePage.jsp.

For Clinicians

American Heart Association: 2013 Prevention Guidelines Tools: CV Risk Calculator. Available at: http://my.americanheart.org/cvriskcalculator.

References

Adams RJ, Appleton S, Wilson DH, et al: Population comparison of two clinical approaches to the metabolic syndrome: implications of the new International Diabetes Federation consensus definition. Diabetes Care 28:2777–2779, 2005

Alberti KG, Zimmet P, Shaw J: Metabolic syndrome—a new world-wide definition. A consensus statement from the International Diabetes Federation. Diabet Med 23:469–480, 2006

Alvarez-Jiménez M, González-Blanch C, Crespo-Facorro B, et al: Antipsychotic-induced weight gain in chronic and first-episode psychotic disorders: a systematic critical reappraisal. CNS Drugs 22:547–562, 2008a

Alvarez-Jiménez M, Hetrick S, González-Blanch C, et al: Non-pharmacological management of antipsychotic-induced weight gain: systematic review and meta-analysis of randomised controlled trials. Br J Psychiatry 193:101–107, 2008b

American Diabetes Association: Diagnosis and classification of diabetes mellitus. Diabetes Care 33 (suppl 1):S62–S69, 2010

American Diabetes Association, American Psychiatric Association, American Association of Clinical Endocrinologists, et al: Consensus development conference on antipsychotic drugs and obesity and diabetes. Diabetes Care 27:596–601, 2004

Appel LJ, Moore TJ, Obarzanek E, et al: A clinical trial of the effects of dietary patterns on blood pressure. DASH Collaborative Research Group. N Engl J Med 336(16):1117–1124, 1997

Azadbakht L, Mirmiran P, Esmaillzadeh A, et al: Beneficial effects of a Dietary Approaches to Stop Hypertension eating plan on features of the metabolic syndrome. Diabetes Care 28:2823–2831, 2005

Barnes T, Paton C, Hancock E, et al: Screening for the metabolic syndrome in community psychiatric patients prescribed antipsychotics: a quality improvement programme. Acta Psychiatr Scand 118:26–33, 2008

Biton V, Mirza W, Montouris G, et al: Weight change associated with valproate and lamotrigine monotherapy in patients with epilepsy. Neurology 56:172–177, 2001

Brand-Miller J, Hayne S, Petocz P, et al: Low-glycemic index diets in the management of diabetes: a meta-analysis of randomized controlled trials. Diabetes Care 26:2261–2267, 2003

Caemmerer J, Correll CU, Maayan L: Acute and maintenance effects of non-pharmacologic interventions for antipsychotic associated weight gain and metabolic abnormalities: a meta-analytic comparison of randomized controlled trials. Schizophr Res 140:159–168, 2012

Chengappa KN, Chalasani L, Brar JS, et al: Changes in body weight and body mass index among psychiatric patients receiving lithium, valproate, or topiramate: an open-label, nonrandomized chart review. Clin Ther 24:1576–1584, 2002

Cicero AF, Tartagni E, Ertek S: Metformin and its clinical use: new insights for an old drug in clinical practice. Arch Med Sci 8:907–917, 2012

Dickstein K, Cohen-Solal A, Filippatos G, et al: ESC Guidelines for the diagnosis and treatment of acute and chronic heart failure 2008: the Task Force for the Diagnosis and Treatment of Acute and Chronic Heart Failure 2008 of the European Society of Cardiology. Developed in collaboration with the Heart Failure Association of the ESC (HFA) and endorsed by the European Society of Intensive Care Medicine (ESICM). Eur Heart J 29:2388–2442, 2008

Dicpinigaitis PV: Angiotensin-converting enzyme inhibitor–induced cough: ACCP evidence-based clinical practice guidelines. Chest 129:169S–173S, 2006

Drugs for psychotic disorders. Treat Guide Med Lett 8:61–64, 2010

Expert Panel on Detection, Evaluation, and Treatment of High Blood Cholesterol in Adults: Executive summary of the third report of the National Cholesterol Education Program (NCEP) (Adult Treatment Panel III). JAMA 285:2486–2497, 2001

Fernandez-Egea E, Miller B, Bernardo M, et al: Parental history of type 2 diabetes in patients with nonaffective psychosis. Schizophr Res 98:302–306, 2008

Ford ES: Prevalence of the metabolic syndrome defined by the International Diabetes Federation among adults in the U.S. Diabetes Care 28:2745–2749, 2005

Ford ES, Giles WH, Dietz WH: Prevalence of the metabolic syndrome among US adults: findings from the third National Health and Nutrition Examination Survey. JAMA 287:356–359, 2002

Grundy SM, Cleeman JI, Daniels SR, et al: Diagnosis and management of the metabolic syndrome: an American Heart Association/National Heart, Lung, and Blood Institute Scientific Statement. Circulation 112:2735–2752, 2005

Hansen T, Ingason A, Djurovic S, et al: At-risk variant in TCF7L2 for type II diabetes increases risk of schizophrenia. Biol Psychiatry 70:59–63, 2011

Jones PH, Davidson MH, Stein EA, et al: Comparison of the efficacy and safety of rosuvastatin versus atorvastatin, simvastatin, and pravastatin across doses (STELLAR* Trial). Am J Cardiol 92:152–160, 2003

Kastorini CM, Milionis HJ, Esposito K, et al: The effect of Mediterranean diet on metabolic syndrome and its components: a meta-analysis of 50 studies and 534,906 individuals. J Am Coll Cardiol 57:1299–1313, 2011

Keaney JF, Curfman GD, Jarcho JA: A pragmatic view of the new cholesterol treatment guidelines. N Engl J Med 370:275–278, 2014

Knowler WC, Barrett-Connor E, Fowler SE, et al: Reduction in the incidence of type 2 diabetes with lifestyle intervention or metformin. N Engl J Med 346:393–403, 2002

Ko YH, Joe SH, Jung IK, et al: Topiramate as an adjuvant treatment with atypical antipsychotics in schizophrenic patients experiencing weight gain. Clin Neuropharmacol 28:169–177, 2005

Lawlor DA, Smith GD, Ebrahim S: Does the new International Diabetes Federation definition of the metabolic syndrome predict CHD any more strongly than older definitions? Findings from the British Women's Heart and Health Study. Diabetologia 49:41–48, 2006

Maayan L, Vakhrusheva J, Correll CU: Effectiveness of medications used to attenuate antipsychotic-related weight gain and metabolic abnormalities: a systematic review and meta-analysis. Neuropsychopharmacology 35:1520–1530, 2010

McEvoy JP, Meyer JP, Goff DC, et al: Prevalence of metabolic syndrome in patients with schizophrenia: baseline results from the Clinical Antipsychotic Trials of Intervention Effectiveness (CATIE) schizophrenia trial and comparison with national estimates from NHANES III. Schizophren Res 80(1):19–32, 2005

Meyer JM, Dollarhide A, Tuan IL: Lithium toxicity after switch from fosinopril to lisinopril. Int Clin Psychopharmacol 20:115–118, 2005

Mirza N, Marson AG, Pirmohamed M: Effect of topiramate on acid-base balance: extent, mechanism and effects. Br J Clin Pharmacol 68:655–661, 2009

Nussberger J, Cugno M, Cicardi M: Bradykinin-mediated angioedema. N Engl J Med 347:621–622, 2002

Osborn DP, Levy G, Nazareth I, et al: Relative risk of cardiovascular and cancer mortality in people with severe mental illness from the United Kingdom's General Practice Research Database. Arch Gen Psychiatry 64:242–249, 2007

Papanastasiou E: Interventions for the metabolic syndrome in schizophrenia: a review. Ther Adv Endocrinol Metab 3:141–162, 2012

Rocha A, Almeida M, Santos J, et al: Metformin in patients with chronic kidney disease: strengths and weaknesses. J Nephrol 26:55–60, 2013

Rosa AR, Fountoulakis K, Siamouli M, et al: Is anticonvulsant treatment of mania a class effect? Data from randomized clinical trials. CNS Neurosci Ther 17:167–177, 2011

Sando KR, Barboza J, Willis C, et al: Recent diabetes issues affecting the primary care clinician. South Med J 104:456–461, 2011

Serretti A, Mandelli L: Antidepressants and body weight: a comprehensive review and meta-analysis. J Clin Psychiatry 71:1259–1272, 2010

Simpson GM, Weiden P, Pigott T, et al: Six-month, blinded, multicenter continuation study of ziprasidone versus olanzapine in schizophrenia. Am J Psychiatry 162:1535–1538, 2005

Thakore JH, Mann JN, Vlahos I, et al: Increased visceral fat distribution in drug-naive and drug-free patients with schizophrenia. Int J Obes Relat Metab Disord 26:137–141, 2002

Thompson PD, Buchner D, Pina IL, et al: Exercise and physical activity in the prevention and treatment of atherosclerotic cardiovascular disease: a statement from the Council on Clinical Cardiology (Subcommittee on Exercise, Rehabilitation, and Prevention) and the Council on Nutrition, Physical Activity, and Metabolism (Subcommittee on Physical Activity). Circulation 107:3109–3116, 2003

Thompson PD, Clarkson PM, Rosenson RS: An assessment of statin safety by muscle experts. Am J Cardiol 97:69C–76C, 2006

Tiihonen J, Lonnqvist J, Wahlbeck K, et al: 11-year follow-up of mortality in patients with schizophrenia: a population-based cohort study (FIN11 study). Lancet 374:620–627, 2009

Venkatasubramanian G, Chittiprol S, Neelakantachar N, et al: Insulin and insulin-like growth factor-1 abnormalities in antipsychotic-naive schizophrenia. Am J Psychiatry 164:1557–1560, 2007

Wu RR, Zhao JP, Jin H, et al: Lifestyle intervention and metformin for treatment of antipsychotic-induced weight gain: a randomized controlled trial. JAMA 299:185–193, 2008

Zipursky RB, Gu H, Green AI, et al: Course and predictors of weight gain in people with first-episode psychosis treated with olanzapine or haloperidol. Br J Psychiatry 187:537–543, 2005

CHAPTER 13

Osteoporosis

Soraya Azari, M.D.
Reena Gupta, M.D.

Case Discussion

Ms. H is a 67-year-old white woman with a history of tobacco dependence, at-risk alcohol use, hypertension, and depression. Three years prior to this follow-up visit, she was hospitalized with a suicide attempt. She has received psychotherapy and has been taking sertraline and bupropion. Her depression has been in clinical remission for the past 1.5 years. She has smoked half a pack of cigarettes daily for the past 40 years (20 pack-year history). She currently drinks three 5-oz glasses of wine nightly, which is significantly decreased from her previous usage of five glasses per night. She has no history of alcohol withdrawal and denies any illicit drug use. Her family history is notable for depression and a hip fracture in her mother. Ms. H is 5′4″ and weighs 54 kg (119 lb). She is well groomed and cooperative, with no specific complaints.

Clinical Overview

Osteoporosis is defined as "a skeletal disorder characterized by compromised bone strength predisposing to an increased risk of fracture" ("Osteoporosis Prevention, Diagnosis, and Therapy" 2000). Patients with osteoporosis may suffer from fragility fractures, which are fractures that occur in the absence of trauma or from falling from standing height. These fractures most commonly occur at three sites: vertebrae, hip, and distal radius. Osteoporosis is

183

classified as primary or secondary: primary disease occurs with aging, specifically following menopause in women, and secondary osteoporosis is due to an alternative etiology (e.g., glucocorticoid use, hypogonadism).

Osteoporosis is a common disorder. An estimated 200 million people worldwide have the disease, and 8.9 million fractures occur annually (World Health Organization 2004). In the United States and Europe, 30% of all postmenopausal women have osteoporosis, and 40% of these women will have one or more fragility fractures in their lifetime (International Osteoporosis Foundation 2013; World Health Organization 2004). Osteoporosis is overrepresented in the psychiatric population. Estimates of prevalence vary depending on the population studied. In psychiatric inpatients, 50%–60% of patients have osteoporosis (Guo et al. 2012; Stubbs et al. 2009). Schizophrenia, schizoaffective disorder, major depression, and bipolar disorder have all been associated with low bone mineral density (De Hert et al. 2011). In a review of studies of osteoporosis in patients with schizophrenia, 15 of 16 studies showed lower bone mineral density in patients with schizophrenia than in healthy control subjects (Kishimoto et al. 2012).

The consequences of an osteoporotic fracture to patients and society are significant. Osteoporotic fractures are known to cause severe, debilitating pain. Quality-of-life studies show a significant difference in pain, physical function, social function, and general health after vertebral or hip fracture (Lips and van Schoor 2005). Hip fracture in particular is associated with high morbidity and mortality. In the first year after a hip fracture, one-third of patients are discharged to a nursing home, one-fifth will die, and only half will walk again, and often not at the same level as prior to the injury. In the United States, osteoporotic fractures cause 500,000 hospitalizations, 800,000 emergency department visits, 2.6 million physician visits, and 180,000 nursing home placements per year. The direct costs to the health care system are estimated to be $10–$15 billion dollars annually in the United States (National Institutes of Health Consensus Development Panel on Osteoporosis Prevention, Diagnosis, and Therapy 2001).

Despite the harm from this disease, osteoporosis is underdiagnosed. In a sample of Medicare claims from 1999 to 2000, only 30% of eligible women over age 65 had had a bone density test (Curtis et al. 2007). Psychiatric patients, particularly those with schizophrenia or substance use disorders, receive even less preventive care and screening for osteoporosis (Bishop et al. 2004; Kelly et al. 2011; Lord et al. 2010).

The increased risk of osteoporosis in psychiatric patients has been variably attributed to the disease itself, the medications used to treat the disease, and certain lifestyle factors associated with mental illness (e.g., tobacco and alcohol use) (Brown and Mezuk 2012). Compared with matched control subjects, patients with mental illnesses, including depression, schizophrenia, schizoaffective states, bipolar disorder, and eating disorders, have an increased risk of low bone mineral density (Kishimoto et al. 2012; Misra et al. 2004; Yirmiya and Bab 2009). Psychiatric medication has also been associated with an increased risk of osteoporosis and fractures. Multiple studies of selective serotonin reuptake inhibitors (SSRIs) have shown negative effects on bone mineral density (Diem et al. 2007; Seifert and Wiltrout 2013). Risk of fracture is increased with use of psychiatric medications, with an estimated relative risk for fracture of 1.6 for all classes of antidepressants, 1.54 for nonbarbiturate antiepileptic drugs (AEDs), 2.17 for barbiturate AEDs, and 1.59 for antipsychotics (Howard et al. 2007; Pouwels et al. 2009; Takkouche et al. 2007; Wu et al. 2012). Finally, potential confounders—including use of tobacco, alcohol, or drugs; nutritional insufficiency; and the effect of chronic stressors—may affect many of these studies.

There is biological plausibility for how certain psychiatric medications disrupt bone metabolism (Table 13–1). Antipsychotics carry the risk of hyperprolactinemia. High prolactin is thought to have a direct effect of increasing bone resorption, and it is known to inhibit the secretion of sex hormones, which are important for bone homeostasis (Wu et al. 2013). Antiepileptic drugs that induce cytochrome P450 enzymes, such as the drugs phenobarbital and carbamazepine, can lead to excessive metabolism of vitamin D, resulting in conversion of 25-hydroxyvitamin D [25(OH)D] into inactive metabolites. Vitamin D deficiency prevents normal calcium absorption, leading to elevations of parathyroid hormone and to bone breakdown (Meier and Kraenzlin 2011). The mechanism for SSRIs affecting bone metabolism is less clear, but serotonin receptors have been found on osteoclasts, osteoblasts, and osteocyte cell lines, suggesting that serotonin may have an important regulatory role in bone (Sansone and Sansone 2012). The direct effects of other psychiatric medications on bone metabolism are similarly not well established.

Given the potential negative impact of psychiatric medications on bone metabolism, the mental health provider should be mindful of additional risk factors that patients may have for osteoporosis (Table 13–2). The most common risk factors, independent of bone mineral density, are age older than 50 years, prior fracture, long-term glucocorticoid therapy (>3 months), history of fracture in a first-degree relative, low body weight (less than 57 kg or 126 lb), current tobacco use, and excess alcohol use (Raisz 2005). The presence of these risk factors should heighten concern for osteoporosis, and screening testing should be pursued in addition to an assessment of any fall risk associated with the psychotropic medication.

TABLE 13–1. Mechanisms of psychiatric medication impact on bone metabolism

Medication class	Impact on bone metabolism
Antipsychotics	Antipsychotics may cause hyperprolactinemia, with resultant increased bone resorption, and may cause inhibition of sex hormones, which are important for bone homeostasis.
Antiepileptics	The antiepileptics that induce cytochrome P450 enzymes lead to increased vitamin D metabolism, resulting in decreased calcium absorption, increased parathyroid hormone, and bone breakdown.
Selective serotonin reuptake inhibitors (SSRIs)	The mechanism of action of SSRIs remains unknown; however, serotonin receptors are found on osteoclasts and osteoblasts, suggesting that serotonin may have an important regulatory role in bone metabolism.

TABLE 13–2. **Risk factors for osteoporosis**

Age >50

Female sex

White or Asian race

Prior fracture

First-degree relative with fracture

Current cigarette smoking

Excess alcohol use

Low body weight (<57 kg or 126 lb)

Medications: glucocorticoid use (e.g., prednisone 5 mg or equivalent for ≥3 months), aromatase inhibitors, androgen deprivation therapy

Conditions associated with bone loss: hyperthyroidism, hyperparathyroidism, hypogonadism, Cushing's syndrome

Psychiatric patients
    Increased risk of fracture associated with psychotropic medications
        Selective serotonin reuptake inhibitors
        Antiepileptic drugs
        Sedatives
    Consider risk of hyperprolactinemia in patients taking antipsychotics
    Consider risk of vitamin D deficiency in patients taking cytochrome P450– inducer antiepileptic drugs, elderly patients, and institutionalized patients

Practical Pointers

- U.S. Preventive Services Task Force (2011) recommends screening the following patients for osteoporosis:
  - Women age 65 years and older
  - Any patient with prior fragility fracture
  - Women under age 65 years whose fracture risk is equal to or greater than that of a 65-year-old white woman (10-year risk of major osteoporotic fracture ≥ 9.3% with the World Health Organization Fracture Risk Assessment Tool (FRAX); see discussion of FRAX in section "Preventive Guidelines")
- Diagnosis of osteoporosis includes the following:
  - Fragility fracture with no alternative explanation
  - Bone mineral density testing (dual-energy X-ray absorptiometry, or DEXA)
    - T-score ≤ –2.5 (any location)

- Treatment of osteoporosis includes the following:
  - Lifestyle modification: tobacco cessation, alcohol reduction, weight-bearing exercise, and proper nutrition
  - Adequate calcium and vitamin D intake
- Pharmacological treatment with bisphosphonate should be considered when the following are present:
  - T-score $\leq$ –2.5 at the lumbar vertebrae, femoral neck, total hip, or distal radius
  - History of fragility fracture
- Fall risks should be reduced.
- If the patient is taking a psychiatric medication with a high fall risk, consider a medication change.

Diagnosis

Osteoporosis is most commonly diagnosed through use of *dual-energy X-ray absorptiometry*. DEXA is used to measure bone mineral density in two locations: the lumbar vertebrae (L1–L4) and the hip, which consists of measures of the femoral neck, Ward's triangle, greater trochanter, and total hip (a composite). T-score and Z-score are generated from this information. The T-score is a comparison of the patient's bone mineral density to that of a healthy 30-year-old female reference, whereas the Z-score compares the patient's bone mineral density to that of a reference matched for age, ethnicity, and sex. The numerical value represents the number of standard deviations above or below the comparison group; for example, a T-score of –1.0 at the hip means that the patient's bone mineral density score is one standard deviation below the mean score for a healthy referent. The T-score is used to make the diagnosis of osteoporosis based on criteria established by the World Health Organization (WHO; 2004), as shown in Table 13–3. Patients with a T-score less than –2.5 have osteoporosis. Those with T-scores between –1.0 and –2.5 have osteopenia. A presumptive diagnosis of osteoporosis may also be made following a fragility fracture (low-trauma fracture), regardless of bone mineral density testing.

Importantly, the provider should review the DEXA results closely. Periodically the T-score for L2–L4 can be normal while the density of an individual vertebra is decreased to the osteoporotic range. The composite score is elevated because of the increased bone mass from arthritic changes. Therefore, it is recommended that providers use the two lowest values to make the diagnosis (Raisz 2005). Also of note, if DEXA is done for a premenopausal woman or man under age 50, the WHO criteria should not be applied. Instead, the Z-score (which compares age-matched controls) should be used

TABLE 13–3. World Health Organization diagnostic classification of osteoporosis

Category	T-score[a]	Bone mineral density
Normal	> −1.0	Within 1 SD of a young normal adult
Low bone mass (osteopenia)	−1.0 to −2.5	Between 1 and 2.5 SD below that of a young normal adult
Osteoporosis	< −2.5	> 2.5 SD below that of a young normal adult
Severe osteoporosis	< −2.5 and ≥1 fragility fracture	> 2.5 SD below that of a young normal adult

Note. SD = standard deviation.

[a]The T-score compares an individual's bone mineral density with the mean value for young healthy individuals and expresses the difference as a SD score.

Source. Adapted from World Health Organization 2004.

for diagnosis; in this case, a score of less than −2.0 is considered abnormal (Lewiecki 2011).

Patients occasionally receive testing with peripheral densitometry due to lower cost and wider availability. These tests include peripheral DEXA, X-ray absorptiometry, and ultrasound of the radius, heel, and hands. These tests may be used to assess whether formal DEXA is indicated. If a patient has a T-score of −1.0 or below on these peripheral studies, it is recommended that referral be made for formal DEXA testing.

When the diagnosis of osteoporosis is being considered, patients should undergo a focused history and physical examination, along with basic laboratory testing. The history should focus on lifestyle factors (diet, exercise, and use of nicotine, alcohol, and drugs), family history of osteoporosis, and any symptoms that may reflect a secondary cause of osteoporosis (e.g., amenorrhea, hyperthyroidism, galactorrhea, low testosterone). The patient's physical examination may be notable for loss of height from prior vertebral fracture, or impaired gait suggesting increased fall risk. Psychiatric patients should be assessed for orthostatic hypotension. Laboratory testing should include a complete blood count, serum calcium, phosphorus, creatinine, liver function, thyroid-stimulating hormone, and, in men with osteoporosis, testosterone. Abnormal laboratory testing may indicate a secondary cause of osteoporosis, such as hyperparathyroidism or hypogonadism (Lewiecki 2011).

Preventive Guidelines

Guidelines for the prevention and management of osteoporosis have been issued by several professional organizations. The most commonly cited guidelines come from the U.S. Preventive Services Task Force (USPSTF; 2011), which recommends screening women over age 65 years, as well as women under age 65 who have a risk greater than or equal to that of their elder counterparts (equivalent to a 10-year risk of a major osteoporotic fracture ≥9.3%) (Figure 13–1). To estimate a patient's risk of a major osteoporotic fracture, WHO has developed the FRAX calculator (Fracture Risk Assessment Tool; www.shef.ac.uk/FRAX). The Web-based calculator takes into account major risk factors for osteoporosis such as age, sex, height, smoking status, and bone mineral density. The National Osteoporosis Foundation (2013) has broader recommendations for screening, including all women older than 65 years and men older than 70 years, postmenopausal women and men ages 50–70 years when risk factors are present, adults with a fracture after age 50, and adults taking a medicine associated with low bone mass or bone loss. Importantly, patients should be tested only if the results will change their management.

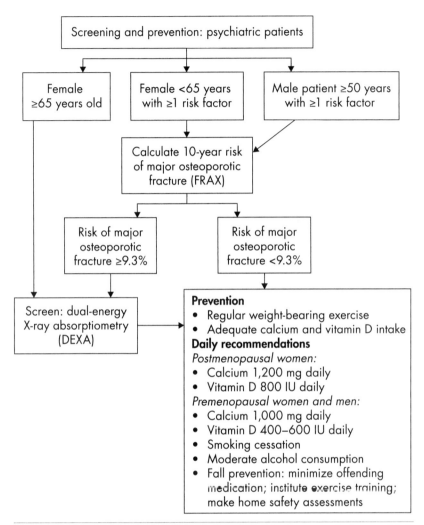

FIGURE 13–1. Screening and prevention of osteoporosis in psychiatric patients.

Note. FRAX = World Health Organization Fracture Risk Assessment Tool (www.shef.ac.uk/FRAX); IU = international units.

All patients should receive education about prevention of osteoporosis, including the importance of regular physical activity, good nutrition, and adequate intake of calcium and vitamin D. Weight-bearing exercise is most effective because it stimulates bone formation. Healthy, balanced diets containing calcium and vitamin D are important. Food sources of calcium include dairy products (yogurt, cottage cheese, milk), tofu, beans, and nuts. Vitamin D is obtained through sunlight exposure and fortified foods, including milk and breakfast cereals.

Use of supplemental calcium and vitamin D for prevention of osteoporosis has been a subject of controversy (Bauer 2013). Regarding the use of these two supplements for prevention of osteoporosis, the USPSTF has stated that insufficient evidence is available to make a recommendation (U.S. Preventive Services Task Force 2011). Differing methodology and confounders complicate studies in this area. Nevertheless, current recommendations are that individuals should consume adequate calcium and vitamin D, preferably through diet and sun exposure, with use of supplements if the person has inadequate intake (Bauer 2013; Institute of Medicine 2010). Postmenopausal women are recommended to have 1,200 mg of calcium and 800 international units (IU) of vitamin D daily. Men and premenopausal women are generally recommended to have 1,000 mg of calcium and 400–600 IU of vitamin D daily (Institute of Medicine 2010; Rosen 2013). Of note, certain patient groups are at risk of vitamin D insufficiency, including the elderly, persons with darker skin pigmentation, institutionalized persons (including those with severe mental illness), individuals with any malabsorptive disorder (or who have gastric bypass surgery leading to malabsorption), persons receiving tube feeding, and those taking AEDs. These individuals should be tested for vitamin D deficiency by obtaining a 25(OH)D level; if the level is less than 20 ng/mL (50 nmol/L), repletion should be given. Repletion doses can be given either with ergocalciferol (vitamin D_2) 50,000 IU once per week for 8 weeks or with 6,000 IU cholecalciferol (vitamin D_3) daily until the 25(OH)D level is above 30 ng/mL, after which a person should be given maintenance therapy of 1,500–2,000 IU daily (Table 13–4) (Holick et al. 2011). Finally, patients who smoke cigarettes or drink unhealthy amounts of alcohol (three or more standard drinks per day) should receive counseling about cessation.

A final preventive measure that is relevant to psychiatric patients is fall prevention. Studies of fall prevention in psychiatric patients have taken place primarily in the inpatient setting. Various risk factors have been identified, including use of benzodiazepines, acute medical conditions, electroconvulsive therapy, extrapyramidal symptoms, and medication changes (Chan et al. 2013; de Carle and Kohn 2001; Estrin et al. 2009). A fall risk assessment tool has been developed for psychiatric inpatients but has not yet been externally validated (Edmonson et al. 2011). Studies in geriatric patients have also shown that psychiatric medications are strongly associated with a 78% increased risk of fall (Bloch et al. 2011; Landi et al. 2005). Most of the understanding about fall prevention is from the geriatric literature. Physical training is very important, including balance and muscle strength training, followed by flexibility and endurance exercises. Patients can also be referred

TABLE 13–4. **Vitamin D repletion**

25(OH) vitamin D level	Repletion dosing
<20 ng/mL	1. Ergocalciferol (vitamin D_2) 50,000 IU once a week for 8 weeks OR 2. Cholecalciferol (vitamin D_3) 6,000 IU daily *Followed by* maintenance therapy 1,500–2,000 IU daily after 25(OH) level increases to >30 ng/mL
20–30 ng/mL	Cholecalciferol (vitamin D_3) 1,500–2,000 IU daily maintenance

Note. 25(OH) vitamin D=25-hydroxyvitamin D, also known as calcidiol; IU=international units.

for a home safety assessment (Karlsson et al. 2013). Multifaceted interventions for fall prevention in psychiatric inpatients have been developed and shown to be effective. Most falls in psychiatric patients are related to getting up or ambulating; therefore, interventions may include checking all patients for orthostatic hypotension, recommending assistive devices such as canes and walkers when appropriate, changing the physical environment to make travel more efficient, educating staff about fall risk, and having increased communication between providers about at-risk patients (Lee et al. 2012). Minimizing medications that cause excessive sedation, dizziness, or hypotension is also extremely important.

Treatment Recommendations

Treatment for osteoporosis includes lifestyle modification and pharmacological treatment. Patients with diagnosed osteoporosis should consume 1,200 mg of calcium and 800 IU of vitamin D daily (National Osteoporosis Foundation 2013; Rosen 2013). Calcium supplementation is available as calcium carbonate or calcium citrate. Calcium carbonate requires the presence of stomach acid to be absorbed, so it should be taken with meals and should be avoided in patients taking antacid medications. Calcium citrate does not require the presence of stomach acid for absorption and is recommended for elderly patients and those taking medications that decrease stomach acidity (Lewiecki 2011). Higher doses of vitamin D may be required for patients with malabsorption or those taking AEDs. Patients should be encouraged to participate in physical activity for at least 30 minutes 3 times per week.

Smoking cessation and a reduction of alcohol use are also important given the deleterious effects of these substances on bone strength.

Pharmacological treatment is recommended for men and women who have osteoporosis as shown by DEXA testing and those who have experienced a fragility fracture (Favus 2010; Qaseem et al. 2008). The National Osteoporosis Foundation (2013) also recommends treatment in postmenopausal women and men over age 50 who have low bone mass (T-score between −1.0 and −2.5, at any location) and a 10-year risk of hip fracture that is 3% or greater or a 10-year major osteoporotic fracture risk that is 20% or greater as determined by the WHO Fracture Risk Assessment Tool, or FRAX (available at: www.shef.ac.uk/FRAX). The American College of Physicians gives the above criteria for treatment a weak recommendation with moderate-quality evidence (Qaseem et al. 2008).

Multiple medications have U.S. Food and Drug Administration (FDA) approval for treatment of osteoporosis, including bisphosphonates (alendronate, ibandronate, risedronate, and zoledronic acid), calcitonin, selective estrogen receptor modulators (raloxifene), estrogen products, parathyroid hormone (teriparatide), and inhibitors of osteoclasts (denosumab). The most commonly used agents with the largest body of evidence supporting their use are the bisphosphonates. Bisphosphonates have been shown to decrease the risk of vertebral and hip fractures in postmenopausal women with osteoporosis (Favus 2010). The mechanism of action is to prevent bone breakdown. The choice between the different bisphosphonates often depends on patient preference and cost. Importantly, bisphosphonates are contraindicated in patients with a creatinine clearance less than 35 mL/min (alendronate) or less than 30 mL/min (risedronate, ibandronate). Because bisphosphonates can cause significant esophageal irritation, the oral forms must be taken first thing in the morning, while fasting, with 6–8 oz of water, and the patient must remain upright and not eat for at least 30–60 minutes after the dose (Lewiecki 2011). Fortunately, these medications can be dosed infrequently: alendronate on a weekly basis, ibandronate on a monthly basis, and risedronate on a weekly or monthly basis, to improved adherence. Finally, the bisphosphonates that have FDA approval for use in men are alendronate and risedronate.

Atypical fractures are an additional side effect associated with long-term use of bisphosphonates. These fractures are "atypical" because they are subtrochanteric or within the femoral shaft as opposed to the more typical osteoporotic fracture that occurs in the femoral neck or intertrochanteric region. These atypical fractures are associated with minimal trauma and prolonged use of bisphosphonates, with an incidence of 78 per 100,000 cases per year after 8 years of bisphosphonate use. These fractures are also more common in Asian females, and the fractures are often bilateral, occasionally with prodromal symptoms of dull or aching pain in the thighs (Desai et al. 2013). Consultation with a primary care physician or endocrinologist is encouraged for patients who have been taking a bisphosphonate for over 3–5 years.

When to Refer

Situations warranting referral to a primary care provider or endocrinologist include the following:

- Recommendations on initial evaluation (e.g., DEXA, laboratory testing)
- Patients taking chronic glucocorticoids
- Concern for secondary cause of osteoporosis (e.g., hypogonadism, hyperparathyroidism, hyperthyroidism, Cushing's syndrome)
- Abnormal laboratory testing that complicates treatment (e.g., elevated creatinine)
- Concern for drug-drug interactions and medication side effects
- History of fragility fracture with normal bone mineral density testing
- Recommendations for initiation of bisphosphonate or other pharmacological treatment for patients with osteoporosis
- Prolonged use of bisphosphonate (more than 3–5 years)
- Patients who experience fragility fractures while taking medication for osteoporosis

Special Treatment Considerations for the Psychiatric Patient Population

The treatment of osteoporosis can be complicated if a patient has complex medical and psychiatric conditions. For example, if a patient is medically complex, a primary care provider should be involved to determine whether the patient may have any secondary causes of osteoporosis and to determine which treatment is best. If the patient has severe psychiatric disease requiring multiple psychiatric medications and is diagnosed with osteoporosis, psychiatry and primary care should work together to consider whether any psychiatric medication changes would be possible for the patient. If not, then close consideration should be given to preventing falls (i.e., balance training, home safety assessment), avoiding medication interactions (i.e., multiple agents that can cause orthostatic hypotension), reducing or eliminating alcohol and tobacco intake, providing vitamin D supplementation if vitamin D level is low, and adhering to osteoporosis treatment if indicated. Dialogue between primary care and mental health providers is also very important for any patient with paranoia, mistrust of providers, and poor social support, so that patients will hear a consistent message.

Case Discussion (*continued*)

Given the patient's age (>65 years) and risk factors for osteoporosis, including postmenopausal status, tobacco dependence, risky alcohol use, and history of depression with antidepressant use, Ms. H was referred for DEXA testing. Her DEXA T-score of the femur was −2.8, consistent with a diagnosis of osteoporosis. Ms. H received counseling about tobacco and alcohol cessation, and her doctor prescribed a nicotine patch along with bupropion. She was advised to conduct weight-bearing exercise and evaluated for fall risk. She was screened for vitamin D deficiency and found to have a 25(OH)D level of 12, consistent with significant vitamin D deficiency. She received vitamin D repletion with ergocalciferol, followed by maintenance vitamin D with calcium. She was counseled about adequate dietary calcium intake. In partnership with her psychiatrist and primary care physician, the decision was made to continue her current antidepressant regimen given her history of severe depression with recent suicide attempt, and Ms. H was initiated on weekly alendronate for treatment of her osteoporosis.

Clinical Highlights

- Osteoporosis is a common disease, and fragility fractures are associated with significant morbidity and mortality.

- Patients with mental illness are at increased risk of osteoporosis, which is likely related to psychotropic medication effects, lifestyle factors, comorbid alcohol and tobacco use, and mental illness itself.

- Screening is recommended for all postmenopausal women over age 65, as well as for women under age 65 who have a calculated risk of fracture that is equivalent to that of a 65-year-old woman (10-year major fracture risk ≥9.3%) by the World Health Organization Fracture Risk Assessment Tool (FRAX) calculator (www.shef.ac.uk/FRAX).

- Screening is done via dual-energy X-ray absorptiometry (DEXA) testing of the hip and vertebrae.

- A diagnosis of osteoporosis is made if a person has suffered a fragility fracture or if DEXA testing shows a T-score less than −2.5 in any of the measurements.

- Causes of secondary osteoporosis that should be considered in psychiatric patients are hyperprolactinemia for patients taking antipsychotics, and vitamin D deficiency for patients taking antiepileptic drugs (AEDs) or those who are institutionalized.

- Treatment of osteoporosis consists of adequate calcium (1,200 mg) and vitamin D (800 IU) intake, discussion of tobacco and alcohol use, weight-bearing exercise, fall prevention, and use of bisphosphonates.

Resources

For Patients

National Osteoporosis Foundation: Resources. Available at: http://nof.org/resources.

Rosen HN: Patient Information: Osteoporosis Prevention and Treatment (Beyond the Basics). UpToDate, 2012. Available at: http://www.uptodate.com/contents/osteoporosis-prevention-and-treatment-beyond-the-basics.

U.S. Department of Health and Human Services: The Surgeon General's Report on Bone Health and Osteoporosis: What It Means to You. Bethesda, MD, U.S. Department of Health and Human Services, Office of the Surgeon General, 2012. Available at: http://www.niams.nih.gov/Health_Info/Bone/SGR/SGRBoneHealth_Eng.pdf

For Clinicians

FRAX WHO Fracture Risk Assessment Tool: http://www.shef.ac.uk/FRAX

National Osteoporosis Foundation: NOF's Clinician's Guide to the Prevention and Treatment of Osteoporosis. Washington, DC, National Osteoporosis Foundation, 2013. Available at: http://nof.org/hcp/resources/913.

U.S. Preventive Services Task Force: Screening for Osteoporosis, Topic Page. Available at: http://www.uspreventiveservicestaskforce.org/uspstf/uspsoste.htm.

References

Bauer DC: Calcium supplements and fracture prevention. N Engl J Med 369:1537–1543, 2013

Bishop JR, Alexander B, Lund BC, et al: Osteoporosis screening and treatment in women with schizophrenia: a controlled study. Pharmacotherapy 24:515 521, 2004

Bloch F, Thibaud M, Duqué B, et al: Psychotropic drugs and falls in the elderly people: updated literature review and meta-analysis. J Aging Health 23:329–346, 2011

Brown MJ, Mezuk B: Brains, bones, and aging: psychotropic medications and bone health among older adults. Curr Osteoporos Rep 10:303–311, 2012

Chan CH, Gau SS, Chan HY, et al: Risk factors for falling in psychiatric inpatients: a prospective, matched case-control study. J Psychiatr Res 47:1088–1094, 2013

Curtis JR, Carbone L, Cheng H, et al: Longitudinal patterns in bone mass measurement among US Medicare beneficiaries. J Bone Miner Res 22(suppl):S193, 2007

de Carle AJ, Kohn R: Risk factors for falling in a psychogeriatric unit. Int J Geriatr Psychiatry 16:762–767, 2001

De Hert M, Cohen D, Bobes J, et al: Physical illness in patients with severe mental disorders, I: prevalence, impact of medications and disparities in health care. World Psychiatry 10:52–77, 2011

Desai PA, Vyas PA, Lane JM: Atypical femoral fractures: a review of the literature. Curr Osteoporos Rep 11:179–187, 2013

Diem SJ, Blackwell TL, Stone KL, et al: Use of antidepressants and rates of hip bone loss in older women: the study of osteoporotic fractures. Arch Intern Med 167:1240–1245, 2007

Edmonson D, Robinson S, Hughes L: Development of the Edmonson Psychiatric Fall Risk Assessment Tool. J Psychosoc Nurs Ment Health Serv 49:29–36, 2011

Estrin I, Goetz R, Hellerstein DJ, et al: Predicting falls among psychiatric inpatients: a case-control study at a state psychiatric facility. Psychiatr Serv 60:1245–1250, 2009

Favus MJ: Bisphosphonates for osteoporosis. N Engl J Med 363:2027–2035, 2010

Guo P, Wang S, Zhu Y, et al: Prevalence of osteopenia and osteoporosis and factors associated with decreased bone mineral density in elderly inpatients with psychiatric disorders in Huzhou, China. Shanghai Archives of Psychiatry 24:262–269, 2012

Holick MF, Binkley NC, Bischoff-Ferrari HA, et al: Evaluation, treatment, and prevention of vitamin D deficiency: an Endocrine Society clinical practice guideline. J Clin Endocrinol Metab 96:1911–1930, 2011

Howard L, Kirkwood G, Leese M: Risk of hip fracture in patients with a history of schizophrenia. Br J Psychiatry 190:129–134, 2007

Institute of Medicine: Dietary Reference Intakes for Calcium and Vitamin D. Washington, DC, National Academies Press, 2010. Available at: http://www.iom.edu/Reports/2010/Dietary-Reference-Intakes-for-calcium-and-vitamin-D.aspx. Accessed October 23, 2013.

International Osteoporosis Foundation: What Is Osteoporosis: Epidemiology. Available at: http://www.iofbonehealth.org/epidemiology. Accessed October 28, 2013.

Karlsson MK, Vonschewelov T, Karlsson C, et al: Prevention of falls in the elderly: a review. Scand J Public Health 41:442–454, 2013

Kelly DL, Myers CS, Abrams MT, et al: The impact of substance abuse on osteoporosis screening and risk of osteoporosis in women with psychotic disorders. Osteoporos Int 22:1133–1143, 2011

Kishimoto T, De Hert M, Carlson HE, et al: Osteoporosis and fracture risk in people with schizophrenia. Curr Opin Psychiatry 25:415–429, 2012

Landi F, Onder G, Cesari M, et al: Psychotropic medications and risk for falls among community-dwelling frail older people: an observational study. J Gerontol A Biol Sci Med Sci 60:622–626, 2005

Lee A, Mills PD, Watts BV: Using root cause analysis to reduce falls with injury in the psychiatric unit. Gen Hosp Psychiatry 34:304–311, 2012

Lewiecki EM: In the clinic: osteoporosis. Ann Intern Med 155:ITCI-1–ITCI-15, 2011

Lips P, van Schoor NM: Quality of life in patients with osteoporosis. Osteoporos Int 16:447–455, 2005

Lord O, Malone D, Mitchell AJ: Receipt of preventive medical care and medical screening for patients with mental illness: a comparative analysis. Gen Hosp Psychiatry 32:519–543, 2010

Meier C, Kraenzlin ME: Antiepileptics and bone health. Ther Adv Musculoskelet Dis 3:235–243, 2011

Misra M, Papakostas GI, Klibanski A: Effects of psychiatric disorders and psychotropic medications on prolactin and bone metabolism. J Clin Psychiatry 65:1607–1618, 2004

National Institutes of Health Consensus Development Panel on Osteoporosis Prevention, Diagnosis, and Therapy: Osteoporosis prevention, diagnosis, and therapy. JAMA 285:785–795, 2001

National Osteoporosis Foundation: NOF's Clinician's Guide to the Prevention and Treatment of Osteoporosis. Washington, DC, National Osteoporosis Foundation, 2013. Available at: http://nof.org/hcp/resources/913. Accessed October 28, 2013.

Osteoporosis prevention, diagnosis, and therapy. NIH Consens Statement Mar 27–29 17(1):1–45, 2000. Available at: http://consensus.nih.gov/2000/2000osteoporosis111html.htm. Accessed on October 23, 2013.

Pouwels S, van Staaa TP, Egberts AC, et al: Antipsychotic use and the risk of hip/femur fracture: a population-based case-control study. Osteoporosis Int 20:1499–1506, 2009

Qaseem A, Snow V, Shekelle P, et al: Pharmacologic treatment of low bone density or osteoporosis to prevent fractures: a clinical practice guideline from the American College of Physicians. Ann Intern Med 149:404–415, 2008

Raisz L: Screening for osteoporosis. N Engl J Med 353:164–171, 2005

Rosen H: Calcium and vitamin D supplementation in osteoporosis. UpToDate, August 28, 2013. Available at: http://www.uptodate.com/contents/calcium-and-vitamin-d-supplementation-in-osteoporosis. Accessed October 28, 2013.

Sansone RA, Sansone LA: SSRIs: bad to the bone? Innov Clin Neurosci 9:42–47, 2012

Seifert CF, Wiltrout TR: Calcaneal bone mineral density in young adults prescribed selective serotonin reuptake inhibitors. Clin Ther 35:1412–1417, 2013

Stubbs B, Zapata-Bravo E, Haw C: Screening for osteoporosis: a survey of older psychiatric inpatients at a tertiary referral centre. Int Psychogeriatr 21:180–186, 2009

Takkouche B, Montes-Martinez A, Gill SS, et al: Psychotropic medications and the risk of fracture: a meta-analysis. Drug Saf 30:171–184, 2007

U.S. Preventive Services Task Force: Screening for Osteoporosis, Topic Page. Rockville, MD, U.S. Preventive Services Task Force, January 2011. Available at: http://www.uspreventiveservicestaskforce.org/uspstf/uspsoste htm. Accessed October 28, 2013.

World Health Organization: WHO Scientific Group on the Assessment of Osteoporosis at Primary Health Care Level, Summary Meeting Report, Brussels, Belgium, 5–7 May, 2004. Geneva, Switzerland, World Health Organization, 2004. Available at: http://www.who.int/chp/topics/Osteoporosis.pdf. Accessed October 28, 2013.

Wu H, Deng L, Zhao L, et al: Osteoporosis associated with antipsychotic treatment in schizophrenia. Int J Endocrinol Apr 17, 2013 [Epub ahead of print]

Wu Q, Bencaz AF, Hentz JG, et al: Selective serotonin reuptake inhibitor treatment and risk of fractures: a meta-analysis of cohort and case-control studies. Osteoporosis Int 23:365–375, 2012

Yirmiya R, Bab I: Major depression is a risk factor for low bone mineral density: a meta-analysis. Biol Psychiatry 66:423–432, 2009

CHAPTER 14

Thyroid Disorders

Alison Semrad, D.O., F.A.C.P.

Christopher A. Bautista, M.D.

Case Discussion

Ms. T is a 30-year-old woman with a history of major depressive disorder and active tobacco use. Her mood symptoms were well controlled at her last session 6 months ago and have been stable over the last several years with fluoxetine and behavioral therapy. She returns now reporting that for 4 months she has been experiencing depressed mood, fatigue, difficulty concentrating, decreased energy, and anxiety.

On further review of systems, she also endorses "feeling cold all the time," constipation, irregular menstrual periods, and a gradually worsening "swollen" feeling in her neck and upper chest over the last 2 months. Her vital signs are normal. Pertinent positive findings on examination include a diffusely enlarged nodular thyroid gland noted on palpation. Her affect is severely blunted, and she exhibits psychomotor retardation. In summary, Ms. T presents with 1) a new thyroid enlargement and 2) decompensation of depression and anxiety, concurrent with symptoms suggestive of hypothyroidism.

Clinical Overview

Structural thyroid disorders present as singular or multiple palpable anterior neck masses or nodules. Thyroid nodules are relatively common and can be palpated in approximately 5% of women and 1% of men in iodine-sufficient areas worldwide, and can be detected in up to 67% of the general population using ultrasound imaging (Cooper et al. 2009). Thyroid nodules may represent a broad spectrum of thyroid disorders, including iodine deficiency, euthyroidism, hypothyroidism, and hyperthyroidism.

Functional thyroid disorders (hypothyroidism and hyperthyroidism) are common. In the United States, the prevalence of hypothyroidism is 4.6% and the prevalence of hyperthyroidism is 1.3% (Hollowell et al. 2002). Thyroid hormone has widely recognized but poorly understood effects on brain metabolism and neurotransmitter function, which helps to explain the complex association between thyroid and neuropsychiatric disorders (Bauer et al. 2008). Of patients with affective disorders, 1%–4% are found to have overt hypothyroidism, and 4%–40% have subclinical hypothyroidism (Hage and Azar 2012). Depression occurs in 30%–60% of patients with hypothyroidism, and anxiety symptoms occur in up to 60% of patients with hyperthyroidism.

Postpartum women and elderly individuals deserve special consideration given the prevalence of comorbid neuropsychiatric symptoms and thyroid disease in these populations. Postpartum thyrotoxicosis occurs in approximately 8% of women after delivery. Studies have shown an association between postpartum depression and postpartum thyrotoxicosis (Stagnaro-Green et al. 2011). In elderly individuals with thyroid disease, one-third present with only weight loss, apathy, and tachycardia (Papaleontiou and Haymart 2012).

Psychiatrists must keep a high index of suspicion for thyroid disorders in their patients for two reasons: psychiatric symptoms commonly occur in patients with thyroid disease, and there is a high prevalence of thyroid disease in patients with psychiatric disorders.

Practical Pointers

- Thyroid hormone as adjunct to antidepressants in the first-line treatment of mood disorder is not recommended for euthyroid patients. However, thyroid hormone has been evaluated to augment antidepressants in nonresponders (second-line treatment), with conflicting results.

- Lithium is known to cause hypothyroidism (Hage and Azar 2012). Between 6% and 52% of patients with antithyroid antibodies go on to develop hypothyroidism while taking lithium, which is a higher rate than for antibody-negative patients. Goiter may also occur with continuous lithium use, with a prevalence of 4%–6% and up to 50% with continuous use for approximately 10 years. While a patient is taking lithium, thyroid-stimulating hormone (TSH) should be obtained at baseline before treatment, annually, and with any symptoms suggestive of a thyroid disorder. Examination of the thyroid should also be done on a regular basis in patients who take lithium.

- Carbamazepine and phenytoin can alter thyroid hormone levels.
- Significant numbers of patients receiving lithium for a bipolar disorder will develop hypothyroidism and goiter.
- In patients with preexisting autoimmune thyroid disease, lithium can stimulate a rise in the thyroid antibody titer. For patients with this disorder, TSH, free thyroxine (T_4), and an antithyroid peroxidase antibody (TPOAb) titer should be checked before the patient takes lithium. Additionally, TSH and free T_4 should be checked regularly while the patient is receiving treatment.
- If hypothyroidism develops, this should be treated with levothyroxine. The development of hypothyroidism is not an indication to discontinue lithium.

Diagnosis

Clinical Features

The clinical presentation of goiters is wide and varied. The severity and constellation of presenting symptoms depend on the size, location, and functional status of the thyroid mass (Bahn and Castro 2011). Patients can be completely asymptomatic and have masses that are incidentally found on physical examination, or patients can present with complaints of enlarging neck masses, choking sensations, swallowing difficulties, or persistent hoarse voice. In any case, it is important for the clinician to perform a thorough neck examination, paying particular attention to the size of the thyroid gland, the presence of any palpable nodules, and any audible bruits over the thyroid gland.

Patients with hyperthyroidism present with symptoms common to anxiety and depressive disorders (Table 14–1), including nervousness and irritability, cognitive impairment, heart palpitations, sleep disturbances, fatigue, exertional intolerance, muscle weakness, alterations in appetite, and weight changes (loss or gain). Other symptoms that suggest hyperthyroidism include frequent bowel movements, heat intolerance, tremor, and symptoms of thyroid eye disease such as proptosis and/or diplopia.

Patients with hypothyroidism also present with neuropsychiatric symptoms, including depressed mood, fatigue, decreased concentration, cognitive impairment, and weight gain (see Table 14–1). Other symptoms include cold intolerance, constipation, dry skin and coarse hair, ataxia, reflex delay, irregular or heavy menses, bradycardia, and hypothermia. The American Association of Clinical Endocrinologists (AACE) recommends consideration of the diagnosis of subclinical or clinical hypothyroidism in every patient

TABLE 14–1. **Common signs and symptoms of thyroid dysfunction**

Hyperthyroidism

   Anxiety, irritability

   Cognitive impairment

   Heart palpitations

   Sleep disturbances

   Fatigue, exertional intolerance

   Muscle weakness

   Frequent bowel movements

   Altered appetite, weight change (loss or gain)

   Heat intolerance

   Tremor

   Eye disease (proptosis or diplopia)

Hypothyroidism

   Depression, fatigue, decreased concentration

   Cognitive impairment

   Weight gain

   Cold intolerance

   Constipation

   Bradycardia

   Hypothermia

   Dry skin, coarse hair

   Ataxia

   Delayed deep tendon reflex

   Irregular or heavy menses

with depression, because hypothyroidism is a potentially reversible cause of depression (Baskin et al. 2002).

   Thyroid disease presents atypically in postpartum women. Postpartum depression can mimic the clinical presentation of postpartum thyroiditis, which can occur as early as 2 months and as late as 1 year after delivery. The natural history of postpartum thyroiditis includes a hyperthyroid phase, followed by a hypothyroid phase, before patients return to a euthyroid state.

   In elderly patients, thyroid disease can present as "apathetic hyperthyroidism," with a paucity of nonspecific symptoms that may suggest primary psychiatric disease, including lethargy and weight loss. Hypothyroidism in elderly patients can present simply with depression, fatigue, weakness, and cold intolerance. Often, symptoms of thyroid disease can be mistakenly attributed to aging, isolated affective disorder, or dementia.

Laboratory Tests and Imaging

As shown in Figure 14–1, the initial laboratory test in any patient with suspected thyroid disease is serum TSH. In the absence of pituitary dysfunction, this test is a good screening tool because it is very sensitive to changes in serum thyroid hormone levels. TSH levels are low in the setting of hyperthyroidism (except in rare cases of a pituitary tumor with excess TSH production) and high in hypothyroid states. Free T_4 further supports the diagnosis and is increased in hyperthyroid states (above the normal range) and decreased in hypothyroid states (below the normal range). Although screening thyroid ultrasound is not recommended for the general population, it should be performed in all patients with thyroid nodules regardless of the method of discovery. For patients with hyperthyroidism (low TSH), radioactive iodine thyroid uptake and scan may help to distinguish the cause of hyperthyroidism (Cooper et al. 2009; Papaleontiou and Haymart 2012). Biopsy of concerning thyroid nodules by fine needle aspiration is highly sensitive for ruling out thyroid malignancy.

Preventive Guidelines

Primary Prevention of Goiter

The primary prevention of the development of goiter involves ensuring adequate intake of iodine, which is not typically a problem in most developed countries. Smoking is a known risk factor for the development of goiter, as well as autoimmune thyroid diseases, including Graves' disease and Hashimoto's thyroiditis (Knudsen et al. 2002; Vestergaard et al. 2002). Thus, smoking cessation counseling is important for patients with thyroid disease.

Screening for Hyperthyroidism or Hypothyroidism

Screening the general population for hyperthyroidism or hypothyroidism using serum TSH is controversial. Recommendations of various professional groups vary. The U.S. Preventive Services Task Force Ratings (2000–2003) makes no recommendation because of "insufficient evidence." The American Thyroid Association (ATA) recommends screening in patients beginning at age 35 and every 5 years thereafter, and the AACE recommends screening in "older patients, especially women." However, recent guidelines from the

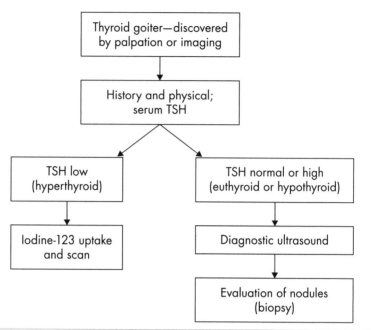

FIGURE 14–1. Assessment of thyroid goiter.

TSH = thyroid-stimulating hormone.

ATA and AACE say that there is "compelling evidence" to support screening for thyroid dysfunction in patients with psychiatric disorders (Garber et al. 2012).

We recommend that a screening TSH be considered in the evaluation of the psychiatric patient, given the significant overlap in clinical presentation between neuropsychiatric disease and thyroid disease. It is particularly important to screen elderly patients who have new or worsening cognitive or psychiatric symptoms. Untreated functional thyroid disease can exacerbate atrial fibrillation and other cardiac disease, osteoporosis, and underlying cognitive impairment. A summary of preventive and screening guidelines for thyroid disorders appears in Table 14–2.

Treatment Recommendations

Treatment of thyroid diseases should be made in consultation with the patient's primary care provider. Endocrine consultation may be helpful in patients with complicated thyroid disease.

TABLE 14–2. **Summary of preventive and screening guidelines for thyroid disorders**

Primary prevention

Ensure adequate iodine intake.

Encourage smoking cessation in active smokers.

Screening guidelines

Obtain a baseline, screening serum TSH level as part of the initial workup of all psychiatric patients, particularly those who have affective and anxiety disorders.

Consider screening TSH in any patient over age 35 and every 5 years thereafter, particularly for women and elderly patients.

Screen elderly patients with any new or worsening cognitive dysfunction or mood symptoms.

Note.   TSH = thyroid-stimulating hormone.

Hyperthyroidism

Hyperthyroidism is treated with antithyroid medications, radioactive iodine ablation, or surgical resection of the thyroid gland. Methimazole and propylthiouracil are the two antithyroid medications used in the United States. For patients who are pregnant, propylthiouracil is the preferred agent due to the teratogenic effects of methimazole in the first trimester (Yoshihara et al. 2012). Symptom control is also important in the treatment of hyperthyroidism. Propranolol, a nonselective β-blocker, improves tachycardia and may decrease the conversion of T_4 to its active form, triiodothyronine (T_3). Corticosteroids may also be used to decrease conversion of T_4 to T_3 but should be used cautiously in psychiatric patients because of adverse effects, including exacerbation of anxiety and psychosis.

Radioactive iodine is frequently used in the United States. Although this treatment is safe, ablative doses of radioactive iodine cause patients to become hypothyroid and thus to require replacement thyroid treatment for life. Thyroid surgery should be considered if patients have a large goiter (> 80 g) with symptomatic compression; documented or suspected thyroid malignancy; or coexisting hyperparathyroidism. Surgery also should be considered for women planning pregnancy within 6 months.

Hypothyroidism

Hypothyroidism is treated with thyroid replacement therapy in the form of levothyroxine (Table 14–3). A small subset of patients may subjectively benefit from $T_4 + T_3$ treatment. T_3 alone for replacement of thyroid hormone is

TABLE 14–3. **Treatment of hypothyroidism**

Start levothyroxine 25–75 µg/day (dosage varies based on degree of thyroid-stimulating hormone elevation and comorbidities); may need to titrate up to 1.6 µg/kg/day over months to years.

Take cardiac comorbidities into account. Thyroid hormone should be started at a low dose and titrated slowly in patients with significant cardiovascular disease.

not recommended (Cooper et al. 2009). The usual full replacement dosage of levothyroxine is approximately 1.6 µg/kg of body weight per day after thyroidectomy. However, nonsurgically hypothyroid patients should start taking lower doses, with the dose titrated up over time due to a varying amount of residual thyroid function early in the course of hypothyroidism. Particular care should be taken with medication titration for patients who are newly hypothyroid and are elderly or have comorbid heart disease.

Serum TSH should be measured 6–8 weeks after the initiation of treatment as well as 6–8 weeks after any dose adjustment, until it falls within the normal range. When patients become euthyroid, follow-up can be spaced out to every 3–6 months, then yearly based on the stability of serum TSH and clinical symptoms. The absorption of levothyroxine can be significantly affected by coadministration with other medications. Therefore, patients should be advised to take levothyroxine on an empty stomach and 1 hour before taking a meal or other medications.

When to Refer

Situations warranting referral to a primary care provider and/or endocrinologist include the following:

- Palpation of an enlarged goiter or thyroid nodule
- Symptoms or signs that are atypical of primary psychiatric disorders, including cardiac dysrhythmias, hot or cold intolerance, bowel dysfunction, skin or nail changes, and neurological abnormalities
- Abnormal serum TSH levels that may require frequent monitoring
- Initiation of pharmacological treatment for thyroid disorders
- High risk for drug-drug interactions

Special Treatment Considerations for the Psychiatric Patient Population

Treating Depressed Patients for Thyroid Disease

Historically, T_3 has been evaluated as an adjunctive treatment to accelerate and potentiate the clinical response of depressed patients to tricyclic antidepressants (TCAs). Some studies have supported this positive association (Altshuler et al. 2001). However, TCAs are no longer first-line treatment for mood disorders; selective serotonin reuptake inhibitors (SSRIs) are now the mainstay of treatment. A meta-analysis of double-blind studies comparing SSRI with coinitiation of T_3 versus SSRI treatment alone revealed no benefit with the addition of T_3 in the treatment of depression (Papakostas et al. 2009).

Empirical treatment with thyroid hormone preparations as adjuncts to antidepressants in the treatment of mood disorder is not routinely recommended for several reasons: 1) there is no conclusive evidence that thyroid hormone augments the efficacy of first-line treatment for depression in the absence of overt hypothyroidism; 2) confirming clinical suspicion of hypothyroidism with a serum TSH level is a sensitive, cost-effective, and quick screening tool for evaluation of patients' thyroid function prior to initiation of treatment; and 3) empirical treatment with thyroid hormone may expose euthyroid patients to the risks and complications of thyrotoxicosis. The recommendation cautioning against empirical use of thyroid hormone is supported by recent professional endocrine organization guidelines (Garber et al. 2012).

Effects of Psychiatric Medications on Thyroid Function

Potential drug-drug interactions between neuropsychiatric medications and thyroid hormone should be considered in all psychiatric patients with comorbid thyroid disease. Lithium is known to potentially cause hypothyroidism and goiter by decreasing the release and synthesis of thyroid hormone, as well as by decreasing the activity of the enzyme responsible for the peripheral conversion of T_4 to T_3 (Kibirige et al. 2013). Carbamazepine and phenytoin alter thyroid hormone levels by increasing hepatic metabolism and displacing thyroid hormone from serum binding proteins (Kundra and Burman 2012).

TCAs have an unclear effect on thyroid function, although some studies have shown a decrease in free T_4 levels in patients treated with TCAs. Likewise, the SSRI effect on thyroid function is controversial, with available studies revealing conflicting results. However, a prospective study of sertraline and fluoxetine revealed no clinically significant effect on thyroid function or thyroid autoimmunity (de Carvalho et al. 2009).

In patients who take any of these medications, it will be important for clinicians to be aware of and monitor any potential drug-drug interactions and effects on thyroid function. For patients starting treatment with lithium, SSRIs, TCAs, or antiepileptics, we recommend obtaining a baseline serum TSH level and monitoring TSH levels and results of thyroid exam by palpation at least annually or more frequently (i.e., every 3–6 months at the initiation of treatment), particularly for patients who have known thyroid disease, a family history of thyroid disease, or any change in symptoms.

Case Discussion (*continued*)

Ms. T presents with a new goiter and symptoms suggestive of hypothyroidism. The first step in the evaluation for possible thyroid disease is to obtain a serum TSH. The patient was found to have a TSH level of 15 mIU/mL, indicating a hypothyroid state. She then underwent thyroid ultrasound, which revealed evidence of inflammation and a diffusely enlarged thyroid gland without any distinct nodules. Serum thyroid antibody testing with TPOAb was suggestive of autoimmune thyroiditis as the etiology of her thyroid dysfunction. She was treated with levothyroxine to achieve a euthyroid state. She continued fluoxetine (SSRI) treatment without complication. She was counseled to quit smoking.

Clinical Highlights

- Thyroid masses represent a wide spectrum of thyroid disease. Thyroid enlargement may be diffuse or focal, with or without thyroid nodules. Single or multiple thyroid nodules may be present in a goiter. These nodules may be benign or malignant. Additionally, some nodules may be hyperfunctioning.

- Functional thyroid disease (hypothyroidism or hyperthyroidism) may present with features of depression, mania, anxiety, or cognitive impairment.

- Once functional thyroid disease has been diagnosed with serum thyroid-stimulating hormone (TSH), imaging may follow (particularly thyroid ultrasound if a thyroid mass is palpated).

- Patients with psychiatric disease should be considered for screening of possible thyroid dysfunction with serum TSH.

- Guidelines from professional endocrine societies do not support empirical treatment of depression with thyroid hormone.

- Thyroid disease presents atypically in two particular groups with comorbid neuropsychiatric diseases: postpartum women and elderly patients. A higher index of suspicion is needed for these two populations, because symptoms may be more insidious in their onset and presentation.

- Lithium is known to potentially cause thyroid dysfunction, particularly hypothyroidism and goiter. Tricyclic antidepressants and selective serotonin reuptake inhibitors have debatable effects on thyroid function.

- The American Association of Clinical Endocrinologists recommends considering the diagnosis of subclinical or clinical hypothyroidism in every patient with depression, because hypothyroidism is a potentially reversible cause of depression.

Resources

For Patients

Endocrine Society Hormone Health Network: http://www.hormone.org

For Clinicians

American Association of Clinical Endocrinologists: https://www.aace.com
American Thyroid Association: http://www.thyroid.org
Endocrine Society: https://www.endocrine.org

References

Altshuler LL, Bauer M, Frye MA, et al: Does thyroid supplementation accelerate tricyclic antidepressant response? A review and meta-analysis of the literature. Am J Psychiatry 158:1617–1622, 2001

Bahn RS, Castro MR: Approach to the patient with nontoxic multinodular goiter. J Clin Endocrinol Metab 96:1202–1212, 2011

Baskin HJ, Cobin RH, Duick DS, et al: American Association of Clinical Endocrinologists medical guidelines for clinical practice for the evaluation and treatment of hyperthyroidism and hypothyroidism. Endocr Pract 8:457–469, 2002

Bauer M, Goetz T, Glenn T, et al: The thyroid-brain interaction in thyroid disorders and mood disorders. J Neuroendocrinol 20:1101–1114, 2008

Cooper DS, Doherty GM, Haugen BR, et al: Revised American Thyroid Association management guidelines for patients with thyroid nodules and differentiated thyroid cancer. Thyroid 19:1167–1214, 2009

de Carvalho GA, Bahls SC, Boeving A, et al: Effects of selective serotonin reuptake inhibitors on thyroid function in depressed patients with primary hypothyroidism or normal thyroid function. Thyroid 19:691–697, 2009

Garber JR, Cobin RH, Gharib H, et al: Clinical practice guidelines for hypothyroidism in adults: cosponsored by the American Association of Clinical Endocrinologists and the American Thyroid Association. Thyroid 22:1200–1235, 2012

Hage MP, Azar ST: The link between thyroid function and depression. J Thyroid Res 2012:590648, 2012

Hollowell JG, Staehling NW, Flanders WD, et al: Serum TSH, T(4), and thyroid antibodies in the United States population (1988 to 1994): National Health and Nutrition Examination Survey (NHANES III). J Clin Endocrinol Metab 87:489–499, 2002

Kibirige D, Luzinda K, Ssekitoleko R: Spectrum of lithium induced thyroid abnormalities: a current perspective. Thyroid Res 6:3, 2013

Knudsen N, Laurberg P, Perrild H, et al: Risk factors for goiter and thyroid nodules. Thyroid 12:879–888, 2002

Kundra P, Burman KD: The effect of medications on thyroid function tests. Med Clin North Am 96:283–295, 2012

Papakostas GI, Cooper-Kazaz R, Appelhof BC, et al: Simultaneous initiation (co-initiation) of pharmacotherapy with triiodothyronine and a selective serotonin reuptake inhibitor for major depressive disorder: a quantitative synthesis of double-blind studies. Int Clin Psychopharmacol 24:19–25, 2009

Papaleontiou M, Haymart MR: Approach to and treatment of thyroid disorders in the elderly. Med Clin North Am 96:297–310, 2012

Stagnaro-Green A, Abalovich M, Alexander E, et al: Guidelines of the American Thyroid Association for the diagnosis and management of thyroid disease during pregnancy and postpartum. Thyroid 21:1081–1125, 2011

U.S. Preventive Services Task Force Ratings: Grade definitions: strength of recommendations and quality of evidence, in Guide to Clinical Preventive Services, 3rd Edition: Periodic Updates, 2000–2003. Available at: www.uspreventiveservicestaskforce.org/3rduspstf/ratings.htm. Accessed August 18, 2014.

Vestergaard P, Rejnmark L, Weeke J, et al: Smoking as a risk factor for Graves' disease, toxic nodular goiter, and autoimmune hypothyroidism. Thyroid 12:69–75, 2002

Yoshihara A, Noh J, Yamaguchi T, et al: Treatment of Graves' disease with antithyroid drugs in the first trimester of pregnancy and the prevalence of congenital malformation. J Clin Endocrinol Metab 97:2396–2403, 2012

SECTION IV

Infectious Disorders
in the Psychiatric
Patient Population

CHAPTER 15

Adult Immunizations

Y. Pritham Raj, M.D.
Lucy Lloyd, M.D.

Case Discussion

Mr. D is a 26-year-old man with schizoaffective disorder, bipolar type, who presents to establish care following a recent hospitalization for psychosis. He provides a poor medical history but expresses delusional ideas about medical providers experimenting on him and implanting a microchip in his brain. His current medications include valproic acid 500 mg bid and olanzapine 10 mg at bedtime. He smokes one pack of cigarettes per day and during his recent hospitalization was noted to have findings consistent with chronic obstructive pulmonary disease (COPD) on chest X ray. He has also been drinking heavily, as evidenced by elevated liver enzymes and mild alcohol withdrawal during the hospitalization. Mr. D does not have a primary care doctor and cannot provide definitive information about his past medical history, including vaccinations. The psychiatrist is very concerned that Mr. D's psychiatric illness will be a barrier to his self-care.

Clinical Overview

Compared with the general population, patients with diagnosable mental illness have higher rates of poverty, poor nutrition, obesity, and smoking—factors that contribute to a stunning 25-year loss in life expectancy among those with severe mental illness (Newcomer and Hennekens 2007). One way to reverse the unacceptable trends for this at-risk population is by improving health care screening and preventive services, including the delivery of potentially life-saving immunizations. Vaccination against preventable diseases remains a fundamental component of the current standard of primary care and preventive medicine, and the delivery of such vaccines is the responsibility of all care providers, including mental health clinicians.

According to the Centers for Disease Control and Prevention (CDC), approximately 45,000 adults die each year from vaccine-preventable diseases, the majority from influenza (Kroger et al. 2006). Immunization guidelines typically do not address psychiatric populations specifically; however, studies suggest that patients with mental illness may indeed be at higher risk for preventable infectious illnesses (Seminog and Goldacre 2013) and may experience increased morbidity and mortality as a result (Cole 2007). Unfortunately, this vulnerable population is known to have lower vaccination rates than the general population (Lord et al. 2010). More specifically, patients with depression are less likely to have influenza vaccination compared with those without depression (Druss et al. 2008) and veterans with diagnosed mental disorders are less likely to have ever received a pneumonia vaccine or an annual flu vaccine (Druss et al. 2002).

Many barriers exist to the delivery of preventive services such as immunizations to patients with mental illness; chief among them are the inherent cognitive, behavioral, and social challenges posed by some disorders. Symptoms of mental illness not only interfere with volition but also make it difficult to engage with primary care physicians in meaningful shared decision making surrounding vaccine administration. More medical visits are often needed to achieve preventive care goals, and precarious insurance coverage issues pose additional challenges. Compared with patients with either psychiatric or substance use disorders alone, patients with both have lower rates of receipt of preventive care (Druss et al. 2002).

Currently, there is a national, incentivized push toward the *patient-centered medical home* (PCMH) model of health care delivery, which relies on a multidisciplinary team approach, especially with the utilization of nurse care managers. Given the success of the PCMH model in improving outcomes in primary medical care settings, some have advocated for similar enhanced care management interventions in psychiatric settings. The use of psychiatric care managers, for example, enhances communication and advocacy between patients and medical providers, and improves the general level of health care understanding by the patients. In fact, the use of such care managers led 58.7% of patients with severe mental illness at an urban community mental health center to receive recommended preventive services, compared with only 21.8% of similar patients in the "usual care" group, which lacked a care manager (Druss et al. 2010). Thus, we recommend that psychiatric practices also take a prominent role in immunization advocacy, similar to the efforts by community pharmacies throughout the United States.

In this chapter we review the major infectious illnesses that are preventable with vaccination and highlight the ways in which psychiatric patients, by virtue of their illness, require special consideration for these vaccinations. We hope that our recommendations will help guide psychiatric providers to deliver preventive care in their patients' best interest. This chapter should not be considered a comprehensive guideline for the general population. For the most up-to-date and complete vaccination recommendations, the reader should refer to the CDC Web site (www.cdc.gov/vaccines/schedules/index.html). Additionally, general immunization information can be found in the General Recommendations on Immunization (Kroger et al. 2011). Most of the following discussion is adapted from materials from the CDC Web site. The American College of Physicians has also published a recent review (Advisory Committee on Immunization Practices 2013). Table 15–1 provides an overview of a recommended adult immunization schedule for key vaccinations.

Practical Pointers

- Smokers, especially those with chronic lung disease, are at risk of pneumococcal- and influenza-related illness and should receive vaccination regardless of age.
- A high-dose influenza vaccine is available for adults age 65 and older; it contains 4 times the typical amount of antigen and is intended to trigger a stronger immune response in older adults.
- Pneumococcal vaccine does not decrease the rate of pneumonia but rather decreases the burden of bacteremia associated with pneumonia, thereby lowering the overall mortality rate.
- Adults ages 19–64 are recommended to have vaccination against pertussis with a single dose of tetanus-diphtheria-pertussis (Tdap) vaccine regardless of their prior immunization against tetanus or diphtheria.
- Patients with high risk sexual behavior (including mania) should be considered for vaccinations for human papillomavirus (HPV), hepatitis B, and hepatitis A.
- HPV vaccination is available for adult women and men younger than age 27 and can help protect against the most oncogenic strains of the virus.
- Any form of immunosuppression renders the varicella zoster vaccine contraindicated because it contains a live form of the virus.
- Patients with alcoholism, with chronic liver disease, or seeking substance abuse treatment should be screened for and vaccinated against hepatitis B.
- Hepatitis A vaccination is recommended for all patients who use illicit drugs, regardless of mode of use.

TABLE 15–1. **Overview of recommended adult immunization schedule**

Human papillomavirus vaccine

All previously unvaccinated women up to age 26

Three doses on 0-, 2-, 6-month schedule

Do not give during pregnancy

Influenza vaccination

All adults in the fall or winter

Pneumococcal vaccine (Pneumovax)

All patients age 65 or older get once

Patients younger than age 65 with a chronic illness that predisposes them to pneumonia: chronic heart disease (e.g., congestive heart failure and coronary artery disease), chronic lung disease (e.g., chronic obstructive pulmonary disease, asthma), diabetes mellitus, chronic liver disease, chronic kidney disease, nephrotic syndrome, immunocompromise (due to disease or drugs)

Active smokers and those who chronically misuse alcohol

Patients living in high-risk settings (e.g., nursing homes, long-term care facilities)

For patients younger than age 65 who receive the vaccine, revaccination is recommended after 5 years or age 65, whichever comes first.

Tetanus-diphtheria (Td) or tetanus-diphtheria-pertussis (Tdap) vaccine

For adults who have had primary series, recommended to get booster of Td every 10 years

For adults younger than age 65 who have not had Tdap before, recommended to get once in place of Td booster

Varicella zoster vaccine (Zostavax)

All patients age 60 and older

Exclude patients with cellular or acquired immunodeficiency (e.g., those who have HIV or who are undergoing chemotherapy)

Infectious Illnesses

Influenza

There is little debate surrounding the recommendation for all persons age 6 months or older, except those individuals who have had an allergic reaction to a vaccine component (including egg protein), to receive annual influenza vaccination. Inactivated influenza vaccine (administered intramuscularly or intradermally) is available to all eligible persons. A live attenuated vaccine is available in a particularly convenient intranasal mist and is safe for healthy, nonpregnant persons ages 2–49 years without high-risk medical conditions.

Case Discussion (*continued*)

For Mr. D, the opportunity to provide or recommend annual influenza vaccination should not be missed, particularly given that he is a smoker with lung disease and is at higher risk to get flu. Because of his comorbid lung disease and alcoholism, he should be offered the inactive form of influenza vaccine.

Starting in 2013, a new quadrivalent vaccine option is now available. Along with the two typical A strains, this vaccine will also incorporate two circulating B strains, which is an upgrade to the current trivalent option.

Pneumococcus

All adults age 65 years and older should be vaccinated against pneumococcal infection with pneumococcal polysaccharide (PPSV23). For these patients, a single dose is sufficient and revaccination is not necessary. For adults younger than 65, the vaccination is still indicated in the presence of chronic lung disease, cardiovascular disease, diabetes mellitus, chronic renal failure, nephrotic syndrome, chronic liver disease, alcoholism, cochlear implants, cerebrospinal fluid leaks, immunocompromising conditions, and functional or anatomic asplenia. Other indications include residency at a nursing home or long-term care facility and smoking.

For younger adults who qualify for pneumococcal vaccination based on presence of a chronic medical condition, a single revaccination with PPSV23 is recommended 5 years after the initial dose. Patients who receive early vaccination with or without revaccination will still need routine vaccination at age 65 with PPSV23, as long as it has been 5 years since the last dose (Table 15–1).

For unvaccinated adults with particular vulnerability due to immunocompromise, chronic renal failure, nephrotic syndrome, asplenia, cerebrospinal fluid leaks, or cochlear implants, initial vaccination with pneumococcal conjugate 13-valent vaccine (PCV13) is indicated, followed by PPSV23 at least 8 weeks later, in order to provide broader coverage of pneumococcal serotypes. If a patient in this category has already had PPSV23, PCV13 is still recommended but should be administered at least 1 year after the past PPSV23 dose.

Case Discussion (*continued*)

In Mr. D's case, his smoking history and evidence of lung disease on X ray are indications for vaccinations against pneumococcal illness despite his young age of 26 years. Assuming he is not immunocompromised and has no other indication for PCV13, administration of PPSV23 is appropriate. He will then need revaccination in 5 years in addition to routine vaccination at age 65 years.

Meningococcus

Meningococcal disease describes the spectrum of infections caused by *Neisseria meningitidis* (meningococcus), including meningitis, bacteremia, and bacteremic pneumonia. Meningococcal disease develops rapidly, typically among previously healthy children and adolescents, and results in high morbidity and mortality. Meningococcal vaccination is routinely recommended in adolescents and is recommended for adults at increased risk for disease based on likelihood of exposure or presence of underlying medical illness.

Adolescents should be routinely vaccinated at age 11 or 12, with a booster at age 16. Any college students living in residence halls should be vaccinated if they did not receive routine immunization at age 16. Two doses of conjugate vaccine (MCV4) are administered at least 2 months apart to adults with asplenia, persistent complement component deficiencies, or HIV. A single dose of vaccine is recommended for microbiologists with exposure to *N. meningitidis,* military recruits, and persons traveling in countries where meningococcal disease is hyperendemic or epidemic. For adults over age 55, meningococcal polysaccharide (MPSV4) is preferred over MCV4. Revaccination every 5 years is recommended for adults at greater risk of infection due to asplenia or persistent complement component deficiencies.

Tetanus-Diphtheria-Pertussis

Although tetanus is quite rare, with a mere 233 tetanus cases reported from 2001 to 2008 in the United States, the case fatality rate was 13.2%, highlighting the importance of ongoing vaccination (Centers for Disease Control and Prevention 2011). For adults who never completed vaccination, a three-dose primary vaccination series should begin or be completed, including one dose of Tdap. The second dose should be at least 4 weeks after the first, and the final dose 6–12 months after the initial dose. Adults with prior vaccination should receive a booster dose every 10 years. The Advisory Committee on Immunization Practices (2013) currently recommends that patients ages 19–64 receive a single dose of Tdap to replace their active booster vaccination, to reduce the morbidity associated with pertussis in adults and reduce the risk for transmitting pertussis to at-risk persons, especially children. In recent years, there has been a resurgence of pertussis in the United States, with many experts blaming attenuation of prior vaccinations, which prompted the recommendation for revaccination against pertussis in adulthood. Pregnant women should receive Tdap for every pregnancy regardless of interval from prior tetanus-diphtheria (Td) or Tdap, preferably during weeks 27–36 of gestation.

Case Discussion (*continued*)

Although Mr. D's vaccination status is unknown, he likely qualifies for adult vaccination against pertussis. A single dose of Tdap is sufficient to provide coverage against pertussis and boost immunity against tetanus and diphtheria. He will need subsequent booster immunizations with the Td vaccine every 10 years.

Human Papillomavirus

The HPV vaccine is now available to both females and males for protection against four strains of HPV (6, 11, 16, and 18) and prevention of HPV-associated diseases, including genital warts and cervical cancer. The Advisory Committee on Immunization Practices (2013) recommends routine vaccination of females ages 11–12 years with three doses of quadrivalent HPV vaccine. The vaccination series can be started as young as age 9 years. The second and third doses should be administered 2 and 6 months after the first dose.

The vaccine, which is also recommended for females ages 13–26 years who have not been previously vaccinated or who have not completed the full series, has been shown to decrease HPV prevalence by 56% among those ages 14–19 since the vaccine was introduced in 2006 (Markowitz et al. 2013). Ideally, the vaccine should be administered before potential exposure to HPV through sexual contact to provide full benefit from vaccination; however, females who are sexually active and who might have HPV based on abnormal Pap results should still be vaccinated because it is impossible to determine which strains they may or may not have contracted and which strains they would still be at risk of acquiring with ongoing sexual activity. Pap testing and screening for HPV DNA or HPV antibody are not needed before vaccination. Because the HPV vaccine does not provide coverage for all 40+ high-risk or low-risk genital strains of the virus, vaccination does not change the important recommendations for cervical cancer screening in women. Women should be advised that results from clinical trials do not indicate that the vaccine will have any therapeutic effect on existing HPV infection or cervical lesions. The vaccine is not recommended during pregnancy, but quantitative human chorionic gonadotropin (hCG) testing is not required prior to vaccination. If pregnancy is discovered after the initial dose has been given, no precautions are necessary but the remaining two doses of vaccine can be postponed until after pregnancy.

The approach to patients with current or past episodes of genital warts is similar. A history of genital warts or clinically evident genital warts indicate infection with HPV, most often type 6 or type 11. Vaccination provides protection against infection by other strains of HPV not already acquired. However, patients should be advised that results from clinical trials do not indicate that the vaccine will have any therapeutic effect on existing HPV infection or genital warts. Because the quadrivalent HPV vaccine is a noninfectious vaccine, it can be administered to patients who are immunosuppressed as a result of disease, including HIV, or medications; however, because the efficacy is based on immune responses, immunization might be less in patients who are immunosuppressed than in persons who are immunocompetent. Vaccination with HPV4 is recommended for males ages 13–21 years who have not been vaccinated previously or who have not completed the three-dose series. Males ages 22–26 years may also elect to be vaccinated and are recommended to do so if they have ever had sex with men, given that they are at increased risk of acquiring conditions associated with HPV types 6, 11, 16, and 18, such as anal intraepithelial neoplasia, anal cancers, and genital warts. It must be noted that the upper age limit is somewhat arbitrary; some physicians elect to offer the vaccine to men even older than age 27.

Case Discussion (*continued*)

Mr. D is eligible to receive the HPV vaccination series should he desire immunity against the high-risk strains of the virus. His sexual history—specifically his history of sexual contact with men—would help inform the clinician's recommendation.

Varicella Zoster

Varicella zoster virus (VZV), which causes chickenpox, can reactivate clinically decades after initial infection to cause shingles, a localized and generally painful cutaneous eruption that occurs most frequently among older adults. Approximately 1 million new cases of zoster occur in the United States annually, and one in three persons in the general population will develop zoster during his or her lifetime. A common complication of zoster is postherpetic neuralgia (PHN), a chronic pain condition that can last months or even years. In May 2006, a live attenuated vaccine (single dose) for prevention of zoster was licensed in the United States for use in persons age 60 or older. The age limit was subsequently lowered to include adults over age 50, although the Advisory Committee on Immunization Practices (2014) continues to recommend that vaccination begin at age 60 years. Older age is the most important risk factor for development of zoster, along with prior infection with VZV or any deficiencies in cell-mediated immunity.

Determination of varicella (chickenpox) history or immune status is not necessary prior to administration of the vaccine. Persons who report a previous episode of zoster and persons with chronic medical conditions (e.g., chronic renal failure, diabetes mellitus, rheumatoid arthritis, COPD) can be vaccinated unless those conditions are contraindications or precautions. Zoster vaccination is not indicated to treat acute zoster, to prevent persons with acute zoster from developing PHN, or to treat ongoing PHN. Zoster vaccine should not be administered to persons with primary or acquired immuno-deficiency from malignancies, HIV/AIDS, or immunosuppressive medications (including high-dose steroids lasting 2 weeks or more), or with evidence of impaired cellular immunity on laboratory testing.

Case Discussion (*continued*)

Mr. D has evidence of COPD and alcoholism; however, the Advisory Committee on Immunization Practices (2014) does not currently recommend vaccinating adults under age 60 years.

Hepatitis B

Viral hepatitis is a potential comorbidity for psychiatric patients who have substance abuse and/or high-risk sexual behaviors. Hepatitis B vaccination is the most effective measure to prevent hepatitis B virus (HBV) infection and its consequences, including cirrhosis of the liver, liver cancer, liver failure, and death. In adults, ongoing HBV transmission occurs primarily among un-vaccinated persons with behavioral risks (e.g., heterosexuals with multiple sex partners, injection drug users, men who have sex with men [MSM], house-hold contacts and sex partners of persons with chronic HBV infection). Patients presenting to a substance abuse treatment facility or seeking care related to HIV or other sexually transmitted infections are recommended to receive vaccination. The three-dose vaccine series is administered intramus-cularly at 0, 1, and 6 months. Prevailing recommendations are to vaccinate anyone seeking protection from hepatitis B and persons at higher risk for in-fection due to medical conditions, behaviors, occupation, and/or travel-related exposure risk. Medical risk factors include diabetes, end-stage renal disease (including patients on hemodialysis), HIV, chronic liver disease, and any present or suspected sexually transmitted diseases. Asians and Pacific Is-landers are at increased risk for acquiring hepatitis B and should be screened and treated accordingly.

Case Discussion (*continued*)

The clinician suspects that Mr. D has alcohol dependence with alcohol-related liver disease, which, if chronic, would indicate a need for vaccination. If there is any additional evidence of behavioral risks, such as multiple sex partners, sex with men, or injection drug use, vaccination against HBV would certainly be indicated.

Hepatitis A

Routine vaccination against hepatitis A virus (HAV) in children has substan-tially decreased rates of infection and community-wide outbreaks. This virus is usually transmitted person to person by fecal-oral routes, often in settings of sexual or household contact with an infected person or by consumption of contaminated food or water. Outbreaks among MSM and users of illicit drugs continue to occur.

The Advisory Committee on Immunization Practices (2014) recommends vaccinating anyone seeking protection from HAV and anyone at higher risk of infection due to medical conditions, behaviors, occupation, and/or travel-related exposure. Medical risk factors include presence of chronic liver disease or clotting deficiencies. Behavioral risk factors include MSM and use of illicit drugs by *any* route (injection or noninjection). Anyone working in a lab with HAV-infected primates or anyone traveling to countries with high or intermediate endemicity of hepatitis A should also be vaccinated.

Measles, Mumps, Rubella

Persons born before 1957 are generally considered immune to measles and mumps. Otherwise, adults should have documentation of at least one dose of measles, mumps, rubella (MMR) vaccine unless medically contraindicated or unless immunity to all three diseases can be verified by serological testing. Documented disease is not considered adequate evidence of immunity. Two doses of vaccine are recommended for patients at high risk for exposure and transmission of measles and mumps, such as students attending colleges or other post–high school educational institutions, health care personnel, and international travelers. The minimum interval between the two doses of MMR vaccine is 28 days, with the first dose administered at age 12 months or older. For women of childbearing age, rubella immunity should be determined, and the vaccine should be administered to women without immunity if they are not pregnant. During pregnancy, the vaccination should be postponed and offered upon completion or termination of pregnancy and prior to discharge from the health care facility.

Special Considerations for the Psychiatric Patient Population

Delivering immunizations to the psychiatric patient population deserves special consideration based on commonly occurring medical diseases and risk factors that impact recommendations for vaccination. Of particular relevance to this topic are HIV, COPD, chronic liver disease, alcoholism, and substance misuse disorders. Substance misuse disorders, which are well-known comorbidities among psychiatric patients, can introduce risk for several preventable diseases. Smoking is twice as common in patients with mental illness as in the general population (Lasser et al. 2000) and is a risk factor for influenza and pneumococcus. Even after controlling for smoking, prevalence studies demonstrate that COPD (mainly from chronic bronchitis) and asthma are more common in patients with schizophrenia and bipolar disorder than in the general population (De Hert et al. 2011). Patients with severe persistent mental illness, such as schizophrenia, have a much higher lifetime prevalence of comorbid substance abuse—as high as 50%, according to some estimates (Thoma and Daum 2013). Although reported prevalence rates have varied, it is generally understood that patients with severe mental illness have higher rates of HIV (as high as 8 times the risk) than those in the general population (De Hert et al. 2011; Rosenberg et al. 2001). The increased risk is likely multifactorial, from higher rates of substance abuse, higher-risk sexual behavior, and lack of awareness about HIV transmission (De Hert et al. 2011). Prevalence rates of hepatitis C are also markedly increased among patients with severe mental illness. Recent studies estimate that 20%–25% of persons with severe mental illness are infected with the hepatitis C virus, most commonly transmitted through intravenous drug use or high-risk sexual behaviors (De Hert et al. 2011; Rosenberg et al. 2001). Hence, the CDC's current recommendation is that anyone born between 1945 and 1965 should receive one-time screening for hepatitis C.

Finally, adverse effects from certain psychiatric medications may lead to conditions that would impact vaccination recommendations. For instance, medications such as clozapine and mirtazapine carry a risk for agranulocytosis and impaired cell-mediated immunity. Patients who develop issues with leukopenia and agranulocytopenia while taking clozapine, as well as patients with HIV, should avoid live forms of vaccine such as the intranasal influenza vaccine, the herpes zoster vaccine, and the MMR vaccine. Chronic lithium use carries a risk for renal impairment and other forms of kidney disease, which would change the recommendations for pneumococcal vaccination. The same is true for patients with diabetes, which is often relevant for patients taking second-generation antipsychotics.

Case Discussion (*continued*)

Mr. D represents a fairly typical clinical scenario for the practicing psychiatrist. The patient has a complex combination of psychiatric and medical pathology, as well as behaviors that are likely to contribute to his morbidity and risk for complications. As his physician, the psychiatrist may have difficulty gathering vital historical information. Also, unfortunately, the likelihood of successfully referring such a patient to a primary care provider (or other specialty service) is often low. All things considered, it is not difficult to imagine how Mr. D might miss opportunities to receive needed vaccines. However, his smoking status, pulmonary and liver disease, alcoholism, and potential complications from olanzapine are all factors that require special attention and warrant delivery of vaccinations to avoid complications from preventable illnesses. He should be screened for HIV and hepatitis B and C, which would further modify the recommendations, as would any history of high-risk sexual behavior. Where possible, consolidating these services with his psychiatric follow-up will enhance adherence and ultimately his health outcomes.

Clinical Highlights

- The following are medical and behavioral risk factors commonly found in psychiatric patients that can impact immunization recommendations:
  - HIV
  - Chronic obstructive pulmonary disease
  - Smoking
  - Alcoholism
  - Substance abuse
  - Residency in facilitated living or substance abuse treatment
  - Viral hepatitis
  - Chronic liver disease
  - Renal disease (potentially related to use of commonly prescribed psychiatric medications)
  - Diabetes (also potentially related to use of commonly prescribed psychiatric medications)

Resources

Centers for Disease Control and Prevention: Recommended Adult Immunization Schedule by Vaccine and Age Group. Atlanta, GA, Centers for Disease Control and Prevention, 2014. Available at: http://www.cdc.gov/vaccines/schedules/hcp/imz/adult.html.

References

Advisory Committee on Immunization Practices: Recommended adult immunization schedule: United States, 2013. Ann Intern Med 158:191–199, 2013

Centers for Disease Control and Prevention: Tetanus surveillance—United States, 2001–2008. MMWR Morb Mortal Wkly Rep 60:365–369, 2011

Centers for Disease Control and Prevention: Recommended Adult Immunization by Vaccine and Age Group. Atlanta, GA, Centers for Disease Control and Prevention, 2014. Available at: http://www.cdc.gov/vaccines/schedules/hcp/imz/adult.html. Accessed January 1, 2014.

Cole MG: Does depression in older medical inpatients predict mortality? Improving the quality of health care for mental and substance use conditions. Am J Psychiatry 29:425–430, 2007

De Hert M, Correll CU, Bobes J: Physical illness in patients with severe mental disorders, I: prevalence, impact of medications and disparities in health care. World Psychiatry 10:52–77, 2011

Druss BG, Rosenheck RA, Desai MM, et al: Quality of preventive medical care for patients with mental disorders. Med Care 40:129–136, 2002

Druss BG, Rask K, Katon W: Major depression, depression treatment and quality of primary medical care. Gen Hosp Psychiatry 30:20–25, 2008

Druss BG, von Esenwein SA, Compton MT, et al: A randomized trial of medical care management for community mental health settings: the Primary Care Access, Referral, and Evaluation (PCARE) study. Am J Psychiatry 167:151–159, 2010

Kroger AT, Sumaya CV, Pickering LK, et al: General recommendations on immunization: recommendations of the Advisory Committee on Immunization Practices (ACIP). MMWR Recomm Rep 55:1–48, 2006

Kroger AT, Sumaya CV, Pickering LK, et al: General recommendations on immunization: recommendations of the Advisory Committee on Immunization Practices (ACIP). MMWR Recomm Rep 60:1–60, 2011. Available at: http://www.cdc.gov/mmwr/preview/mmwrhtml/rr6002a1.htm. Accessed April 28, 2014.

Lasser K, Boyd J, Woolhandler S, et al: Smoking and mental illness: a population-based prevalence study. JAMA 284:2606–2610, 2000

Lord O, Malone D, Mitchell AJ: Receipt of preventive medical care and medical screening for patients with mental illness: a comparative analysis. Gen Hosp Psychiatry 32:519–543, 2010

Markowitz LE, Hariri S, Lin C, et al: Reduction in human papillomavirus (HPV) prevalence among young women following HPV vaccine introduction in the United States, National Health and Nutrition Examination Surveys, 2003–2010. J Infect Dis 208:385–393, 2013

Newcomer JW, Hennekens CH: Severe mental illness and risk of cardiovascular disease. JAMA 298:1794–1796, 2007

Rosenberg SD, Goodman LA, Osher FC, et al: Prevalence of HIV, hepatitis B, hepatitis C in people with severe mental illness. Am J Public Health 91:31–37, 2001

Seminog OO, Goldacre MJ: Risk of pneumonia and pneumococcal disease in people with severe mental illness: English record linkage studies. Thorax 68:171–176, 2013

Thoma P, Daum I: Comorbid substance use disorder in schizophrenia: a selective overview of neurobiological and cognitive underpinnings. Psychiatry Clin Neurosci 67:367–383, 2013

CHAPTER 16

Sexually Transmitted Infections

Christopher A. Kenedi, M.D., M.P.H., F.R.A.C.P., F.A.C.P.

Stephanie Collier, M.D., M.P.H.

Chinthaka Bhagya Samaranayake, M.B.Ch.B.

Thomas Daniel Sapsford, M.B.Ch.B. (Hons.), M.Sc., B.Sc. (Hons.)

Case Discussion

Ms. K, A 25-year-old woman with bipolar disorder, presents to the community psychiatrist with lower abdominal pain. She has recently recovered from a manic episode and has started to reintegrate with the community mental health team. She has been maintained on lithium monotherapy. Ms. K refused to see her general practitioner and was adamant that she wished to see her psychiatrist, the only doctor with whom she has rapport. On further history, she reports lower abdominal pain for 3–4 days and fever for 1 day. The pain is dull in character. She denies any diarrhea, vomiting, or urinary symptoms but on further questioning reveals new-onset foul-smelling vaginal discharge without vaginal bleeding. Her menstrual cycle is usually regular, but her last menstrual period occurred 2 months ago. In terms of her past medical history, she had an appendectomy at age 10 years and she is a current cigarette smoker. The clinical notes from the time of her manic episode revealed high-risk behavior, including having unprotected sexual intercourse with multiple partners. On examination, Ms. K is febrile and tachycardic with a tender lower abdomen.

Clinical Overview

Sexually transmitted infections (STIs) continue to be a significant public health problem with potential serious complications (Fenton and Lowndes 2004). The incidence of STIs, including viral STIs, in the United States alone is estimated to be 19 million cases per year (Trigg et al. 2008). *Chlamydia trachomatis* infection remains the most common reportable bacterial STI, with an estimated annual incidence of 2.8 million cases in the United States and 50 million worldwide. Infection with *Neisseria gonorrhoeae* is the second most common. Herpes simplex virus (HSV) is one of the most common viral STIs, and the incidence of human papillomavirus (HPV), which is associated with cervical cancer, has steadily increased worldwide (Frenkl and Potts 2008; Gilson and Mindel 2001). Young people ages 15–24 years are at highest risk of acquiring new STIs, with almost 50% of new cases of STIs reported among this age group (Weinstock et al. 2004). STIs can have serious complications and sequelae. For example, 20%–40% of women with chlamydia infections and 10%–20% of women with gonococcal infections develop pelvic inflammatory disease (PID) (Trigg et al. 2008). Women with a previous episode of PID are at risk for subsequent ectopic pregnancy, infertility, and chronic pelvic pain.

Patients with mental illness are at high risk of acquiring STIs. In the United States, the prevalence of human immunodeficiency virus (HIV) among the psychiatric patient population is 10–20 times higher than in the general population (King et al. 2008; Rosenberg et al. 2001). Factors contributing to increased vulnerability to STIs in the psychiatric patient population include impaired autonomy, increased impulsivity, and increased susceptibility to coerced sex (King et al. 2008). Furthermore, a higher incidence of poverty, placement in risky environments, and overall poor health and medical care also contribute to the high prevalence of STIs and their complications in this population. Because of various unique risk factors in the psychiatric patient population (Table 16–1), standard STI prevention interventions are not always successful, and novel, innovative behavioral approaches are necessary (Erbelding et al. 2004). Her psychiatrist refers her to the emergency department.

Practical Pointers

- Those with severe mental illness are at particular risk for sexually transmitted infections (STIs), which are likely to increase morbidity.
- Conditions such as herpes simplex and human immunodeficiency virus (HIV) are chronic conditions with no known cure, and both have a higher incidence in those with severe mental illness.
- Psychiatrists are well positioned to screen for STIs, as well as to educate patients about prevention.

TABLE 16–1.	Factors that place patients with mental illness at high risk for sexually transmitted infections

Impulsivity

Risky behavior

Impaired autonomy

Poverty

Stigma around sexual orientation

Poor access to medical care

Chronic physical illness

Medication nonadherence

Impaired judgment

Impaired self-esteem

Trauma

Poor social support

Substance use

Lower educational level

Diagnosis

To make a diagnosis of STI, the clinician must first consider its likelihood. A sexual history allows assessment of the need for further investigation and provides an opportunity for risk reduction. In line with recent guidelines (Workowski et al. 2010), we encourage all health care providers to consider the sexual history a routine aspect of the clinical encounter. The Centers for Disease Control and Prevention's (CDC's) "Five P's" approach (Centers for Disease Control and Prevention 2010b) is an excellent tool for guiding further investigation and counseling (Table 16–2). A summary of the initial diagnostic tests and treatment options is presented in Table 16–3.

Modern laboratory techniques have greatly improved the ease with which STIs can be diagnosed. Analysis of urine or serum reduces the need for invasive sampling. If swabs are required for diagnosis, self-collection by the patient of urethral, vulvovaginal (Schoeman et al. 2012), rectal, or pharyngeal specimens is accurate and better tolerated than clinician-collected samples (Freeman et al. 2011). Because of local variation in diagnostic assays, we recommend contacting the laboratory prior to sending nonstandard samples to ensure accurate collection and analysis.

Chlamydia and Gonorrhea

In most circumstances, the diagnosis of chlamydia and gonorrhea can be made using nucleic acid amplification testing (NAAT), which is highly sensi-

TABLE 16–2. The "Five P's" approach to a patient's sexual history

Partners

Do you have sex with men, women, or both?

How many sexual partners have you had in the past year?

Could any of those partners have been in another sexual relationship while they were with you?

Pregnancy

What are you doing to prevent pregnancy?

Protection

How do you protect yourself from STIs and HIV?

Practices

To understand your risk for STI, I need to ask about the type of sex you have had recently:

Have you had vaginal sex?

Have you had oral sex?

Have you had anal sex?

Do you use condoms? Are there any times you do not use a condom?

Past history of STI

Have you or your partners ever had an STI?

Have you ever injected drugs?

Have any of your partners exchanged money or drugs for sex?

Is there anything else that I need to know about your sexual experiences?

Note.   HIV=human immunodeficiency virus; STI=sexually transmitted infection.
Source.   Adapted from Erbelding et al. 2004.

tive and specific. These techniques can confirm the diagnosis using first-void urine or urethral, vaginal, and rectal swabs. Diagnosis of oropharyngeal gonorrhea varies by local laboratory. It is always sensible to send appropriate samples for microscopy and culture, especially in atypical or treatment-resistant cases. Although NAAT urine techniques are good at detection, they cannot provide information on the sensitivity of the pathogen.

Trichomoniasis

Trichomoniasis is an STI caused by the organism *Trichomonas vaginalis.* This protozoan parasite causes vaginal discharge and urethritis. It is traditionally diagnosed at bedside with microscopy and testing of wet mount specimens. In the psychiatric setting, self-collected vaginal or urethral samples can be

TABLE 16–3. Summary of initial diagnostic tests and treatments for sexually transmitted infections (STIs)

Infection	Initial diagnostic test	Treatment	
		First-line	Second-line (if available)
Chlamydia (*Chlamydia trachomatis*)	NAAT using 1) first-void urine or 2) urethral, vaginal, and rectal swabs	Azithromycin 1 g orally, single dose	Doxycycline 100 mg orally bid for 7 days
Gonorrhea (*Neisseria gonorrhoeae*)	NAAT using 1) first-void urine or 2) urethral, vaginal, and rectal swabs	Ceftriaxone 250 mg intramuscularly, single dose, plus either azithromycin 1 g orally, single dose, or doxycycline 100 mg orally bid for 7 days	
Trichomoniasis (*Trichomonas vaginalis*)	Culture, PCR, or antigen testing (depending on local availability) using self-collected vaginal or urethral samples	Metronidazole 2 g orally, single dose	Tinidazole 2 g orally, single dose
Syphilis (*Treponema pallidum*)	Dark-field microscopy or direct fluorescent antibody testing on exudate or tissue from the chancre; serology (VDRL) is useful 6 weeks after infection	Benzathine penicillin 2.4 million units (1.44 g) intramuscularly, single dose (see section "Treatment Recommendations" for details)	
Bacterial vaginosis (not exclusively an STI)	Gram staining and presence of clue cells in vaginal fluid	Metronidazole 500 mg bid orally for 7 days	
Herpes simplex virus	Viral PCR of ulcer swabs	Acyclovir 400 mg tid orally for 7–10 days	Valacyclovir or famciclovir

Note. NAAT = nucleic acid amplification testing; PCR = polymerase chain reaction; VDRL = Venereal Disease Research Laboratory.

sent for culture, polymerase chain reaction (PCR), or antigen testing, depending on local availability.

Syphilis

Primary syphilis, the first stage of the disease caused by the spirochete bacterium *Treponema pallidum,* occurs on average 3 weeks after initial exposure and results in a painless ulcer (chancre) at the site of infection, usually on the penis, anus, or cervix. Primary syphilis is usually diagnosed and treated empirically based on a history of unprotected sex and clinical examination. The diagnosis can be confirmed with dark-field microscopy or direct fluorescent antibody testing on exudate or tissue from the chancre. Serology becomes useful 6 weeks after infection. Initial nontreponemal screening tests include the Venereal Disease Research Laboratory (VDRL) slide test and the rapid plasma reagin (RPR) test; these tests are similar, and most labs choose to provide one or the other. Although sensitive, these tests are not specific; many conditions, including autoimmune disorders, pregnancy, malaria, tuberculosis, and endocarditis, can result in false-positive results. A positive nontreponemal screening test should be confirmed with treponemal tests such as *T. pallidum* particle agglutination (TPPA) or fluorescent treponemal antibody absorption (FTA-ABS) tests.

A clinical suspicion of neurosyphilis can be confirmed by cerebrospinal fluid (CSF) analysis for white cells and protein in conjunction with VDRL testing. The VDRL test is relatively insensitive on CSF and cannot rule out infection. FTA-ABS testing of CSF is more sensitive and may be useful to rule out disease (Ratnam 2005). Some centers offer treponemal PCR, which can be performed on both ulcer swabs and CSF.

Bacterial Vaginosis

Bacterial vaginosis is the most common cause of vaginal discharge and results from the replacement of the normal vaginal flora by a high concentration of anaerobes. Diagnosis is through Gram staining of vaginal swabs or a positive "whiff test," where a strong fishy odor results from the addition of potassium hydroxide to the discharge on a slide.

Herpes Simplex Virus

Painful anogenital ulcers are usually caused by HSV type 1 or 2. Diagnosis can be confirmed on viral PCR of ulcer swabs. In unclear cases, type-specific serological assays can be requested.

Human Papillomavirus

Tests are available for confirming HPV infection, but they are only approved in women over age 30 who are undergoing cervical cancer screening. They are not validated for STI screening or in men. The primary importance of HPV is that infection is associated with a significantly higher risk of cervical cancer. HPV infection is believed to cause 70% of all cervical cancers, as well as a subset of vulvar, vaginal, anal, and oral cavity cancers (Centers for Disease Control and Prevention 2010a).

Preventive Guidelines

There are no specific guidelines for prevention of STIs in the psychiatric population, although there is a clear need for focused intervention in this vulnerable patient group (Rein et al. 2004). Rates of STI screening are generally low in the psychiatric setting, which results in a considerable burden of disease (Rosenberg et al. 2001; Rothbard et al. 2009; Satriano et al. 2007). All psychiatric patients should be encouraged to engage with STI screening programs in line with national guidelines. In the inpatient psychiatric or medical environment, clinicians have a responsibility to ensure that STI screening is considered for each patient.

Patients with mental illness should be presumed to be sexually active, even if they do not overtly disclose this to clinicians. There should be a low threshold for the encouragement of safe sex practices (including condom use). Women should be encouraged to develop a relationship with a family practitioner, internist, or gynecologist. Men who have sex with men (MSM) should be encouraged to regularly visit a doctor for screening for HIV and rectal, anal, or oral STIs as behavior and symptoms dictate.

Notwithstanding some small differences, there is general agreement about STI screening among the U.S. Preventive Services Task Force (USPSTF), CDC, American Academy of Family Physicians, American Academy of Pediatrics, and American College of Obstetricians and Gynecologists. The USPSTF guidelines (Meyers et al. 2008) are summarized in Table 16–4.

In addition to these guidelines, the CDC suggests that all adults and adolescents be tested at least once for HIV (Branson et al. 2006). The CDC also recommends at least annual testing of MSM for HIV, syphilis, chlamydia, and gonorrhea. In MSM who have multiple partners or who have sex while using illicit drugs, testing should occur more frequently (every 3–6 months) (Centers for Disease Control and Prevention 2013).

HPV screening is not recommended, but there are two vaccines available that prevent oncogenic HPV (types 16 and 18). All females ages 13–26 should have three doses of HPV vaccine over a 6-month period (Centers for Disease Control and Prevention 2010a). The quadrivalent vaccine (Gardasil) also protects against HPV types 6 and 11, which cause 90% of genital warts. It can be used in males ages 9–26, although ideally it should be given before sexual activity begins (Centers for Disease Control and Prevention 2011). It

TABLE 16–4. **Summary of U.S. Preventive Services Task Force guidelines on sexually transmitted infection screening**

Sexually active women under age 25 should be screened annually for chlamydia and gonorrhea.

All women who engage in high-risk sexual behavior (multiple partners, new partners, inconsistent condom use, having sex under the influence of alcohol or drugs, having sex in exchange for money or drugs) should be routinely screened for chlamydia, gonorrhea, human immunodeficiency virus (HIV), and syphilis.

Pregnant women should be screened for syphilis, HIV, chlamydia, and hepatitis B at the first prenatal visit, as well as gonorrhea if at risk.

Men engaging in high-risk sexual behavior should be screened for syphilis and HIV.

There is no benefit to screening the general population for hepatitis B, herpes simplex virus, or human papillomavirus.

Source.   Adapted from Meyers et al. 2008.

is important to emphasize that women should still attend routine cervical cancer screening because 30% of cervical cancers are not caused by HPV 16 and 18 (Centers for Disease Control and Prevention 2010a).

Practical Application

Figure 16–1 provides health care providers with an algorithm to guide testing for STIs in the psychiatric population. Clinicians should be aware that chlamydia, gonorrhea, syphilis, viral hepatitis, and HIV are notifiable diseases and must be reported to state public health agencies and the CDC.

Treatment Recommendations

In this section we discuss treatment of most of the STIs covered in this chapter. The treatment of HIV and HPV is covered in Chapter 18, "HIV/AIDS," and Chapter 23, "Cervical Cancer," respectively.

Chlamydia and Gonorrhea

Prompt treatment should be provided to the patient with chlamydia or gonorrhea and to all sexual partners to prevent reinfection. Sexual abstinence is recommended for 1 week after commencement of treatment. Those with gonorrhea are frequently coinfected with chlamydia and should therefore receive treatment for both infections. For patients who may have difficulty

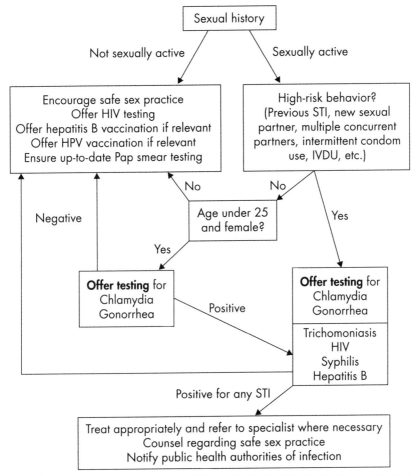

FIGURE 16–1. An algorithm for assessing and diagnosing sexually transmitted infections in the psychiatric patient population.

Note. HIV=human immunodeficiency virus; HPV=human papillomavirus; IVDU=intravenous drug user; STI=sexually transmitted infection.

completing longer courses of antibiotics, single-dose directly observed therapy is recommended. All patients should be retested after 3 months or as soon as practicable to minimize harm from reinfection by an untreated or new partner (Fung et al. 2007; Hosenfeld et al. 2009).

Chlamydial infection is best treated with a single dose of azithromycin 1 g. Doxycycline 100 mg bid for 7 days is an alternative. Gonorrhea is treated with a single dose of ceftriaxone 250 mg intramuscularly. Other treatments are not currently recommended due to increasing drug resistance of *N. gonorrhoeae.*

Trichomoniasis

Metronidazole (2-g single dose orally) is the first-line treatment for trichomoniasis. Patients must abstain from alcohol for 72 hours postingestion to avoid a disulfiram-like reaction, which can result in nausea, vomiting, and significant abdominal discomfort. Because reinfection can occur from untreated partners, retesting is advised in sexually active women 3 months after treatment. Low-level resistance to metronidazole does occur; therefore, in cases where reinfection is ruled out, tinidazole treatment (2-g single dose orally) is suggested (Forna and Gulmezoglu 2003).

Syphilis

For syphilis, the treatment of choice is penicillin G. The preparation varies with disease stage. Physicians should be careful to prescribe the correct preparation of the drug, because names of different preparations are similar. Standard benzathine penicillin (Bicillin L-A) should be used rather than the combination product benzathine-procaine penicillin (Bicillin C-R).

Primary and secondary syphilis are treated with a single 1.44-g dose (2.4 million units) of standard benzathine penicillin intramuscularly. Early latent syphilis, defined as asymptomatic seropositive disease in patients infected within the last year, is treated in the same way. True latent syphilis, or latent syphilis of unknown duration, should be treated with a prolonged course of 7.2 million units of benzathine penicillin in three intramuscular doses of 2.4 million units weekly. This treatment also applies to those with tertiary syphilis without neurological involvement.

Neurosyphilis or syphilitic eye disease often requires inpatient treatment for 10–14 days with aqueous crystalline penicillin G 18–24 million units daily, either in divided doses or as continuous infusion. If compliance is a certainty, the CDC recommends a 10- to 14-day course of intramuscular procaine penicillin 2.4 million units daily with probenecid 500 mg orally qid to reduce renal excretion (Workowski et al. 2010).

Treatment of infection at any disease stage may provoke a Jarisch-Herxheimer reaction as endotoxins are released from the dying spirochetes. Patients should be warned of the possibility of headache, malaise, fever, hyperventilation, and myalgias, which usually occur within 24 hours of treatment. If unsure about how to diagnose or treat syphilis, mental health providers should refer the patient to a primary care provider or infectious disease specialist.

Bacterial Vaginosis

Treatment of bacterial vaginosis should be given to all symptomatic women. Metronidazole 500 mg bid for 7 days is the first-line therapy. Alternatives include topical treatment with metronidazole or clindamycin. Women should avoid vaginal douching to reduce the risk of relapse.

Herpes Simplex Virus

First episodes of genital herpes should be treated with oral antivirals. Acyclovir 400 mg tid for 7–10 days is a reasonable option. Valacyclovir or famciclovir can also be used. If ulcers have not healed after 10 days of therapy, the treatment course can be prolonged. In patients with recurrent disease, suppressive or episodic therapy should be considered. Suppression with acyclovir 400 mg bid can reduce recurrence by 70%–80% (Workowski et al. 2010). Episodic therapy consists of a 5-day course of acyclovir at treatment dose, which must be started immediately once symptoms begin.

When to Refer

Situations warranting referral to a primary care provider or specialist include the following:

- All new diagnoses of HIV, hepatitis B, or hepatitis C
- All cases of complicated STI (e.g., PID, epididymitis, proctitis)
- Patients diagnosed with syphilis who have significant penicillin allergy
- Treatment-resistant cases of gonorrhea or trichomoniasis
- Nonhealing ulcers or lesions
- Cases for which specialist input would improve patient outcome

Special Treatment Considerations for the Psychiatric Patient Population

Treatment of STIs in people with mental illness is of great importance to prevent medical complications and to reduce transmission. There are several questions to consider regarding the treatment of a person with mental illness:

1. Does the patient have a primary psychiatric disorder, or is the patient's current psychiatric presentation a result of the infection?

   Certain STIs can manifest with psychiatric symptoms (neurosyphilis, HIV dementia) and pose a diagnostic challenge. Obtaining a longitudinal history of the patient's mental health, age at onset, and family history may help clarify the cause.

2. Are there any psychiatric side effects of STI treatment?

   With the exception of treatment for hepatitis C or HIV (covered in Chapter 17, "Viral Hepatitis," and Chapter 18, "HIV/AIDS," respectively), most drugs used for treatment of common STIs are not known to cause psychiatric side effects. The exceptions are the fluoroquinolones, which may be prescribed for PID if cephalosporin therapy is not feasible. Possible side effects of fluoroquinolones include insomnia, restlessness, confusion, and in rare cases hallucinations, psychosis, and related delirium.

3. What are potential medication interactions to keep in mind when treating a patient with mental illness?

Nonsteroidal anti-inflammatory drugs (NSAIDs), with the exception of sulindac, may increase lithium levels in the blood. Although NSAIDs are not contraindicated in patients taking lithium, other pain relievers, such as acetaminophen, may be preferred as a first-line choice. Carbamazepine may decrease levels of doxycycline (Neuvonen et al. 1975). Azithromycin may have QT_c prolonging effects and has been associated with torsades de pointes (Huang et al. 2007). Numerous psychiatric medications, including atypical antipsychotics, may also prolong the QT_c interval. This may be a consideration in patients with underlying long QT intervals at baseline or a family history of sudden death.

As with any prescribed medication, the potential for overdose in a patient with mental illness must be considered. Medication nonadherence or refusal may be seen in the psychiatric population. Refusals may be the result of grandiose delusions (e.g., "I don't need treatment") or paranoia (e.g., "The doctor is trying to poison me"). One-time doses of antibiotics that can be given in the clinic are the preferred treatment for uncomplicated infections when compliance is an issue. Because patients with mental illness are at higher risk for acquiring STIs, education and counseling (especially substance abuse counseling) are paramount in both primary and secondary prevention strategies. Treatment of the STI should be accompanied by referrals for social work and psychotherapy, when indicated.

The clinician should consider hospitalization if medically indicated or if there is suspicion for nonadherence to therapy. It is important to remember that all kinds of systemic infections (including PID) can result in dehydration and derange renal metabolism, leading to lithium accumulation.

Finally, as with proposed treatment for any patient, it is important to consider whether the patient has capacity to consent to or refuse treatment. To assess for capacity, the clinician must determine that the patient is able to communicate a choice, understands the relevant information, appreciates the medical consequences of the decision, and demonstrates the ability to reason about treatment choices (Appelbaum 2007).

Case Discussion (*continued*)

On Ms. K's presentation to the emergency department, her vital signs are as follows: temperature 39.5°C, heart rate 110 beats per minute, blood pressure 96/67, and respiratory rate 20 breaths per minute. She complains of nausea and two episodes of emesis. She allows for a complete physical examination, including a pelvic exam. Her cervix is inflamed, and she is noted to have adnexal and cervical motion tenderness.

What Is the Differential Diagnosis? The differential diagnosis includes PID, ovarian torsion, ovarian cysts, ectopic pregnancy, and endometriosis. Labs and imaging confirm a diagnosis of PID due to gonorrhea. Ms. K is admitted to the hospital for further treatment. She continues to experience nausea and vomiting, but now also complains of dizziness and diarrhea. Her speech is slurred and a coarse tremor is noticed in her hands.

Providers should have a low threshold of suspicion for PID in a sexually active young woman who presents with abdominal pain and adnexal or cervical motion tenderness. A classic finding in a young patient is "shuffling" while walking; this is a natural attempt to reduce cervical irritation and is commonly associated with PID.

Which Additional Labs Should Now Be Ordered? A lithium level should be ordered. Also, Ms. K should have testing for other STIs that would not show up on swabs from a pelvic exam, such as HIV and syphilis.

Lithium is held given concerns for lithium toxicity. The patient's nausea, vomiting, and diarrhea resolve quickly, and she requests to leave. When she is told that she is not ready for discharge, she becomes upset and rips out her intravenous catheter while yelling, "I don't need treatment from you guys!" A psychiatry consult is called to assess for capacity to refuse treatment. The patient is found to have capacity to refuse treatment, but she becomes agreeable to remaining in the hospital after a phone conversation with her community psychiatry team.

The patient improves with antibiotic treatment. HIV and syphilis serology tests are negative. Prior to her discharge, both her community psychiatrist and primary care provider are informed that lithium was held during hospitalization and restarted prior to discharge. The patient is also educated about the signs and symptoms of lithium toxicity, as well as common STIs.

Clinical Highlights

- Because patients with mental illness are at high risk of acquiring sexually transmitted infections (STIs), the clinician should ask about sexual history and symptoms of STIs.
- The clinician should rule out STIs in men presenting with urinary tract infections.
- Because chlamydia and gonorrhea often co-occur, patients diagnosed with one should be treated for both.

- A patient with an STI should be assessed for human immuno-deficiency virus, hepatitis B, and hepatitis C.
- Treatment with single-dose medications can be effective in patients who have mental illness.
- Risk of STIs is increased during episodes of mania or psychosis.

Resources

For Patients

Association of Reproductive Health Professionals: Sexually Transmitted Diseases/Infections Patient Resources. Available at: http://www.arhp.org/topics/stis/patient-resources.

Centers for Disease Control and Prevention: Sexually Transmitted Diseases (STDs). Available at: http://www.cdc.gov/std.

For Clinicians

Association of Reproductive Health Professionals: Sexually Transmitted Diseases/Infections Patient Resources. Available at: http://www.arhp.org/topics/stis/patient-resources.

STD Awareness Resource Site: Clinic Tools and Resources. Available at: http://www.cdcnpin.org/stdawareness/tools.aspx.

World Health Organization: Sexual and Reproductive Health: Training Modules for the Syndromic Management of Sexually Transmitted Infections. Available at: http://www.who.int/reproductivehealth/publications/rtis/9789241593407/en/index.html.

References

Appelbaum PS: Clinical practice: assessment of patients' competence to consent to treatment. N Engl J Med 357:1834–1840, 2007

Branson BM, Handsfield HH, Lampe MA, et al: Revised recommendations for HIV testing of adults, adolescents, and pregnant women in health-care settings. MMWR Recomm Rep 55:1–17, 2006

Centers for Disease Control and Prevention: FDA licensure of bivalent human papillomavirus vaccine (HPV2, Cervarix) for use in females and updated HPV vaccination recommendations from the Advisory Committee on Immunization Practices (ACIP). MMWR Morb Mortal Wkly Rep 59:626–629, 2010a

Centers for Disease Control and Prevention: Sexually transmitted diseases treatment guidelines, 2010b. Available at: http://www.cdc.gov/std/treatment/2010/clinical.htm. Accessed July 14, 2014.

Centers for Disease Control and Prevention: Recommendations on the use of quadrivalent human papillomavirus vaccine in males—Advisory Committee on Immunization Practices (ACIP), 2011. MMWR Morb Mortal Wkly Rep 60:1705–1708, 2011

Centers for Disease Control and Prevention: CDC Fact Sheet: Incidence, Prevalence, and Cost of Sexually Transmitted Infections in the United States. Atlanta, GA, Centers for Disease Control and Prevention, February 2013. Available at: http://www.cdc.gov/std/stats/sti-estimates-fact-sheet-feb-2013.pdf. Accessed February 22, 2014.

Erbelding EJ, Hutton HE, Zenilman JM, et al: The prevalence of psychiatric disorders in sexually transmitted disease clinic patients and their association with sexually transmitted disease risk. Sex Transm Dis 31:8–12, 2004

Fenton KA, Lowndes CM: Recent trends in the epidemiology of sexually transmitted infections in the European Union. Sex Transm Infect 80:255–263, 2004

Forna F, Gulmezoglu AM: Interventions for treating trichomoniasis in women. Cochrane Database Syst Rev (3):CD000218, 2003

Freeman AH, Bernstein KT, Kohn RP, et al: Evaluation of self-collected versus clinician-collected swabs for the detection of Chlamydia trachomatis and Neisseria gonorrhoeae pharyngeal infection among men who have sex with men. Sex Transm Dis 38:1036–1039, 2011

Frenkl TL, Potts J: Sexually transmitted infections. Urol Clin North Am 35:33–46, 2008

Fung M, Scott KC, Kent CK, et al: Chlamydial and gonococcal reinfection among men: a systematic review of data to evaluate the need for retesting. Sex Transm Infect 83:304–309, 2007

Gilson RJ, Mindel A: Recent advances: sexually transmitted infections. BMJ 322:1160–1164, 2001

Hosenfeld CB, Workowski KA, Berman S, et al: Repeat infection with chlamydia and gonorrhea among females: a systematic review of the literature. Sex Transm Dis 36:478–489, 2009

Huang BH, Wu CH, Hsia CP, et al: Azithromycin-induced torsade de pointes. Pacing Clin Electrophysiol 30:1579–1582, 2007

King C, Feldman J, Waithaka Y, et al: Sexual risk behaviors and sexually transmitted infection prevalence in an outpatient psychiatry clinic. Sex Transm Dis 35:877–882, 2008

Meyers D, Wolff T, Gregory K, et al: USPSTF recommendations for STI screening. Am Fam Physician 77:819–824, 2008

Neuvonen PJ, Pentikainen PJ, Gothoni G: Inhibition of iron absorption by tetracycline. Br J Clin Pharmacol 2:94–96, 1975

Ratnam S: The laboratory diagnosis of syphilis. Can J Infect Dis Med Microbiol 16:45–51, 2005

Rein DB, Anderson LA, Irwin KL: Mental health disorders and sexually transmitted diseases in a privately insured population. Am J Manag Care 10:917–924, 2004

Rosenberg SD, Goodman LA, Osher FC, et al: Prevalence of HIV, hepatitis B, and hepatitis C in people with severe mental illness. Am J Public Health 91:31–37, 2001

Rothbard AB, Blank MB, Staab JP, et al: Previously undetected metabolic syndromes and infectious diseases among psychiatric inpatients. Psychiatr Serv 60:534–537, 2009

Satriano J, McKinnon K, Adoff S: HIV service provision for people with severe mental illness in outpatient mental health care settings in New York. J Prev Interv Community 33:95–108, 2007

Schoeman SA, Stewart CM, Booth RA, et al: Assessment of best single sample for finding chlamydia in women with and without symptoms: a diagnostic test study. BMJ 345:e8013, 2012

Trigg BG, Kerndt PR, Aynalem G: Sexually transmitted infections and pelvic inflammatory disease in women. Med Clin North Am 92:1083–1113, 2008

Weinstock H, Berman S, Cates W Jr: Sexually transmitted diseases among American youth: incidence and prevalence estimates, 2000. Perspect Sex Reprod Health 36:6–10, 2004

Workowski KA, Berman S; Centers for Disease Control and Prevention: Sexually transmitted diseases treatment guidelines, 2010. MMWR Recomm Rep 59:1–110, 2010

CHAPTER 17

Viral Hepatitis

Jeffrey Rado, M.D.
Pravir Baxi, M.D.

Case Discussion

Mr. P is a 44-year-old black man with a long history of schizophrenia (first diagnosed at age 19). He also has hypertension and diabetes. He has not worked for more than 20 years and was previously incarcerated for selling heroin. He intermittently binges on crack cocaine. Several years ago, he completed a drug rehabilitation program and maintained sobriety for nearly 2 years. He currently is receiving disability insurance and lives with his elderly mother. She locks him out of the house when he is using drugs. During these times, he ends up staying with his girlfriend, who is also a drug abuser and who sometimes uses intravenous heroin.

He presents to the clinic because he wants some alprazolam, because he is very "anxious and depressed." Risperidone adequately controls his auditory hallucinations and paranoid delusions. He admits to having used freebase crack cocaine 2 days earlier. During this time he stopped his insulin. He does not know his most recent blood glucose readings. He is staying with his girlfriend right now because his mother will not let him return home until he "gets cleaned up."

Clinical Overview

Hepatitis refers to inflammation of the liver, which may be due to different etiologies, including viral infections, alcohol, and autoimmune disease. *Viral hepatitis* refers to infection from five distinct groups of virus, designated A through E (Centers for Disease Control and Prevention 2013).

Infection with hepatitis A virus (HAV) occurs worldwide. Its incidence has been decreasing in the United States since the implementation of vaccination. In the year 2010 (the last year for which data have been reported), about 1,600 cases of HAV were reported by the Centers for Disease Control and Prevention (CDC; 2013), with an incidence of 0.6 per 100,000. HAV is transmitted via the fecal-oral route. The virus is spread more easily in lower socioeconomic areas, due to lack of adequate sanitation, and is more common among U.S. residents who travel abroad to endemic areas (Klevens et al. 2010). The incubation period for HAV averages approximately 30 days, after which prodromal symptoms begin. These include fatigue, malaise, fever, abdominal pain, and anorexia. Nausea and vomiting are also common. Patients can develop jaundice, typically after about 2 weeks, with noted dark urine and pale stools (Klevens et al. 2010). Overall, the course of HAV is self-limited, and treatment is supportive. Furthermore, immunoglobulin G antibodies provide lifelong protection after recovery (Centers for Disease Control and Prevention 2013; Lednar et al. 1985).

The rate of infection with hepatitis B virus (HBV) in the United States is also on the decline, with 2,890 cases reported to the CDC in 2011 (Centers for Disease Control and Prevention 2014). HBV is spread via contact with infectious blood and body fluids. Perinatal transmission is common in high-prevalence regions, and sexual transmission is common in developed countries (Alter et al. 1990). The incubation period for the virus is typically about 90 days. Most patients develop subclinical or anicteric hepatitis (without jaundice); fewer develop icteric hepatitis (Alter et al. 1990). Fulminant hepatitis is a rare form of HBV. About 95% of adult patients recover and do not develop chronic HBV, whereas about 25%–50% of child patients develop chronic infection (Centers for Disease Control and Prevention 2013).

An estimated 2.7–3.9 million patients in the United States have chronic hepatitis C virus (HCV). The CDC reported 1,229 new cases of acute HCV in 2011 (Centers for Disease Control and Prevention 2014). Transmission is via the parenteral route, most commonly via intravenous drug use and blood transfusions. Perinatal transmission has also been reported. The majority of patients with HCV are asymptomatic, although some do develop symptoms of acute hepatitis. In contrast to the other forms of viral hepatitis, 75%–85% of infections with HCV become chronic, with a high incidence of liver failure requiring liver transplantation (Centers for Disease Control and Prevention 2013). HCV is generally not considered a sexually transmitted disease.

Hepatitis D virus (HDV), in comparison to other viruses, is a defective RNA virus that can only duplicate in the presence of coexisting HBV. HDV carriers are common in central Africa, the Middle East, and parts of Asia

(Centers for Disease Control and Prevention 2013). Rates of infection with HDV are common in regions where HBV is endemic, with about 15 million persons with serological evidence of HDV (Hughes et al. 2011). As with HBV, HDV is spread via the parenteral route, specifically through sexual intercourse and intravenous drug use. Superinfection of HDV presents as acute hepatitis that is sometimes misdiagnosed as HBV or worsening chronic HBV. HDV in a patient with chronic HBV results in chronic HDV (Hughes et al. 2011).

Although relatively uncommon in the United States, hepatitis E virus (HEV) is very widespread in developing countries, with an estimated 2.3 billion persons infected globally (Khuroo et al. 2004). Like HAV, it is spread primarily via the fecal-oral route, although some believe that transmission via blood transfusions can occur in endemic areas (Khuroo et al. 2004). Symptoms, which usually begin about 40 days after exposure to the virus, include nonspecific complaints of fever, nausea, abdominal pain, malaise, and fatigue (Centers for Disease Control and Prevention 2013). Although young adults and older men may have symptomatic illness, pregnant women are at increased risk to develop fulminant hepatic failure from HEV. In most cases, however, the illness is self-limited, with no data suggesting chronic HEV (Teshale and Hu 2011).

HCV occurs more frequently in patients with chronic mental illness than in the general population. The seroprevalence of HCV among patients hospitalized in a psychiatric hospital was found to be 8.5%, compared with 1.8% in the general population (Dinwiddie et al. 2003). Compared with the rate of HCV in the general population (0.8%), the rate among patients surveyed in a Canadian clozapine clinic (N=110) was higher (2.7%) (Sockalingam et al. 2010). Patients in four public sector clinics for patients with chronic mental illness (N=668) underwent HIV and hepatitis laboratory evaluation (Osher et al. 2003). HCV was found in 122 (18%), of whom 53 (9%) had only HCV, 56 (8%) had HBV and HCV, and 3 (1%) had HCV and HIV. Risk factors for having HCV were common and included use of injection drugs (>20%), sharing needles (14%), and crack cocaine use (>20%). Similarly, higher than normal rates of HCV (prevalence: 9.1%) were described in hospitalized patients with schizophrenia and comorbid psychoactive substance abuse in Japan (Nakamura et al. 2004).

Patients with schizophrenia in a large Veterans Affairs (VA) database were two times more likely than control subjects (patients without schizophrenia) to get tested for HCV but also 2 times more likely to be infected (Huckans et al. 2006). Patients in this study were not less likely than controls to receive treatment for HCV. Butterfield et al. (2003) found that HCV in patients with chronic mental illness occurred twice as often in men as in women. Men had higher rates of needle sharing and crack cocaine use, whereas women had higher rates of unprotected sexual intercourse. Two years after a screening for HCV in a cohort of 98 patients with schizophrenia, none of the 8 patients who tested positive for HCV antibody had received any treatment (Freudenreich et al. 2007).

Patients with chronic mental illness should be screened for HCV risk factors such as unprotected intercourse with a high-risk person and sharing needles for illicit drug use. Patients frequently underreport these activities. Patients with any of these risk factors should undergo laboratory testing for antibodies against HIV-1, HCV, and HBV.

It is crucial that mental health providers counsel patients on risk reduction (e.g., avoiding unprotected sexual intercourse and sharing of drug paraphernalia) and complications of viral hepatitis to motivate them to change risky behaviors. A survey of 236 patients with serious mental illness found that only 175 (70%) were able to demonstrate basic knowledge about HCV on a standardized questionnaire (Goldberg et al. 2009). A brief intervention to increase screening and treatment in patients with chronic mental illness was undertaken by Rosenberg et al. (2010) in four community-based mental health clinics. Patients with chronic mental illness ($N=236$) were randomized to either the intervention group, which consisted of on-site education, screening, blood draws, and vaccine administration, or the treatment-as-usual group (referral to local community health sources). Testing for HBV and HCV was more likely in the intervention group patients, who also increased their knowledge about hepatitis and reduced their substance use. High-risk behaviors, however, did not decrease; patients were not more likely to be referred for specialty care, and HIV knowledge did not increase (Rosenberg et al. 2010).

Practical Pointers

- Because patients with chronic mental illness are at increased risk of hepatitis B virus and hepatitis C virus infections, they should be screened for risk factors (i.e., sharing of drug paraphernalia, unprotected intercourse).
- Patients should be counseled on risk factor reduction (i.e., condom use, avoiding of shared needles for illicit drug use).
- Patients with substance use disorders (abuse or dependence) should be referred for specialized treatment of chemical dependency, such as that provided by an addiction medicine specialist.

Diagnosis

Acute viral hepatitis is often preceded by a prodrome of symptoms, which are systemic and may be variable. Although each form of viral hepatitis has its

TABLE 17–1. Diagnosis of acute and chronic hepatitis

Diagnosis of acute hepatitis

Hepatitis A	+IgM anti-HAV
Hepatitis B	+HBsAg, +IgM anti-HBc, +HBV DNA ±HBeAg
Hepatitis C	+Anti-HCV
Hepatitis D*	+HDAg, +HDV RNA
Hepatitis E*	+HEV PCR, +IgM anti-HEV

Diagnosis of chronic hepatitis

Hepatitis B	+HBsAg, +IgG anti-HBc, +HBV DNA ±HBeAg, IgM anti-HBc
Hepatitis C	+Anti-HCV, +HCV RNA

Note. Anti-HAV=antibody to hepatitis A; Anti-HBc=antibody to hepatitis B core; anti-HCV=antibodies to HCV; anti-HEV=antibody to HEV; HBV=hepatitis B virus; HBeAg=hepatitis B e antigen; HBsAg=hepatitis surface antigen; HCV= hepatitis C virus; HDAg=Hepatitis D antigen; HDV=hepatitis D virus; HEV=hepatitis E virus; IgG=immunoglobulin G; IgM=immunoglobulin M; PCR=polymerase chain reaction.
*Not routinely tested in the United States.
Source. Adapted from Centers for Disease Control and Prevention 2013. http://www.cdc.gov/hepatitis/Statistics/SurveillanceGuidelines.htm#GenCA.

own unique characteristics, the symptoms of acute and chronic viral hepatitis are similar in these different infections. Most often, nonspecific constitutional symptoms, consisting of fever, fatigue, headache, cough, nausea, and vomiting, appear first. Jaundice, commonly associated with hepatic diseases, develops in the next 7–14 days, often with associated pain in the right upper quadrant of the abdomen. In severe cases of acute viral hepatitis, fulminant hepatic failure is possible, with rapid clinical deterioration and death. In contrast, chronic hepatitis is often asymptomatic, and clinical examination may reveal stigmata of chronic liver disease (e.g., jaundice, ascites, peripheral edema) (Longo et al. 2012).

Although elevated serum transaminases are associated with acute viral hepatitis, levels may vary in chronic cases. Serological tests, as outlined in Table 17–1, are used to establish the diagnosis.

If there is clinical suspicion of viral hepatitis, psychiatrists can initiate the laboratory evaluation. Testing for viral hepatitis is done when clinical symptoms and clinical history indicate possible hepatitis. Commonly, patients with symptoms or with elevated transaminases undergo workup with testing for HAV, HBV, and HCV. HDV testing is not routinely done and is reserved for cases in which specific risk factors are present or in cases of hepatitis with unusual courses (Center for Substance Abuse Treatment 1993). HEV serology testing is done only in special cases through the CDC, because no commercial testing exists (Emerson and Purcell 2007).

Preventive Guidelines

Screening

The U.S. Preventive Services Task Force (USPSTF) published guidelines in 2004 on routine screening for HBV and HCV. The USPSTF recommended against routine screening for chronic HBV in the general asymptomatic population (U.S. Preventive Services Task Force 2004b). Similarly, for HCV, the USPSTF recommended against routine screening in asymptomatic persons who are not at increased risk; however, for persons at increased risk for infection, the USPSTF found insufficient evidence to recommend for or against screening for HCV (U.S. Preventive Services Task Force 2004a). In June 2013, the USPSTF published a revision of this statement for HCV, now recommending that physicians conduct a onetime screening for HCV in adults born between 1945 and 1965 (U.S. Preventive Services Task Force 2013). The CDC also endorses this recommendation (Centers for Disease Control and Prevention 2013). Furthermore, the USPSTF recommends screening for HCV in persons at high risk, including those with a history of intravenous drug use or a blood transfusion prior to 1992 (U.S. Preventive Services Task Force 2004a). The CDC, on the other hand, recommends screening for both HBV and HCV in high-risk individuals. HBV screening is also recommended in Asians and Pacific Islanders due to the remarkably high prevalence of HBV in this population (Centers for Disease Control and Prevention 2013). These screening recommendations are summarized in Table 17–2.

Vaccinations

Currently, vaccinations for HAV and HBV exist and are routinely given in the outpatient setting. The CDC recommends that all infants receive both vaccines at age 1 year. There is no vaccine for HCV. High-risk groups should also receive the vaccine for HAV. This includes men who have sex with men, injection drug users, patients with chronic liver disease, persons who are traveling to or working in countries with high rates of HAV, and persons with occupational risk factors for infection. The vaccine for HAV is an inactivated vaccine that is given in a two-dose schedule (Centers for Disease Control and Prevention 2013).

The vaccine for HBV, like that for HAV, is an inactivated vaccine. Adults who should receive the vaccine include men who have sex with men, injec-

TABLE 17–2. **Screening recommendations for hepatitis B and C**

Centers for Disease Control and Prevention

Hepatitis B   Asymptomatic or low-risk patients—should not be screened

High-risk patients[a]—should be screened

Asian Americans and Pacific Islanders[b]—should be screened

Hepatitis C   Asymptomatic or low-risk patients—onetime screening for adults born between 1945 and 1965; otherwise, no screening indicated

High-risk patients[c]—should be screened

U.S. Preventive Services Task Force

Hepatitis B   Asymptomatic or low-risk patients—should not be screened

High-risk patients[a]—no evidence for or against, no specific recommendations

Hepatitis C   Asymptomatic or low-risk patients—onetime screening for adults born between 1945 and 1965; otherwise, no screening indicated

High-risk patients[c]—should be screened

[a]Sex partners of hepatitis B–infected persons, HIV patients, men who have sex with men, injection drug users, people born in countries with prevalence >2%, persons receiving immunosuppressive therapy.
[b]Anyone born in Asia (except Japan) or the Pacific Islands (except New Zealand and Australia); anyone born in the United States who was not vaccinated at birth and who has at least one parent born in East or Southeast Asia (except Japan) or the Pacific Islands (except New Zealand and Australia).
[c]Injection drug users, persons with recognizable exposure such as needle stick, persons who received blood transfusions before 1992, persons with medical conditions such as long-term dialysis.
Source. Adapted from Centers for Disease Control and Prevention 2013; U.S. Preventive Services Task Force 2004a, 2004b.

tion drug users, health care and public safety workers, and persons with end-stage renal disease, chronic liver disease, HIV infection, or diabetes mellitus. Both single-antigen HBV and combination vaccines (i.e., with *Haemophilus influenzae* type B, tetanus) exist in the current market. The most common vaccination schedule used is three intramuscular injections over a 4- to 6-month period (Centers for Disease Control and Prevention 2013).

Treatment Recommendations

In most clinical cases, acute viral hepatitis does not necessitate immediate treatment. Excluding cases of fulminant hepatitis, which frequently lead to intensive care unit admissions, acute viral hepatitis is managed by supportive care in an outpatient setting (Longo et al. 2012). Recent clinical studies have shown that implementing treatment in cases of severe acute HCV is beneficial in reducing the rate of chronic infections; however, no general consensus exists in terms of duration and optimum regimen (European Association for the Study of the Liver 2011). Treatment options for chronic viral hepatitis are an ongoing topic of considerable research. Goals of therapy are to reduce complications from chronic viral hepatitis, including cirrhosis and hepatic failure. Currently, first-line therapies for chronic HBV include pegylated interferon (IFN), entecavir, and tenofovir (Lok and McMahon 2009). Although pegylated IFN is usually finite in duration of therapy, duration and treatment end points for oral medications are still not well established, with ranges of 4 years to indefinite therapy (Lok and McMahon 2009). Some parameters used to assess the treatment response in chronic HBV include decrease in HBV DNA, and loss of hepatitis B e antigen (HBeAg) (Lok and McMahon 2009). Given the complexity of monitoring and medication choices, treatment is typically managed by a hepatologist.

Chronic HCV treatment consists of pegylated IFN in addition to oral ribavirin (Ghany et al. 2009). The optimal regimen and its duration depend on the HCV genotype and have been well studied in the literature (Longo et al. 2012). Treatment results are followed by virological parameters, including serum transaminases, HCV RNA levels, and histology. Most important in treatment of chronic HCV is the sustained virological response, which is the absence of HCV RNA 24 weeks after discontinuation of therapy (Ghany et al. 2009).

When to Refer

- Patients with acute hepatitis should be urgently evaluated to determine need for intravenous rehydration or other higher levels of care.
- Asymptomatic patients who test positive for HBV should see their primary care provider or a hepatologist.
- All patients who test positive for HCV should be evaluated and treated by a hepatologist. Also, patients with HCV should be routinely vaccinated against HBV.

Special Treatment Considerations for the Psychiatric Patient Population

Pegylated IFN is associated with various neuropsychiatric symptoms, including depression, anxiety, and hostility (Kraus et al. 2003). The spectrum of reported symptoms includes slowness, fatigue, hypersomnia, lethargy, depressed mood, irritability, emotional lability, social withdrawal, and poor concentration (Lotrich et al. 2007; Raison et al. 2005). Depressive symptoms can present as early as 1 month after starting treatment (Raison et al. 2005). Udina et al. (2012) conducted a systematic review and meta-analysis of 26 observational studies and found a cumulative 25% risk of IFN-induced depression in the general HCV-positive population. In addition, the following risk factors for IFN-induced depression were identified: female gender, history of major depression episode, history of a psychiatric disorder, low educational level, and presence of subthreshold depressive symptoms at baseline.

Concern about inducing depression and other psychiatric symptoms initially led to a general hesitation at providing IFN treatment to patients with psychiatric disorders. Several studies by Huckans and colleagues, however, indicate that antiviral treatment can be safely delivered to patients with psychiatric disorders, with results similar to those in nonpsychiatric populations. Patients with schizophrenia in a VA database ($n = 30$) who received antiviral treatment for HCV were followed over an 8-year period (Huckans et al. 2010a). Compared with controls, these patients did not experience higher rates of symptoms from schizophrenia, depression, or mania. Huckans et al. (2010b) reviewed a VA database of patients with schizophrenia who received HCV antiviral treatment ($n = 30$) and compared them with patients who had HCV but not schizophrenia from the same database. Patients with and without schizophrenia were equally likely to reach end-of-treatment response and sustained viral response, indicating no differential in outcome of adverse effects. Similarly, another VA database review found that patients with schizophrenia were as likely to get screened and receive notification of their results as were patients without psychiatric illness (Huckans et al. 2010b).

Positive outcomes in patients with a history of depression have also been reported. Rates of completion and sustained viral response of patients with a history of major depressive disorder were not different from those of controls (Hauser et al. 2009). Furthermore, frequency of neuropsychiatric side effects did not differ between groups. Finally, patients treated with low-dose pegylated IFN over an average of 3.5 years did not experience higher rates of depression symptoms compared with a no-treatment group (Kronfol et al. 2011).

As a result of the studies discussed previously in this section, presence of a psychiatric disorder is no longer an absolute contraindication to antiviral treatment for HCV. However, close clinical monitoring is necessary. In unstable patients, psychiatric symptom control should be optimized prior to starting treatment for HCV. Sockalingam and Abbey (2009) reviewed nine studies of antidepressants in patients with HCV and found the medications useful for patients with elevated baseline depression or a history of IFN-induced depression. Although most studies are small, the largest amount of evidence supports the safety and efficacy of selective serotonin reuptake inhibitors (SSRIs) for the treatment of IFN-induced depression. Although no SSRIs have received U.S. Food and Drug Administration approval for this indication, citalopram, escitalopram, sertraline, and paroxetine are the best-studied agents.

Prevention of IFN-induced depression has also been studied. For example, Diez-Quevedo et al. (2011) randomized a general population of HCV-positive individuals to either escitalopram or placebo prior to initiating IFN therapy. After 12 weeks of treatment, depression scores increased similarly in both active and placebo groups. The authors concluded that prophylaxis with antidepressants was not useful but that it did warrant further study in subjects at high risk of psychiatric illness. In a review of six prevention studies using antidepressants, Galvao-de Almeida et al. (2010) concluded there was inadequate evidence to support this approach. However, in a study of pre-IFN treatment with escitalopram, the medication did reduce the rates of incidental depression (32%) versus placebo (58%) (Schaefer et al. 2012). Others have taken a more measured approach, suggesting pretreatment only in those patients with elevated depressive symptoms at baseline or those with a history of IFN-induced depression (Udina et al. 2012). The prevailing approach to IFN-induced depression assessment, prevention, and treatment is summarized in Table 17–3.

Case Discussion (*continued*)

Despite counseling by his psychiatrist and other providers, Mr. P resists any intervention for his drug use, claiming, "I can stop whenever I want." After being counseled on risk reduction, he decides to stop sharing needles with his girlfriend. Two months later he agrees to get tested for HCV antibody and HIV-1 antibody. HIV is negative, but HCV is positive. He agrees to an outpatient rehabilitation program for his drug use. It takes several more months before he agrees to an evaluation by a hepatologist. Treatment with IFN and ribavirin is recommended. Given his recurrent depression and anxiety, sertraline 25 mg/day is prescribed, and the dose is titrated to achieve meaningful clinical benefit. With his mood symptoms better controlled, Mr. P begins antiviral treatment. During this period he is followed closely by his psychiatrist for any treatment-emergent mood symptoms.

TABLE 17–3. **Interferon-induced depression**

Clinical concern	Interferon treatment of hepatitis C is associated with a 25% risk of depression.
Risk factors	Being female, history of major depressive episode, history of psychiatric disorder, low educational level, and presence of subthreshold depression symptoms at baseline present risks.
Prevention	Prophylactic use of antidepressants in average-risk patients is not indicated. Also, for patients who present with mood changes, it is important to assess acute risk for suicide.
Management	Optimal stabilization of psychiatric symptoms is advised prior to starting interferon therapy. Selective serotonin reuptake inhibitors (citalopram, escitalopram, sertraline, paroxetine) are safe and effective to treat interferon-induced depression.

Clinical Highlights

- Patients with chronic mental illness have higher rates of hepatitis B virus and hepatitis C virus (HCV) infection.

- Patients should be counseled on risk factors for transmission (e.g., intravenous drug abuse, unprotected intercourse) and be referred, when appropriate, for laboratory evaluation and/or substance abuse treatment.

- All patients born between 1945 and 1965, whether risk factors are present or not, should be screened once for HCV.

- Treatment of HCV with interferon (IFN) is associated with increased risk of depression. Patients at a higher risk of IFN-induced depression (e.g., history of major depression or other psychiatric disorder, presence of baseline depressive symptoms) should have their psychiatric symptoms stabilized prior to initiation of IFN and undergo close psychiatric monitoring throughout treatment. SSRIs are safe and effective for IFN-induced depression.

Resources

For Patients

California Department of Public Health: Viral Hepatitis Resources. Available at: http://www.cdph.ca.gov/programs/Pages/ViralHepatitisResources.aspx.

Centers for Disease Control and Prevention: Viral Hepatitis—Resource Center. Available at: http://www.cdc.gov/hepatitis/resources.

For Clinicians

Centers for Disease Control and Prevention: Hepatitis C Information for Health Professionals. Available at: http://www.cdc.gov/hepatitis/hcv.

Centers for Disease Control and Prevention: Viral Hepatitis—Resource Center. Available at: http://www.cdc.gov/hepatitis/resources.

U.S. Department of Veterans Affairs: Management of Interferon Side Effects. Available at: http://www.hepatitis.va.gov/pdf/treatment-side-effects.pdf.

References

Alter MJ, Hadler SC, Margolis HS, et al: The changing epidemiology of hepatitis B in the United States: need for alternative vaccination strategies. JAMA 263:1218–1222, 1990

Butterfield MI, Bosworth HB, Meador KG, et al: Gender differences in hepatitis C infection and risks among persons with severe mental illness. Psychiatr Serv 54:848–853, 2003

Center for Substance Abuse Treatment: Viral hepatitis D, in Screening for Infectious Diseases Among Substance Abusers [web book]. Rockville, MD, U.S. Substance Abuse and Mental Health Services Administration, 1993. Available at: http://www.ncbi.nlm.nih.gov/books/NBK64706/. Accessed August 1, 2014.

Centers for Disease Control and Prevention: Viral Hepatitis. Atlanta, GA, Centers for Disease Control and Prevention, March 12, 2013. Available at: http://www.cdc.gov/hepatitis/. Accessed August 2013.

Diez-Quevedo C, Masnou H, Planas R, et al: Prophylactic treatment with escitalopram of pegylated interferon alfa-2a-induced depression in hepatitis C: a 12-week, randomized, double-blind, placebo-controlled trial. J Clin Psychiatry 72:522–528, 2011

Dinwiddie SH, Shicker L, Newman T: Prevalence of hepatitis C among psychiatric patients in the public sector. Am J Psychiatry 160:172–174, 2003

Emerson SU, Purcell RH: Hepatitis E. Pediatr Infect Dis J 26:1147–1148, 2007

European Association for the Study of the Liver: EASL Clinical Practice Guidelines: management of hepatitis C virus infection. J Hepatol 55:245–264, 2011

Freudenreich O, Gandhi RT, Walsh JP, et al: Hepatitis C in schizophrenia: screening experience in a community-dwelling clozapine cohort. Psychosomatics 49:405–411, 2007

Galvao-de Almeida A, Guindalini C, Batista-Neves S, et al: Can antidepressants prevent interferon-alpha-induced depression? A review of the literature. Gen Hosp Psychiatry 32:401–405, 2010

Ghany MG, Strader DB, Thomas DL, et al: Diagnosis, management, and treatment of hepatitis C: an update. Hepatology 49:1335–1374, 2009

Goldberg RW, Tapscott SL, Calmes CA, et al: HIV and hepatitis C knowledge among individuals with serious mental illness. Psychiatr Rehabil J 33:47–49, 2009

Hauser P, Morasco BJ, Linke A, et al: Antiviral completion rates and sustained viral response in hepatitis C patients with and without preexisting major depressive disorder. Psychosomatics 50:500–505, 2009

Huckans MS, Blackwell AD, Harms TA, et al: Management of hepatitis C disease among VA patients with schizophrenia and substance use disorders. Psychiatr Serv 57:403–406, 2006

Huckans M, Mitchell A, Pavawalla S, et al: The influence of antiviral therapy on psychiatric symptoms among patients with hepatitis C and schizophrenia. Antivir Ther 15:111–119, 2010a

Huckans M, Mitchell A, Ruimy S, et al: Antiviral therapy completion and response rates among hepatitis C patients with and without schizophrenia. Schizophr Bull 36:165–172, 2010b

Hughes SA, Wedemeyer H, Harrison PM: Hepatitis delta virus. Lancet 378:73–85, 2011

Khuroo MS, Kamili S, Yattoo GN: Hepatitis E virus infection may be transmitted through blood transfusions in an endemic area. J Gastroenterol Hepatol 19:778–784, 2004

Klevens RM, Miller JT, Igbal K, et al: The evolving epidemiology of hepatitis A in the United States: incidence and molecular epidemiology from population-based surveillance, 2005–2007. Arch Intern Med 170:1811–1818, 2010

Kraus MR, Schafer A, Faller H, et al: Psychiatric symptoms in patients with chronic hepatitis C receiving interferon alfa-2b therapy. J Clin Psychiatry 64:708–714, 2003

Kronfol Z, Litman HJ, Back-Madruga C, et al: No increase in depression with low-dose maintenance peginterferon in prior non-responders with chronic hepatitis C. J Affect Disord 129:205–212, 2011

Lednar WM, Lemon SM, Kirkpatrick JW, et al: Frequency of illness associated with epidemic hepatitis A virus infections in adults. Am J Epidemiol 122:226–233, 1985

Lok A, McMahon B: Chronic hepatitis B: update 2009. Hepatology 50:661–662, 2009

Longo DL, Fauci AS, Kasper DL: Harrison's Principles of Internal Medicine, 18th Edition. New York, NY, McGraw-Hill, 2012

Lotrich FE, Rabinowitz M, Gironda P, et al: Depression following pegylated interferon-alpha: characteristics and vulnerability. J Psychosom Res 63:131–135, 2007

Nakamura Y, Koh M, Miyoshi E, et al: High prevalence of the hepatitis C virus infection among the inpatients of schizophrenia and psychoactive substance abuse in Japan. Prog Neuropsychopharmacol Biol Psychiatry 28:591–597, 2004

Osher FG, Goldberg RW, McNary SW, et al: Substance abuse and the transmission of hepatitis C among persons with severe mental illness. Psychiatr Serv 54:842–847, 2003

Raison CL, Borisov AS, Broadwell SD, et al: Depression during pegylated interferon-alpha plus ribavirin therapy: prevalence and prediction. J Clin Psychiatry 66:41–48, 2005

Rosenberg S, Goldberg RW, Dixon LB, et al: Assessing the STIRR model of best practices for blood-borne infections of clients with serious mental illness. Psychiatr Serv 61(9):885–891, 2010

Schaefer M, Sarkar R, Knop V, et al: Escitalopram for the prevention of peginterferon-alpha2-associated depression in hepatitis C virus–infected patients without previous psychiatric disease: a randomized trial. Ann Intern Med 157:94–103, 2012

Sockalingam S, Abbey SE: Managing depression during hepatitis C treatment. Can J Psychiatry 54:614–615, 2009

Sockalingam S, Shammi C, Powel V, et al: Determining rates of hepatitis C in a clozapine treated cohort. Schizophr Res 124:86–90, 2010

Teshale EH, Hu DJ: Hepatitis E: epidemiology and prevention. World J Hepatol 3:285–291, 2011

Udina M, Castellví P, Moreno-España J, et al: Interferon-induced depression in chronic hepatitis C: a systematic review and meta-analysis. J Clin Psychiatry 73:1128–1138, 2012

U.S. Preventive Services Task Force: Screening for hepatitis B virus infection: recommendation statement. Rockville, MD, U.S. Preventive Services Task Force, February 2004a. Available at: http://www.uspreventiveservicestaskforce.org/3rduspstf/hepbscr/hepbrs.htm. Accessed July 2013.

U.S. Preventive Services Task Force: Screening for hepatitis C in adults: recommendation statement. Am Fam Physician 70:1113–1116, 2004b

U.S. Preventive Services Task Force: Screening for hepatitis C virus infection in adults. Task Force final recommendation. Rockville, MD, U.S. Preventive Services Task Force, February 2013. Available at: http://www.uspreventiveservicestaskforce.org/uspstf12/hepc/hepcfact.pdf. Accessed July 2014.

CHAPTER 18

HIV/AIDS

John Onate, M.D.

Case Discussion

Mr. H, a 56-year-old man, is referred to a psychiatry clinic for the treatment of depression and comorbid methamphetamine misuse. The patient has a past psychiatric history of bipolar disorder and compulsive use of methamphetamine. Mr. H has had episodes of major depression lasting several weeks to months since age 18. He has also experienced mood swings and severe irritability between his episodes of depression. He did not graduate from high school and failed twice while trying to pass the GED high school equivalency test. He started using amphetamine at age 22 to improve his energy and focus in construction work; however, the use quickly increased in frequency, and he switched to intravenous methamphetamine for more intense intoxication. The patient identifies himself as heterosexual but during treatment reveals that he traded sex with men for drugs and alcohol, including receptive anal intercourse without condom use. The periods of irritability and impulsivity increased in intensity, and the patient began a pattern of being arrested and spending months to years in jail for substance-related charges until his mid-40s. While in jail, Mr. H was treated by psychiatrists for bipolar disorder and responded to both valproic acid and the periods of sobriety enforced by being incarcerated. At age 41, he married a friend he met at Narcotics Anonymous. He has struggled for the past 15 years with sobriety and has relapsed many times. He and his wife are inconsistent with condom use, but she has tested negative for HIV several times, most recently 1 month ago. The patient was recently diagnosed with type 2 diabetes and during routine screening at the county primary clinic, he was found positive for HIV with a viral load of 55,000 and a CD4 count of 350 cells/mm^3. At the current evaluation, it has been 2 months since his diagnosis of HIV, and he is being treated at a university-associated comprehensive HIV clinic.

Clinical Overview

Human immunodeficiency virus (HIV) continues to be a serious public health risk, with little reduction in the rates of new infections in the United States for the past 10 years despite guidelines that target HIV as a priority for preventive health care screening. Since the first HIV cases were identified in the early 1980s, over 1 million individuals have been infected in the United States and nearly 600,000 have died as a result. The Centers for Disease Control and Prevention (2013) estimates that approximately 50,000 new cases of HIV are diagnosed each year and that an estimated 207,000 individuals are not aware that they are infected. Because of an unprecedented investment of health care resources over the past 30 years, HIV-positive patients who have access to antiviral medication and appropriate prophylaxis can maintain a near-normal quality of life. Vaccine research and attempts at sustained viral remission (without antiviral medication) have had some promising findings but unfortunately have not yet been effective. HIV is a chronic illness that requires access to antiviral medication to prevent disease progression. Research has found that the earlier in the course of the infection a patient can be diagnosed, the better the outcome. Diagnosis can be challenging because HIV is often asymptomatic for many years after the initial infection. Additionally, in the United States, the highest-risk populations have limited or no access to the health care system (Chou et al. 2012). The involvement of psychiatrists and other mental health care providers is crucial to efforts to both expand screening for HIV and reduce the risk factors for transmission. Patients with severe mental illness and illicit drug use have a much higher prevalence of HIV and should be a focus for preventive health collaborations within the mental health care system. The purpose of this chapter is to review the risk factors for HIV and approaches to both screening and HIV transmission risk reduction in patients with mental illness.

HIV/AIDS Rates of Illness and Transmission

As shown in Table 18–1, men who have sex with men (MSM), regardless of ethnic background, share the highest burden of disease. This pattern is found both in the percentage of existing cases and in the rates of new infections, with over 50% of those living with HIV in the United States being MSM. Notably, 45% of new HIV infections in the population of MSM occur among young black MSM. Black women follow MSM among minority populations

TABLE 18–1. Minority U.S. populations that share a disproportionate burden of HIV/AIDS

Men who have sex with men (MSM)

African American men (particularly young MSM)

African American women

Latino women

Injection drug users

Source. Adapted from Centers for Disease Control and Prevention 2013; Chou et al. 2012.

with disproportionate rates of new HIV infections compared with other groups. Hispanics also have increasing rates of HIV infection as an ethnic minority. Since 2010, about 16% of new HIV cases were among Latinos, with women in the group having twice the rate of infection as men. As a whole, those who identify themselves as heterosexual make up 25% of new HIV cases. Injection drug use accounts for 16% of those living with HIV/AIDS and 8% of new cases. The cause of minority populations having the highest rates of disease is multifactorial and still not fully understood. Poverty, lack of access to screening and public health information, language barriers, and substance misuse are certainly factors related to the steady rates of transmission in this population (Centers for Disease Control and Prevention 2012).

HIV has a relatively long, initial dormant phase. The majority of people infected have a brief viral syndrome and are then asymptomatic for many years before experiencing significant loss of immune function. One of the challenges for preventive health interventions is that a newly infected person can start infecting others shortly after the initial infection or seroconversion. The transmission of HIV requires intimate sharing of blood, semen, or saliva intravenously or through damaged mucosa. Table 18–2 lists routine risk factors for transmission. HIV is not transmitted through the air or by touching. For reasons that will be discussed later in this chapter (see "Preventive Guidelines"), the reduction of transmission is complex.

HIV in Individuals With Mental Illness

Even in the early days of the HIV pandemic, studies indicated higher rates of HIV/AIDS in persons with severe mental illness than in other populations. Some studies found double-digit prevalence rates in this population. These early studies were limited by relatively low sample size and comorbid injection drug use. In 2001, a multisite prospective study examined prevalence rates for HIV among individuals with severe mental illness in both inpatient

TABLE 18–2. **Risk factors for transmission of HIV**

Receptive anal intercourse without barrier protection with high-risk partner(s)

Receptive vaginal intercourse without barrier protection with high-risk partners(s)

Injection drug use

Noninjection illicit drug use (particularly stimulants)

Multiple sexual partners

Sex trade work

Exposure by health worker via hollow-bore needle-stick injury

Source.   Adapted from Centers for Disease Control and Prevention 2012.

and outpatient settings and in urban and suburban populations. The results showed increased rates of HIV compared with the general population. Of the population studied, the prevalence was found to be 3.1%—over 3 times the rate of HIV in the general population. Having severe mental illness coupled with engaging in specific behaviors was associated with markedly higher risk of HIV infection and transmission. These behaviors included injection drug use, crack cocaine use, history of sexually transmitted diseases (STDs), and working in the sex trade (Table 18–3). As in other epidemiological studies, African Americans had disproportionately higher rates of infection (Meade and Sikkema 2005; Rosenberg et al. 2001).

Individuals who are at risk for HIV and have mental illness are not always offered HIV testing and counseling. Studies have found that about 60% of mental health patients with risk factors are offered HIV testing. Patients in nonurban settings were less likely to be offered testing. Recognizing and documenting risk factors such as injection drug use, sex without barrier protection, and past sexually transmitted infection did not significantly affect the number of patients offered testing (Goldberg et al. 2005).

Relying on identifying risk factors to trigger HIV testing does narrow the testing to patients with higher risk; however, this practice requires that health care providers use consistent protocols for screening and develop the trust of patients so as to obtain accurate information. A stable rate of new infections has been occurring for over 10 years, and large populations of patients who are infected continue to be unaware of HIV-associated risks despite broad understanding by and training of health care providers on the risk factors as well as increased access to HIV testing. These epidemiological results support the idea that relying on risk factors for initial screening misses many infected patients (Centers for Disease Control and Prevention 2013; Chou et

TABLE 18–3. Populations with risk factors for HIV transmission and severe mental illness comorbidity

Injection drug users

Smokers of crack cocaine

Individuals with history of sexually transmitted disease

Sex trade workers

Source. Adapted from Rosenberg et al. 2001.

al. 2012; Goldberg et al. 2005). Identifying and being aware of risk factors are very important for ongoing screening and planning interventions to reduce the risk of transmission. HIV screening should be a formal and universal part of mental health clinics, regardless of location, population, or insurance status. All adult patients should be tested initially at intake if they have not been tested before or if there is any question on past testing. Risk factors should be documented, and clinic policy and procedures should be developed to review and update the documentation for risk factors throughout the time the patient is an open patient in the clinic setting. The reasoning for universal testing of adults for HIV will be discussed in the following section of this chapter, "Diagnosis." There is clinical utility for evaluating patients for HIV risk factors. Factors such as illicit drug use, sex trade affiliation, multiple anonymous sexual partners, and barriers to condom use can influence or be an integral part in understanding and effectively treating mental illness. A skilled provider can incorporate information about HIV risk factors into a mental health evaluation in a manner that will enhance the relationship with the patient and aid in making a patient-centered treatment plan (Chou et al. 2012; Goldberg et al. 2005; Trivedi et al. 2013).

Practical Pointers

- All adults should be offered human immunodeficiency virus (HIV) screening at least once regardless of risk factors.
- Adults with risk factors should be tested regularly and interventions should be done to reduce risky behavior.
- Adults with mental illness and high-risk behavior, especially men who have sex with men, should have culturally sensitive, patient-centered and empathic asssesments of the behavior(s), and risk reduction and regular testing should be a key part of their treatment plan.
- Coordination of care with a multidisciplinary team is key in the management of HIV-positive patients with mental illness. Treatment plans should pay careful attention to adherence to antiviral medications,

drug interaction, substance use, and high-risk behaviors for sexually transmitted diseases.

Diagnosis

HIV testing has been made widely accessible through one-use in-home testing kits. These over-the-counter kits, available at many pharmacies, can provide results within an hour to a few days and range in retail price from about $20 to $40. Free testing is available at public health settings, and rapid oral testing can be done at point-of-care sites and mobile testing centers. Mental health practitioners should become familiar with local testing centers. Regional public health centers are a great resource for clinicians. If a patient screens negative after a high-risk occurrence, a repeat test should be recommended at least 1–3 months later, because seroconversion usually takes place within 2–4 weeks after exposure but may take as long as 3 months. After a positive screening test, a confirmatory test is automatically performed. After a patient's positive test is confirmed, the severity of HIV infection is largely determined by three factors: viral load, CD4 count, and presence of opportunistic infections (Centers for Disease Control and Prevention 2013; Chou et al. 2012).

Preventive Guidelines

HIV is not curable, and no vaccine is currently available to prevent infection or transmission. Reducing the risk of transmission is a complex and difficult process because of the long asymptomatic period and the fact that prevention requires reducing high-risk sexual behavior and risk practices, such as intravenous drug use. However, some countries with high rates of transmission have been able to significantly reduce HIV transmission through large and well-supported public health interventions.

Some studies support the use of antiretroviral medications as prophylactic interventions in populations with high rates of HIV or in discordant HIV couples (in which one partner is HIV negative). A number of field trials and studies show decreased HIV transmission in targeted groups. More research is needed in the widespread population-based use of antiretrovirals in HIV-negative patients, however, before this will be common practice (Anglemyer et al. 2013; Rausch et al. 2013). In three trials, male circumcision in African countries significantly reduced HIV transmission in treated men. This may be the most cost-effective intervention in areas with high prevalence of HIV (Piot and Quinn 2013).

In patients with mental illness, modified cognitive-behavioral therapy (CBT) to include HIV and STD risk reduction has been shown to have some

TABLE 18–4. **Effective interventions and approaches to reducing HIV transmission**

Single-session sexually transmitted disease risk reduction interventions

Male circumcision

Treatment of depression, anxiety, and substance misuse

Cognitive-behavioral therapy addressing high-risk behavior or
  motivational interview(s)

impact on increasing awareness and understanding of transmission. Motivational interviewing techniques and CBT may also be effective in combination with behavioral change that reduces HIV transmission. Comorbid depression in African American women has been shown to increase risk of HIV transmission. Effective treatment of depression along with education on HIV risk reduction has been shown to decrease risky behavior in high-risk groups (Lennon et al. 2012; Malow et al. 2012).

The most effective behavioral interventions, supported by randomized clinical trials and meta-analysis, are evidence-based, single-session interventions. These trials showed significant reductions in STD risk behaviors. Effective interventions addressed both education of the patient on transmission of STDs and skill building to improve the likelihood of behavioral change, such as condom use (Eaton et al. 2012) (Table 18–4).

Treatment Recommendations

HIV treatment is complicated and requires coordination of care between the primary care provider, infectious disease specialist, and other medical providers. In comprehensive HIV treatment centers, an infectious disease specialist often acts as the primary care provider. Psychiatrists, psychologists, social workers, and substance abuse specialists are very important in the comprehensive treatment of HIV. Because significant mental health problems, social stressors, and substance misuse issues are highly prevalent among patients with HIV, integration of treatment is the standard of care for HIV treatment. The pharmacological treatment of HIV is broken down into two parts: antiretroviral combinations and prophylactic medications to prevent opportunistic infections (World Health Organization et al. 2010).

Highly active antiretroviral therapy (HAART) is the cornerstone of HIV treatment and has greatly reduced the morbidity and mortality from HIV/AIDS and the opportunistic infections associated with the loss of immune function. The specific combinations of antiretroviral medications are beyond the scope of this book, but the reader should be able to recognize the

TABLE 18–5. HIV antiviral medications

Nucleoside reverse transcriptase inhibitors	Abacavir
	Didanosine
	Emtricitabine
	Lamivudine
	Stavudine
	Zidovudine
Nucleotide reverse transcriptase inhibitor	Tenofovir
Nonnucleoside reverse transcriptase inhibitors	Efavirenz
	Etravirine
	Nevirapine
Protease inhibitors	Atazanavir
	Darunavir
	Fosamprenavir
	Indinavir
	Lopinavir
	Saquinavir
	Ritonavir
Integrase strand transfer inhibitor	Raltegravir
Chemokine receptor 5 antagonist	Maraviroc

medications (Table 18–5) and assess any interactions with psychiatric medications (Table 18–6).

Adherence to HAART is key. Because of the slow replication in the HIV life cycle, the virus has a high mutation rate and resistance quickly develops to antiviral medications when taken alone or intermittently. A coordinated and integrated approach to HIV care is important because once a patient starts a HAART regimen, adherence to the first combination can influence greatly the individual's course of illness (Thompson et al. 2012; World Health Organization et al. 2010).

Opportunistic infections are infections by microorganisms that normally are easily repelled by the intact immune system. Untreated HIV progressively causes the immune system to fail, and at certain CD4 levels, the patient becomes more susceptible to infection. HAART is the most important intervention in preventing opportunistic infections, but patients with advanced disease and low CD4 counts require additional medications (Table 18–7). In addition to medications, appropriate adult vaccinations should be maintained under guidance of infectious disease specialists (Kaplan et al. 2009; Piot and Quinn 2013).

TABLE 18–6. Important drug-drug interactions between psychiatric and HIV medications

Psychiatric medication class	HIV medication	Potential interaction	
NNRTI	Efavirenz	*decreases*	levels of bupropion
NNRTI	Nevirapine	*decreases*	levels of fluoxetine and fluvoxamine
Protease inhibitor	Fosamprenavir	*decreases*	levels of paroxetine
Protease inhibitor	Indinavir	*increases*	levels of nortriptyline
Protease inhibitor	Lopinavir	*decreases*	levels of lamotrigine
Protease inhibitor	Darunavir	*decreases*	levels of paroxetine and sertraline
Protease inhibitor	Darunavir	*increases*	levels of trazodone
Protease inhibitor	Nelfinavir	*increases*	levels of desipramine
Protease inhibitor	Ritonavir	*increases*	serum levels of carbamazepine, sertraline, citalopram, paroxetine, nortriptyline, desipramine, imipramine, amitriptyline, clomipramine, and doxepin
Protease inhibitor	Ritonavir	*decreases*	levels of lamotrigine and olanzapine
Protease inhibitor	Tipranavir	*decreases*	levels of bupropion
Azole antifungal	Fluconazole	*increases*	levels of nortriptyline

TABLE 18–6. Important drug-drug interactions between psychiatric and HIV medications *(continued)*

Psychiatric medication class	HIV medication	Potential interaction	
SSRI	Fluoxetine	*increases*	serum levels of amprenavir, delavirdine, efavirenz, indinavir, nelfinavir, ritonavir, and saquinavir
SSRI	Fluvoxamine	*increases*	serum levels of amprenavir, delavirdine, efavirenz, indinavir, nelfinavir, ritonavir, and saquinavir
Phenylpiperazine antidepressant	Nefazodone	*increases*	serum levels of efavirenz and indinavir

Note. NNRTI=nonnucleoside reverse transcriptase inhibitor; SSRI=selective serotonin reuptake inhibitor.
Source. Adapted from Repetto et al. 2008; Watkins et al. 2011.

TABLE 18–7. **Prophylaxis medications in HIV treatment**

CD4 count (cells/mm^3)	Illness	Preventive treatment
<200	*Pneumocystis jirovecii* pneumonia	TMP-SMX
<100	*Toxoplasma gondii* infection	TMP-SMX
<50	Disseminated *mycobacterium avium* complex	Azithromycin

Note. TMP-SMX = trimethoprim-sulfamethoxazole.

When to Refer

- Patients should be referred to an infectious disease specialist upon initial diagnosis and with any concerns about the development of opportunistic infections or worsening immunocompromise.
- An infectious disease specialist should follow patients who have AIDS.
- Patients with multiple medical comorbidities should be referred to a primary care provider.

Special Treatment Considerations for the Psychiatric Patient Population

Patients who have severe mental illness are more likely to be exposed to and to acquire HIV and AIDS. Therefore, it is critical for mental health care providers to screen all patients for HIV at least once and diligently monitor for risk factors and screen accordingly thereafter. It is outside the scope of this chapter to detail the medication management for HIV and AIDS. However, psychiatrists must be mindful about possible common side effects encountered in those taking medications for the treatment of HIV and psychiatric disorders (see Table 18–6).

Case Discussion (*continued*)

The case of Mr. H illustrates a discordant couple—the patient's wife is HIV negative. She will need ongoing HIV testing every 6 months, and the couple should be educated on HIV transmission risk reduction (Anglemyer et al. 2013; Centers for Disease Control and Prevention 2012).

The patient has a number of risk factors that could have been the source of his infection. The intravenous drug use and sex trade affiliation are the most likely behaviors that led to his infection. It is not possible from the lab tests to determine when he was infected. He will need a comprehensive medical examination to see if he has any opportunistic infections and to evaluate whether his diabetes is controlled. The psychiatrist's role is to stabilize the mood disorder and determine whether there is an indication for formal substance use treatment. Additionally, the psychiatrist can aid the infectious disease specialist in assessing the patient's capacity and motivation for HAART. The psychiatrist should have a treatment goal that includes adherence to antiviral medication. Psychiatric consultations involving patients with HIV differ from those in which the focus is on the mental health problem alone. In the comprehensive treatment of HIV, effective treatment of medical, psychiatric, and substance use problems is necessary because the consequence of nonadherence to HAART is antiviral medication resistance that leads to increased viral load and damage to the immune system (Kaplan et al. 2009; Thompson et al. 2012).

Clinical Highlights

- Human immunodeficiency virus (HIV) is more prevalent and has higher rates of transmission among individuals with mental illness, especially among those with comorbid intravenous drug use or multiple sexual partners.

- All patients should be offered HIV testing; those with high-risk behavior should be tested annually or as clinically indicated.

- In patients with HIV, treatment with HAART under the care of expert clinicians is key to reducing morbidity and mortality from infection.

- HIV/AIDS patients with advanced disease must be given appropriate prophylactic medication.

- Integration and collaboration among HIV specialists, primary care providers, and mental health providers are crucial to long-term treatment of HIV in patients with comorbid medical, mental health, and substance abuse problems.

- Psychiatrists are recommended to document all medications used in the treatment of a patient with HIV and consider drug-drug interactions and side effects when choosing psychiatric medications.

- Evidence-based single-intervention risk-reduction sessions can reduce risk factors for HIV and other sexually transmitted diseases. Mental health treatment centers and clinics are ideal sites for these sessions.

Resources

For Patients

AIDS.gov: HIV/AIDS basics. http://aids.gov/hiv-aids-basics

AIDS Info: Fact Sheets. Available at: http://aidsinfo.nih.gov/education-materials/fact-sheets.

HIV InSite: Available at: http://hivinsite.ucsf.edu.

UCSF Medical Center: FAQ: HIV Testing. Available at: http://www.ucsf-health.org/education/hiv_testing.

For Clinicians

American Psychiatric Association: HIV Psychiatry. Available at: http://www.psychiatry.org/practice/professional-interests/hiv-psychiatry.

Centers for Disease Control and Prevention: HIV/AIDS. Available at: http://www.cdc.gov/hiv.

HIV InSite. Available at: http://hivinsite.ucsf.edu.

Johns Hopkins Medicine: Johns Hopkins HIV Guide. Available at: http://www.hopkinsguides.com/hopkins/ub/index/Johns_Hopkins_HIV_Guide/All_Topics/A.

References

Anglemyer A, Rutherford GW, Horvath T, et al: Antiretroviral therapy for prevention of HIV transmission in HIV-discordant couples. Cochrane Database Syst Rev 4:CD009153, 2013

Centers for Disease Control and Prevention: Integrated prevention services for HIV infection, viral hepatitis, sexually transmitted diseases, and tuberculosis for persons who use drugs illicitly: summary guidance from CDC and the U.S. Department of Health and Human Services. MMWR Recomm Rep 61:1–40, 2012

Centers for Disease Control and Prevention: HIV in the United States: At a Glance. Atlanta, GA, Centers for Disease Control and Prevention, April 23, 2013. Available at: http://www.cdc.gov/hiv/statistics/basics/ataglance.html. Accessed June 27, 2013.

Chou R, Selph S, Dana T: Screening for HIV: systematic review to update the 2005 U.S. Preventive Services Task Force recommendation. Ann Intern Med 157:706–718, 2012

Eaton LA, Huedo-Medina HA, Kalichman SC, et al: Meta-analysis of single-session behavioral interventions to prevent sexually transmitted infections: implications for bundling prevention packages. Am J Public Health 102:34–44, 2012

Goldberg RW, Himelhock S, Kreyenbuhl J, et al: Predictors of HIV and hepatitis testing and related service utilization among individuals with serious mental illness. Psychosomatics 46:573–577, 2005

Kaplan JE, Benson C, Holmes KK, et al: Guidelines for prevention and treatment of opportunistic infections HIV-infected adults and adolescents: recommendations from CDC, the National Institutes of Health, and the HIV Medicine Association of the Infectious Diseases Society of America. MMWR Recomm Rep 58:1–207, 2009

Lennon CA, Huedo-Medina TB, Gerwien DP, et al: A role for depression in sexual risk reduction for women? A meta-analysis of HIV prevention trials with depression outcomes. Soc Sci Med 75:688–698, 2012

Malow RM, McMahon RC, Devieux J, et al: Cognitive behavioral HIV risk reduction in those receiving psychiatric treatment: a clinical trial. AIDS Behav.16:1192–1202, 2012

Meade CS, Sikkema KJ: HIV risk behavior among adults with severe mental illness: a systematic review. Clin Psychol Rev 25:433–457, 2005

Piot P, Quinn TC: Response to the AIDS pandemic—a global health model. N Engl J Med 368:2210–2218, 2013

Rausch DM, Grossman CI, Erbelding EJ: Integrating behavioral and biomedical research in HIV interventions: challenges and opportunities. J Acquir Immune Defic Syndr 63 (suppl 1):S6–S11, 2013

Rosenberg SD, Goodman LA, Osher FC, et al: Prevalence of HIV, hepatitis B, and hepatitis C in people with severe mental illness. Am J Public Health 91:31–37, 2001

Thompson MA, Aberg JA, Hoy JA, et al: Antiretroviral treatment of adult HIV infection: 2012 recommendations of the International Antiviral Society–USA panel. JAMA 308:387–402, 2012

Trivedi JK, Tripathi A, Dhanasekaran S, et al: Preventive psychiatry: concept appraisal and future directions. Int J Soc Psychiatry June 19, 2013 [Epub ahead of print]

World Health Organization: Antiretroviral Therapy for HIV Infection in Adults and Adolescents: Recommendations for a Public Health Approach, 2010 Revision. Geneva, Switzerland, World Health Organization, 2010

SECTION V

Oncological Disorders
in the Psychiatric
Patient Population

CHAPTER 19

Breast Cancer

Helen K. Chew, M.D.

Mili Arora, M.D.

Radha Verman, M.D.

Case Discussion

Ms. G is a 54-year-old postmenopausal black woman with schizophrenia who presents with a lump in her right breast. She first noticed this lump 3 months earlier while showering. The lump is nonpainful and has not grown in size. She has never had a screening mammogram. She takes risperidone for schizophrenia and sees her psychiatrist every 4 months. She has not seen a primary care doctor in over 2 years. She drinks one glass of wine weekly and smokes one pack of cigarettes a day. She is married but does not have any children. She has a maternal aunt with a history of breast cancer.

On physical examination, the clinician palpates a 2-cm, hard, mobile nodule in the upper outer quadrant of the patient's right breast. There are no overlying skin changes and no regional lymphadenopathy.

Clinical Overview

Breast cancer is the most common invasive cancer diagnosed in women in the United States, and it is the second leading cause of cancer death in women. The American Cancer Society estimates that over 232,000 new cases of invasive breast cancer and approximately 39,700 deaths occurred in 2013 (Siegel

276 Preventive Medical Care in Psychiatry

et al. 2013). Overall, one in eight women will develop breast cancer during her lifetime.

More than 90% of breast cancers occur in the epithelial lining of the duct lobular unit and are referred to as carcinomas or adenocarcinomas. Many types of changes can occur within the duct lobular unit, including benign conditions, such as hyperplasia or fibrocystic disease; precancerous findings, such as atypical hyperplasia; noninvasive breast cancer, also referred to as in situ carcinoma or intraductal carcinoma; and invasive breast cancer (Hayes 2000).

Invasive adenocarcinoma of the breast, which is the main focus of this chapter, has many histological subtypes (Hayes 2000). The most common subtype is infiltrating ductal carcinoma, not otherwise specified, which makes up 75%–80% of invasive breast cancers. Infiltrating lobular carcinomas and other uncommon subtypes make up the majority of the remaining 20% of histologies.

The most important risk factors for breast cancer are gender and age. Women are 100 times more likely than men to develop breast cancer. The median age at diagnosis is 61 years, and approximately 66% of cases are diagnosed in women age 55 years and older (Siegel et al. 2013). The risk for breast cancer increases with age. There are many other risk factors, including reproductive factors such as early menarche and late menopause, nulliparity, or delaying childbirth until after age 30; family or personal history of breast cancer; history of chest wall radiation; increased breast tissue density; history of proliferative breast disease, particularly with atypia; use of exogenous estrogens; and race (lower incidence in Asian Americans than in whites and blacks). Among patients with a particularly strong family history, inherited genetic mutations in the breast cancer susceptibility gene *BRCA1* or *BRCA2* confer a high lifetime risk of breast cancer. With the exception of gender and age, most people diagnosed with breast cancer do not have other identifiable risk factors.

The independent prognostic factors for breast cancer include tumor size and nodal status (both determine the cancer stage), histological grade, the presence or absence of hormone receptors, and human epidermal growth factor receptor 2 gene (*HER2*) amplification or protein overexpression. Over 90% of patients are diagnosed with early-stage disease—that is, breast cancer confined to the breast (over 60%) or involving the regional lymph nodes (over 30%). Less than 10% of patients with newly diagnosed breast cancer have evidence of distant disease at presentation.

Most of the studies on breast cancer in patients with mental illness report on the incidence of cancer compared to the general population. These are heterogeneous studies in regard to the definition and inclusion of "mental illness," the severity of the condition, and the patient setting. There is no clear consensus regarding a causal or temporally linked association between breast cancer and severe mental illness. Halbreich et al. (1996) evaluated mammograms and charts of 275 female patients over age 40 in a state psychiatric hospital and 928 women of comparable age at a general hospital radiology clinic. They found that the incidence of breast cancer documented by pathology reports among the psychiatric patients was more than 3.5 times that of nonpsychiatric inpatients and 9.5 times the reported incidence in the general population. Similar findings were reported when Catts et al. (2008) performed a meta-analysis on the standardized incidence ratios (SIRs) of cancer in patients with schizophrenia and first-degree relatives and compared the incidence of cancer with that in the general public. Although they found an overall decreased incidence of cancer in patients with schizophrenia and their first-degree relatives compared with the general public, breast cancer rates were significantly increased in females with schizophrenia (SIR 1.12; 95% confidence interval, 1.02–1.23). In contrast, a study by Oksbjerg Dalton et al. (2003) evaluated 7,541 Danish women with schizophrenia and found that the overall relative risk for breast cancer was not higher than in the general population. Finally, a study by Barak et al. (2005) demonstrated a reduced cancer risk in patients with schizophrenia; the SIR was 0.60 for female breast cancer compared with the expected incidence in the age-matched and gender-matched general population.

Several theories regarding the potential protective effect of mental illness on breast cancer have been suggested. One theory is that patients in the hospital for prolonged periods of time are exposed to a better diet and are not permitted to smoke, which may lead to decreasing risk factors for cancer (Fox and Howell 1974). Alternatively, the increased incidence of breast cancer among patients with mental illness has been attributed to hyperprolactinemia, a common side effect of treatment with many antipsychotics, which is particularly associated with the so-called typical agents as well as the atypical antipsychotic risperidone. Hyperprolactinemia has been associated with an increased risk for breast cancer (Halbreich et al. 2003). Patients with mental illness also have increased rates of smoking, alcohol abuse, and low parity, which may modestly increase the risk for breast cancer.

There are limited data on the prognosis of patients with mental illness and specific cancers. Tran et al. (2009) followed 3,470 patients with schizophrenia for 11 years and found a higher risk of mortality by cancer among the patients than expected in the general population. For women, the breast was the most frequent cancer locale.

The prognosis of breast cancer patients with mental illness may potentially be worsened by a delay in diagnosis secondary to decreased attention to symptoms, as well as by treatment challenges, such as drug interactions, lack of capacity, coexisting medical comorbidities, and inadequate compliance with treatment. The overall evidence suggests that such patients are less likely than other groups to receive screening for cancer (Howard et al. 2010). Conversely, some research groups cite increased cancer screening due to constant contact with the health care provider/system (Carney and Jones 2006). It is important for health care providers to conduct appropriate screening tests, to be attentive to the medical care of patients with mental illness, and to provide continued evaluation of their compliance to treatment.

Practical Pointers

- Breast cancer is the most common invasive cancer diagnosed in women and the second leading cause of cancer death.
- The co-occurrence of breast cancer and mental illness has been evaluated in many studies, with conflicting results.
- The prognosis of breast cancer in patients with mental illness may be worse than in the general public.
- It is important for health care providers to conduct appropriate screening tests and to monitor compliance to treatment.

Diagnosis

Breast cancer is initially detected because of a breast mass found on clinical examination or self-examination or because of an abnormality on a screening mammogram. In either case, tissue biopsy for a definitive diagnosis is required (Figure 19–1).

Women can present with the classic characteristics of breast cancer, including a new breast mass or lump that is hard, often painless, and mobile, and that has irregular borders. Other clinical presentations include breast swelling, nipple retraction or discharge, and overlying skin changes such as erythema, thickening, or dimpling (*peau d'orange*). Some patients may have axillary lymphadenopathy that suggests spread to regional lymph nodes. Women presenting with these clinical findings need to undergo diagnostic imaging, including a mammogram and possibly an ultrasound. Depending on the clinical findings, patients may undergo either a fine needle aspiration (FNA) or a core needle biopsy (CNB). FNAs can be done quickly and do not require imaging. However, FNAs require an experienced cytopathologist to make the diagnosis. Because of the scant specimen and the lack of architecture, FNAs often cannot differentiate between noninvasive and invasive cancers. In contrast, CNB often results in a more definitive diagnosis, reduces false-negative sampling, and can differentiate between noninvasive and invasive cancers. If invasive cancer is diagnosed, then the CNB provides enough tissue so that prognostic markers, including histological grade and hormone receptor and *HER2* status, can be determined.

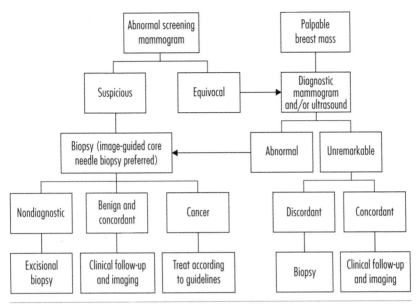

FIGURE 19–1. Breast cancer diagnosis.

Women who present with abnormal imaging findings alone (e.g., have nonpalpable abnormalities) should undergo image-guided biopsy; this procedure is usually done with mammography, although ultrasound or magnetic resonance imaging (MRI) may also be used. Stereotactic CNB is often performed on lesions only seen with mammography and is the standard approach for abnormal calcifications. Ultrasound-guided biopsies can be performed on lesions initially diagnosed with mammography that are also seen on ultrasound, as well as for palpable lesions. If the biopsy result is negative, and there is good correlation between imaging and pathological results, then the patient can be observed with future serial imaging studies. On the other hand, if a patient has a clinically suspicious finding on breast examination, the lesion should be surgically biopsied even if imaging is unremarkable.

Preventive Guidelines

The American Cancer Society (2013) guidelines for early cancer detection are summarized in Table 9–1. High-risk women, who should undergo breast MRI in addition to annual mammograms, include those who have known *BRCA1* and *BRCA2* mutations, who have first-degree relatives with *BRCA1* or *BRCA2* mutations, or who have had radiation therapy to the chest in earlier years.

Not receiving annual screening mammograms appears to be the greatest limitation to early breast cancer detection among the psychiatric population

TABLE 19–1. **Preventive guidelines for breast cancer**

Annual mammograms are recommended beginning at age 40 and
continuing for as long as the woman is in good health.

Clinical breast exams by a health professional are recommended every 3
years starting for women in their 20s and annually for women age 40 or
over.

Breast self-examinations are an option for women in their 20s.

Women at high risk should undergo breast magnetic resonance imaging in
addition to annual mammograms.

Source.   Adapted from American Cancer Society 2013.

(Aggarwal et al. 2013). Although reports are not consistent, the majority of
larger studies report lower rates of breast cancer screening among those
with mental illness. Limitations of these studies include varying population
sizes, definitions of mental illness, and patient settings. In the meta-analysis
by Aggarwal et al. (2013), studies showed that females considered to have
"low-severity mental illness" are more likely to undergo screening tests than
are females without mental illness, due to the former group's close relationship with health care providers. Patients with "severe mental illness" were the
least likely to undergo basic cancer screening tests. Howard et al. (2010) reported that up to 32% of females with mental health conditions do not
undergo screening mammograms. Reasons for noncompliance include lack
of understanding of the susceptibility to develop the disease, lack of access
to annual exams with health care professionals, lack of referral for screening
mammograms by the health care team, and patients' distraction by their
mental illness (Friedman et al. 1999, 2005).

The mental health provider should determine whether a patient is healthy
enough to undergo cancer screening. Furthermore, if an abnormality is
found as a result of screening, the provider must determine whether the patient is able to undergo the necessary diagnostic procedures and possible
systemic therapy. Overcoming the disparities that exist for individuals with
mental illness is an ongoing battle; however, open communication with their
health care providers is the first step in providing appropriate care.

Treatment Recommendations

Treatment of breast cancer often requires a multidisciplinary approach. Options primarily are dependent on the stage of disease (Figure 19–2). Local
disease control can be established with surgery with or without radiation.
Systemic therapy with cytotoxic chemotherapy, endocrine therapy, and/or

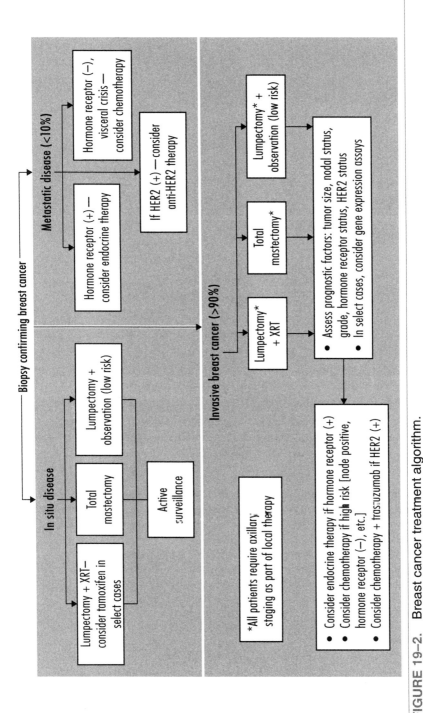

FIGURE 19–2. Breast cancer treatment algorithm.

Note. HER2 = human epidermal receptor 2; XRT = radiation therapy.

targeted biologics may be offered. These treatment decisions are based on multiple factors, including the presence or absence of distant metastatic disease. More than 90% of women present with early-stage disease. In these patients, the independent prognostic factors are tumor size, lymph node positivity, tumor grade, hormone (estrogen or progesterone) receptor status, and HER2 protein overexpression or gene amplification. Tumor gene expression assays may provide further prognostic information in specific patient populations (Paik et al. 2004, 2006). In addition to the tumor characteristics, the overall health of the patient and her willingness or ability to tolerate therapy must be considered.

Treatment decisions are individualized and include local and systemic options. The National Comprehensive Cancer Network (NCCN) provides general guidelines (Gradishar et al. 2014). The following treatment recommendations summarize the authors' approach to localized breast cancer (ductal carcinoma in situ and early-stage invasive breast cancer) and metastatic disease:

1. *Ductal carcinoma in situ:* The goal of treatment is to avoid progression to invasive disease.

   Local therapy: Treatment of choice is generally surgery, either breast-conserving therapy (lumpectomy followed by breast radiation) or total mastectomy.

   Systemic therapy: Tamoxifen, a selective estrogen receptor modulator, can decrease the chance of ipsilateral and contralateral breast cancer recurrence, in either in situ or invasive disease (Fisher et al. 1999). Because the prognosis with in situ disease is excellent, systemic treatment does not reduce overall mortality. The risks and benefits of endocrine therapy should be discussed with a medical oncologist prior to starting therapy.

2. *Invasive breast cancer* (with or without nodal involvement): The goal of treatment is to prevent any local or distant recurrence after surgery by way of "adjuvant" therapy if indicated.

   Local therapy: Disease control must be obtained with surgery, either breast-conserving therapy or total mastectomy (Fisher et al. 2002). With invasive cancer, the lymph node status must also be determined, usually by a sentinel lymph node biopsy or axillary lymph node dissection. A select group of older patients may be treated by lumpectomy alone (Hughes et al. 2004).

   Systemic therapy: Treatment is generally based on the risk of distant recurrence. This risk is determined by the size of the tumor, lymph node involvement, tumor grade, hormone receptor status, and *HER2* status. For select patients, tumor gene assays may provide additional prognostic and predictive information (Paik et al. 2006). Depending on these factors, adjuvant therapy may be recommended.

For women with estrogen and/or progesterone receptor–positive tumors, antihormonal or "endocrine" therapy is offered. Options include 1) selective estrogen receptor modulators (SERMs), such as tamoxifen, for both pre- and postmenopausal females and 2) aromatase inhibitors for postmenopausal women. Other options for premenopausal women include the use of a gonadotropin-releasing hormone agonist or therapeutic oophorectomy. The side-effect profile differs for each endocrine therapy, although the goal of such strategies is to stop estrogen stimulation of potential micrometastases. These antiestrogen effects include hot flashes/flushes and vaginal dryness. Side effects of SERMs also include an increased incidence of venous thromboembolism and endometrial cancer due to selective stimulation of the receptors in these tissues. Aromatase inhibitors are also associated with myalgias, arthralgias, and decreased bone mineral density. Endocrine therapy typically is given for 5 years following surgery, chemotherapy (if administered), and radiation (if administered). Davies et al. (2012) reported a survival benefit for continuing tamoxifen for 10 years rather than stopping at 5 years. These positive data have not been confirmed with aromatase inhibitors.

Patients with high-risk breast cancer may receive adjuvant chemotherapy. Any of the following generally indicate high risk: node positivity, lack of hormone receptors, HER2 positivity, a high grade, or a large tumor. Chemotherapy is generally given for four to six cycles. General side effects are acute, including cytopenias, risk for infection and death, nausea, and fatigue, among others.

Approximately 15% of patients have breast cancers that are HER2 positive, and this population benefits from adjuvant trastuzumab, a monoclonal antibody to HER2 (Romond et al. 2005).

3. *Metastatic disease:* The goal of systemic therapy is not to cure the cancer but rather to improve the patient's quality of life and prolong survival.

Local therapy: There is no proven role for the removal of the primary breast tumor in women who present with distant metastatic disease at the time of diagnosis. Local therapy, including surgery and radiation therapy, may be used to palliate symptoms.

Systemic therapy: For hormone receptor–positive disease, sequential endocrine therapies (e.g., SERMs, aromatase inhibitors, other antiestrogens) are often used. In patients with rapidly symptomatic disease or endocrine-resistant breast cancer, chemotherapy is used. HER2-directed therapies should be used in HER2-positive metastatic breast cancer.

The most common site of metastases is the bones. For patients with osseous involvement, bisphosphonates or a RANK ligand monoclonal antibody, denosumab, is recommended to decrease skeletal-related events. These events include bony pain, need for pain medications and interventions, and progression of bony disease. Both of these medications can lead to rare osteonecrosis of the jaw; therefore, a dental examination is required prior to use.

When to Refer

Situations warranting referral to a primary care provider include the following:

- Nipple discharge
- Breast pain
- Breast cyst or lump
- Persistent breast skin changes
- Strong family history of breast cancer

The patient should be referred to a surgical oncologist/medical oncologist if the biopsy shows any of the following:

- Atypia
- In situ cancer (ductal carcinoma or lobular carcinoma)
- Invasive cancer

Special Treatment Considerations for the Psychiatric Patient Population

There are numerous barriers and challenges for psychiatric patients who are receiving treatment for breast cancer. Cole and Padmanabhan (2012) outline various considerations, such as suboptimal treatment of psychiatric disease, inability to keep scheduled visits, refusal of adjuvant chemotherapy and radiation due to lack of understanding of disease, poor adherence to therapy, and unreliable transportation to and from visits. In addition, patients with severe mental illness are more likely to have other comorbidities, such as cardiovascular disease, pulmonary disease, and obesity, that further complicate treatment, particularly postoperatively (Howard et al. 2010). Regardless of these challenges, these studies comment on the necessity of continuing treatment for mental illness while patients undergo treatment for cancer, although doing so can present additional adverse sequelae.

Psychotropic medications introduce a variety of confounding factors for breast cancer treatment. The role of estrogen therapy in the management of schizophrenia is investigational (Kulkarni et al. 2012). However, the use of antiestrogens is considered for the majority of patients with breast cancer who have hormone receptor–positive disease. Interactions with psychotropic medications and oncological therapies (e.g., chemotherapy, endocrine therapies, antiemetics) can result in adverse side effects. For example, certain antipsychotic medications, such as clozapine, can cause blood dyscrasias; when used in combination with cytotoxic therapy, these medications can lead to profound myelosuppression, causing life-threatening infections. Other examples include pharmacodynamic interactions between antiemetics and psychotropic medications, both of which independently prolong QT_c, which can lead to ventricular tachycardia. Pharmacokinetic interactions must also be considered, including altered metabolism of oncological therapies due to a psychotropic medication.

These complex interactions must all be carefully considered prior to implementing a treatment plan, underscoring the need for close collaboration between the treating oncologist and the psychiatric health care provider.

Case Discussion (*continued*)

Ms. G has a diagnostic mammogram, which reveals a highly suspicious 2.5-cm spiculated mass in her right breast. An ultrasound confirms a hypoechoic mass, and ultrasound-guided core biopsy reveals an intermediate-grade invasive ductal carcinoma that is estrogen and progesterone receptor positive and *HER2* nonamplified.

Her psychiatrist appropriately refers Ms. G to a surgical oncologist, who discusses surgical options. The patient initially defers any type of surgery but eventually agrees to a lumpectomy and sentinel lymph node biopsy after involving her psychiatric care team. Pathology reveals a 2.2-cm tumor and negative lymph nodes. Ms. G subsequently sees medical oncology to discuss adjuvant therapy recommendations. Cytotoxic chemotherapy is not recommended. Because her tumor is hormone receptor positive and she is postmenopausal, Ms. G is advised to start 5 years of aromatase inhibitor therapy. Postlumpectomy radiation therapy is also recommended, and she is referred to a radiation oncologist.

Initially, Ms. G is very cautious of additional therapy due to issues with transportation and fear of side effects and complications with proposed treatment. A multidisciplinary meeting is held with Ms. G's psychiatrist and medical oncologist to better explain the risks and benefits of further treatment. A social worker provides additional support options. Pharmacists thoroughly review the patient's medications to confirm that there will be no interactions with her antipsychotics. Ms. G agrees to a trial of the aromatase inhibitor and to radiation therapy. She will see her medical oncologist at 3- to 6-month intervals while on therapy, and will continue to see her mental health care team regularly.

Clinical Highlights

- Annual screening mammograms are recommended for women age 40 and over as long as good health is maintained.
- Women with mental health problems are often underscreened for breast cancer.
- Treatment options vary according to extent of disease. Most women are diagnosed with early-stage disease.
- General treatment strategies may include surgery, radiation, chemotherapy, and/or endocrine therapy.
- Treatment can be significantly complicated due to psychiatric disease, and treatment plans should be reviewed and discussed with all health care providers involved with the patient's care.

Resources

For Patients

American Cancer Society: http://www.cancer.org
Susan G. Komen for the Cure: http://www.komen.org

For Clinicians

American Cancer Society: http://www.cancer.org
National Comprehensive Cancer Network: http://www.nccn.org

References

Aggarwal A, Pandurangi A, Smith W: Disparities in breast and cervical cancer screening in women with mental illness: a systematic literature review. Am J Prev Med 44:392–398, 2013

American Cancer Society: American Cancer Society Guidelines for the Early Detection of Cancer. Atlanta, GA, American Cancer Society, May 3, 2013. Available at: http://www.cancer.org/healthy/findcancerearly/cancerscreeningguidelines/american-cancer-society-guidelines-for-the-early-detection-of-cancer. Accessed February 27, 2014.

Barak Y, Achiron A, Mandel M, et al: Reduced cancer incidence among patients with schizophrenia. Cancer 104:2817–2821, 2005

Carney CP, Jones LE: The influence of type and severity of mental illness on receipt of screening mammography. J Gen Intern Med 21:1097–1104, 2006

Catts VS, Catts SV, O'Toole BI, et al: Cancer incidence in patients with schizophrenia and their first-degree relatives—a meta-analysis. Acta Psychiatr Scand 117:323–336, 2008

Cole M, Padmanabhan A: Breast cancer treatment of women with schizophrenia and bipolar disorder from Philadelphia, PA: lessons learned and suggestions for improvement. J Cancer Educ 27:774–779, 2012

Davies C, Pan H, Godwin J, et al: Long-term effects of continuing adjuvant tamoxifen to 10 years versus stopping at 5 years after diagnosis of oestrogen receptor-positive breast cancer: ATLAS, a randomised trial. Lancet 381:805–816, 2012

Fisher B, Dignam J, Wolmark N, et al: Tamoxifen in treatment of intraductal breast cancer: National Surgical Adjuvant Breast and Bowel Project B-24 randomised controlled trial. Lancet 353:1993–2000, 1999

Fisher B, Anderson S, Bryant J, et al: Twenty-year follow-up of a randomized trial comparing total mastectomy, lumpectomy, and lumpectomy plus irradiation for the treatment of invasive breast cancer. N Engl J Med 347:1233–1241, 2002

Fox BH, Howell MA: Cancer risk among psychiatric patients: a hypothesis. Int J Epidemiol 3:207–208, 1974

Friedman LC, Moore A, Webb JA, et al: Breast cancer screening among ethnically diverse low-income women in a general hospital psychiatry clinic. Gen Hosp Psychiatry 21:374–381, 1999

Friedman LC, Puryear LJ, Moore A, et al: Breast and colorectal cancer screening among low-income women with psychiatric disorders. Psychooncology 14:786–791, 2005

Gradishar WJ, Anderson BO, Blair SL, et al: Breast cancer version 3.2014. J Natl Compr Canc Netw 12(4):542–590, 2014

Halbreich U, Shen J, Panaro V: Are chronic psychiatric patients at increased risk for developing breast cancer? Am J Psychiatry 153:559–560, 1996

Halbreich U, Kinon BJ, Gilmore JA, et al: Elevated prolactin levels in patients with schizophrenia: mechanisms and related adverse effects. Psychoneuroendocrinology 28(suppl):53–67, 2003

Hayes DF: Atlas of Breast Cancer, 2nd Edition. Maryland Heights, MO, Mosby, 2000

Howard LM, Barley EA, Davies E, et al: Cancer diagnosis in people with severe mental illness: practical and ethical issues. Lancet Oncol 11:797–804, 2010

Hughes KS, Schnaper LA, Berry D, et al: Lumpectomy plus tamoxifen with or without irradiation in women 70 years of age or older with early breast cancer. N Engl J Med 351:971–977, 2004

Kulkarni J, Gavrilidis E, Worsley R, et al: Role of estrogen treatment in the management of schizophrenia. CNS Drugs 26:549–557, 2012

Oksbjerg Dalton S, Munk Laursen T, Mellemkjaer L, et al: Schizophrenia and the risk for breast cancer. Schizophr Res 62:89–92, 2003

Paik S, Shak S, Tang G, et al: A multigene assay to predict recurrence of tamoxifen treated, node-negative breast cancer. N Engl J Med 351:2817–2826, 2004

Paik S, Tang G, Shak S, et al: Gene expression and benefit of chemotherapy in women with node-negative, estrogen receptor–positive breast cancer. J Clin Oncol 24:3726–3734, 2006

Romond EH, Perez EA, Bryant J, et al: Trastuzumab plus adjuvant chemotherapy for operable HER2-positive breast cancer. N Engl J Med 353:1673–1684, 2005

Siegel R, Naishadham D, Jemal A: Cancer statistics, 2013. CA Cancer J Clin 63:11–30, 2013

Tran E, Rouillon F, Loze JY, et al: Cancer mortality in patients with schizophrenia: an 11-year prospective cohort study. Cancer 115:3555–3562, 2009

CHAPTER 20

Prostate Cancer

Zachary Holt, M.D., F.A.C.P.

Case Discussion

Mr. L, a 52-year-old black man with schizoaffective disorder, presents for psychiatric follow-up. He has contact with no other health care providers. Near the conclusion of the visit, he brings up that his grandfather, age 96, recently died of metastatic prostate cancer. Mr. L has no lower urinary tract symptoms but seems quite anxious about the possibility of having prostate cancer.

Clinical Overview

Prostate cancer is the second most common malignancy diagnosed in men, after nonmelanoma skin cancer. An estimated 238,590 new cases of prostate cancer occur per year. It is the second most common cause of cancer death, after lung cancer. Prostate cancer is a disease of age. One in six men will develop prostate cancer, with the risk of invasive prostate cancer rising in each successive decade of life (Siegel et al. 2013). Additionally, roughly half of men have occult prostate cancer at the time of their death (Delongchamps et al. 2006). Despite its large prevalence, the annual death rate from prostate cancer is low (Mohler et al. 2013). Men with prostate cancer confined to the organ at diagnosis can expect a nearly 100% rate survival at 5 years, whereas those with distant metastases have only a 29.3% survival rate (Howlader et al. 2013).

Excluding age, risk factors for prostate cancer include African American ethnicity (Platz et al. 2000); family history (Bruner et al. 2003); *BRCA1* or *BRCA2* mutation (Risch et al. 2006; Thompson and Easton 2002); Lynch syndrome (Raymond et al. 2013); and, to a lesser extent, diet (Chan et al. 2005), insulin resistance (Albanes et al. 2009), and obesity (Stewart and Freedland 2011). Perhaps of particular importance to psychiatric care is the increased risk of prostate cancer in veterans exposed to Agent Orange (Chamie et al. 2008). Because mortality is higher among individuals with psychiatric illness, incidence estimates of prostate cancer in this population have skewed toward younger patients. However, one large retrospective study suggested that the incidence of prostate cancer is lower in patients with schizophrenia. This may be due to the relatively low percentage of older patients with schizophrenia (Lin et al. 2013). Other data show no significant difference between psychiatric patients and control subjects but suggest a similar trend (Hippisley-Cox et al. 2007). A high cumulative dose of phenothiazine may be protective against prostate cancer (Mortensen 1992).

Patients who receive a diagnosis of prostate cancer are vulnerable to developing psychiatric conditions. Clinicians are advised to keep this in mind as their patients proceed through workup and treatment. One study found that up to 4.3% of patients with prostate cancer develop posttraumatic stress disorder (Mehnert et al. 2010).

Practical Pointers

- Prostate cancer may be less common in patients with schizophrenia, but risk assessment for prostate cancer should be the same as it is in patients without mental illness, given the dearth of prostate cancer data in older patients with schizophrenia.
- Prostate-specific antigen (PSA)–based screening for prostate cancer should not be routinely offered to patients with severe mental illness.
- If prostate cancer is diagnosed in a person with psychiatric illness, he should be followed closely by his mental health team.

Diagnosis

Diagnosis of prostate cancer is made by transrectal biopsy of the prostate, usually in response to an elevated PSA level or abnormality on digital rectal examination (DRE). Despite the current controversy about prostate cancer screening, the majority of men who undergo prostate biopsy do so because of an elevated PSA level obtained for screening purposes (Hodgson et al. 2012).

Early prostate cancer is often asymptomatic. Symptoms may include nocturia and urination frequency, urgency, and hesitancy (Abrams et al. 2009);

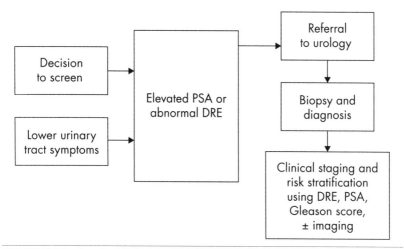

FIGURE 20–1. Prostate cancer diagnosis.

Note. DRE = digital rectal examination; PSA = prostate-specific antigen.

hematuria (Cohen and Brown 2003); and hemospermia (Ahmad and Krishna 2007). Patients with advanced disease may have bladder outlet obstruction or painful metastases. A patient with these symptoms should undergo DRE and, in close discussion with his primary provider, may undergo PSA testing (Abrams et al. 2009) (Figure 20–1).

The traditional cutoff for an abnormal PSA test is 4.0 ng/mL, denoting a positive likelihood ratio of 2.3 for any prostate cancer and 5.6 for high-grade carcinoma. Lowering the cutoff point increases sensitivity but increases false-positive rates, owing to other conditions that can also create an elevated PSA, including benign prostatic hyperplasia and prostatitis (Wolf et al. 2010). There is no PSA value below which a patient can be assured of not having prostate cancer. Some authors suggest using other PSA-derived methods, such as PSA concentration or velocity, or age-adjusted PSA cutoff points; these methods are not standard of care and are not discussed in this chapter.

Any patient with an abnormal PSA test or DRE should be referred to a urologist for discussion of a transrectal ultrasound-guided biopsy. Biopsy specimens positive for carcinoma are assigned a Gleason score based on histological characteristics. Patients next undergo stratification into a risk group based on anatomic stage, Gleason score, and PSA level. Risk in this context is that of recurrence. Risk strata include the following (Mohler et al. 2013):

- Clinically localized disease, further divided into the following:
    Very low risk
    Low risk
    Intermediate risk
    High risk

- Clinically locally advanced disease
- Metastatic disease

Initial risk stratification following diagnosis is important, because it informs clinicians and their patients which treatment options are reasonable. We strongly advise that any psychiatrists or related primary medical providers who make a diagnosis of prostate cancer, even if it is seemingly very low risk, refer the patient to a urology practice or cancer center. That said, there is evidence that primary care physicians who remain involved in the care of their cancer patients can have a beneficial impact (Jang et al. 2010). This is of particular importance for psychiatric patients.

Screening

Although PSA was initially developed as a tumor marker for use after prostate cancer treatment, primary care physicians have also used it for prostate cancer screening. This usage has led to a significant increase in the diagnosis of prostate cancer, primarily due to the detection of early-stage disease. This practice, however, is unsupported by evidence (Brett and Ablin 2011).

Two trials published in 2009 further complicated the issue. A large European trial demonstrated a reduction in prostate cancer mortality in subjects who underwent screening, but indicated that 1,410 patients would have to be screened and 48 prostate cancers treated to prevent just one death from prostate cancer (Schroder et al. 2009). A U.S. study published the same year showed no mortality benefit due to screening (Andriole et al. 2009). Although considerable controversy remains, the U.S. Preventive Services Task Force has recommended against screening for prostate cancer with PSA, citing the many harms of overdiagnosis (Moyer 2012), with others cautiously supporting a shared decision-making approach. Recommendations from several large organizations are summarized in Figure 20–2.

Psychiatric illness adversely affects the likelihood of screening. Patients with depression are less likely to be screened than nondepressed patients. Patients with anxiety are more likely to be screened than nonanxious patients, and how much more they are screened is proportionate to the number of their office visits (Kotwal et al. 2012).

The basic points of prostate cancer screening could be summarized as follows:

1. PSA-based screening for prostate cancer does lead to the early detection of prostate cancer and likely reduces mortality related to prostate cancer, albeit to a small degree.

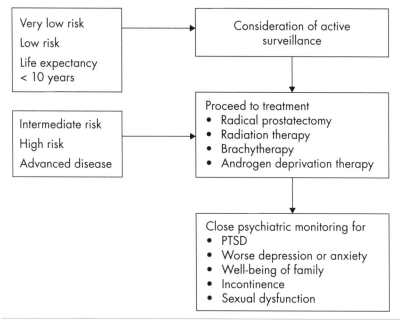

FIGURE 20–2. Prostate cancer treatment in patients with psychiatric illness (simplified).

Note. PTSD = posttraumatic stress disorder.

2. A significant number of prostate cancers detected by screening will not be fatal, or even symptomatic during the life of the patient.
3. The treatment of early prostate cancer can cause harm to the patient.

For patients with mental illness, I recommend that mental health professionals 1) do not routinely offer PSA-based screening for prostate cancer to average-risk individuals and 2) have a thorough risk-benefit discussion with individuals at increased risk. This position is based on the potential for further accrual of psychiatric illness due to overdiagnosis and the aggressive treatment of low-risk cancers (see later section "Treatment Recommendations").

Some patients may be candidates for chemoprevention of prostate cancer with 5α-reductase inhibitors (e.g., finasteride). Although the overall incidence of prostate cancer seems to be reduced by these agents, some data suggest that they may encourage the development of high-grade carcinoma. Additionally, they cause significant side effects (Kramer et al. 2009). Because there is no definitive information regarding chemoprevention, a decision to proceed should be based on a complete discussion of risks and benefits with the patient.

Preventive Guidelines

- *U.S. Preventive Services Task Force:* Do not use PSA-based screening for prostate cancer (Moyer 2012).
- *American Cancer Society:* Discuss risks and benefits of screening starting at age 50, or at age 40–45 in patients with increased risk. Do not screen patients with a life expectancy of less than 10 years. Screening is PSA testing with or without DRE every 1–2 years (Wolf et al. 2010).
- *American Urological Association:* Discuss risks and benefits of screening with patients ages 55–69 who are at average risk, and starting at age 40 with patients who are at high risk. Do not screen patients before age 40, patients age 70 or older, or patients with a life expectancy of less than 10 years. Screening involves PSA testing every 2 years (Carter et al. 2013).
- *American College of Physicians:* Discuss risks and benefits of screening from age 50 through 69 for patients at average risk. Screening involves PSA testing every 1–4 years depending on the PSA level (Qaseem et al. 2013).

Treatment Recommendations

All patients with a diagnosis of prostate cancer should be referred to a specialist for ongoing management. However, it behooves psychiatrists and other primary care providers to be aware of the basics of treatment guidelines so they may provide timely input.

Several guidelines for the treatment of prostate cancer exist. The recommendations in this chapter are based on those of the National Comprehensive Cancer Network (Mohler et al. 2013), which place emphasis on avoiding overtreatment, a consideration that is important in the psychiatric population.

Patients who have a limited life expectancy (less than 20 years for those with very low risk and less than 10 years for those with low or intermediate risk), or who have a longer life expectancy and have very low risk or low risk, are candidates for active surveillance, which includes monitoring PSA levels at short intervals and repeated DREs and prostate biopsies to monitor for disease progression. Patients in this category who elect to receive treatment may proceed to external beam radiation therapy, brachytherapy, or radical prostatectomy. Patients at higher risk are candidates for androgen deprivation therapy (ADT).

Prostatectomy and radiation therapy may lead to troubling complications, including bladder or bowel incontinence and sexual dysfunction (Wilt et al. 2008). The psychological effects of these adverse events cannot be understated, and the burden is felt by both patients and their families. Patients who experience psychological effects benefit from the involvement of mental health professionals (De Sousa et al. 2012).

When to Refer

Situations warranting referral to a primary care provider include the following:

* The patient has just been diagnosed with prostate cancer.
* The patient has significant medical comorbidities.
* The patient is undergoing active surveillance for low-risk prostate cancer.
* The patient has been treated for prostate cancer by surgery or radiation therapy.
* The patient is undergoing current treatment with ADT.

Special Treatment Considerations for the Psychiatric Patient Population

Psychiatric comorbidities are an important consideration during prostate cancer treatment. Patients with depression and prostate cancer are older, more likely to be single, more likely to live in urban settings, more likely to be diagnosed at a later stage, more likely to have undergone radical prostatectomy, more likely to use medical resources, and more likely to die (Jayadevappa et al. 2012). Depression has a higher incidence in patients diagnosed with prostate cancer, with anhedonia being the most prominent symptom (Sharpley et al. 2013).

Patients receiving ADT may experience new or worsening depression, although this may be confounded by the worse prognosis for these patients who are candidates for ADT (Van Tol-Geerdink et al. 2011). A recent trial found no additional risk of depression in patients receiving ADT, but the sample size was small. Until further studies become available, ADT should be viewed as a risk factor for mood disturbance (Hervouet et al. 2013).

Treatment of depression in patients with prostate cancer is similar to that in the general population. Selective serotonin reuptake inhibitors have benefit, as does cognitive-behavioral therapy (Williams and Dale 2006). Patients with advanced prostate cancer, depression, and appetite disturbances may find relief with mirtazapine (Theobald et al. 2002). Patients with depression and end-stage prostate cancer are candidates for psychostimulants (Fernandez et al. 1987).

Case Discussion (*continued*)

On further questioning by his psychiatrist, Mr. L reveals that both of his brothers were diagnosed with prostate cancer in their 40s. After a careful discussion of the risks and benefits of PSA testing, the patient elects to undergo screening for prostate cancer, whereupon he is found to have a PSA of 6. He undergoes biopsy by a community urologist and is found to have low-risk prostate cancer. Mr. L establishes care with a local primary care physician, and in close consultation with his team at the cancer center he begins active surveillance.

Clinical Highlights

- Prostate cancer is a disease of aging. Other risk factors include genetic, lifestyle, and environmental factors, including exposure to Agent Orange.
- Screening for prostate cancer is not recommended in average-risk individuals who have significant psychiatric disease.
- Individuals at increased risk for prostate cancer or those with lower urinary symptoms may undergo prostate-specific antigen (PSA) testing after a careful risk-benefit discussion.
- Patients with an abnormal PSA test or digital rectal exam (DRE) should be referred to urology for biopsy.
- Patients who are diagnosed with prostate cancer should be referred to a primary care physician in addition to a cancer specialist.
- Patients who undergo treatment for prostate cancer should continue close psychiatric monitoring.

Resources

For Patients

American Cancer Society: http://www.cancer.org

For Clinicians

National Comprehensive Cancer Network: http://www.nccn.org
UpToDate: http://www.uptodate.com

References

Abrams P, Chapple C, Khoury S, et al: Evaluation and treatment of lower urinary tract symptoms in older men. J Urol 181:1779–1787, 2009

Ahmad I, Krishna N: Hemospermia. J Urol 177:1613–1618, 2007

Albanes D, Weinstein SJ, Wright ME, et al: Serum insulin, glucose, indices of insulin resistance, and risk of prostate cancer. J Natl Cancer Inst 101:1272–1279, 2009

Andriole GL, Crawford ED, Grubb RL 3rd, et al: Mortality results from a randomized prostate-cancer screening trial. N Engl J Med 360:1310–1319, 2009

Brett A, Ablin R: Prostate-cancer screening—what the U.S. Preventive Services Task Force left out. N Engl J Med 365:1949–1951, 2011

Bruner DW, Moore D, Parlanti A, et al: Relative risk of prostate cancer for men with affected relatives: systematic review and meta-analysis. Int J Cancer 107:797–803, 2003

Carter HB, Albertsen PC, Barry MJ, et al: Early Detection of Prostate Cancer: AUA Guideline. Linthicum, MD, American Urological Association, April 2013. Available at: http://www.auanet.org/education/guidelines/prostate-cancer-detection.cfm. Accessed July 20, 2013.

Chamie K, DeVere White RW, Lee D, et al: Agent Orange exposure, Vietnam War veterans, and the risk of prostate cancer. Cancer 113:2464–2470, 2008

Chan J, Gann P, Giovannucci E: Role of diet in prostate cancer development and progression. J Clin Oncol 23:8152–8160, 2005

Cohen R, Brown R: Clinical practice. Microscopic hematuria. N Engl J Med 348:2330–2338, 2003

Delongchamps N, Singh A, Haas G: The role of prevalence in the diagnosis of prostate cancer. Cancer Control 13:158–168, 2006

De Sousa A, Sonavane S, Mehta J: Psychological aspects of prostate cancer: a clinical review. Prostate Cancer Prostatic Dis 15:120–127, 2012

Fernandez F, Adams F, Holmes VF, et al: Methylphenidate for depressive disorders in cancer patients. An alternative to standard antidepressants. Psychosomatics 28:455–461, 1987

Hervouet S, Savard J, Ivers H, et al: Depression and androgen deprivation therapy for prostate cancer: a prospective controlled study. Health Psychol 32:675–684, 2013

Hippisley-Cox J, Vinogradova Y, Coupland C, et al: Risk of malignancy in patients with schizophrenia or bipolar disorder: nested case-control study. Arch Gen Psychiatry 64:1368–1376, 2007

Hodgson F, Obertova Z, Brown C, et al: PSA testing in general practice. J Prim Health Care 4:199–204, 2012

Howlader N, Noone AM, Krapcho M, et al: SEER Cancer Statistics Review, 1975–2010. Bethesda, MD, National Cancer Institute, June 14, 2013. Available at: http://seer.cancer.gov/csr/1975_2010. Accessed July 27, 2013.

Jang TL, Bekelman JE, Liu Y, et al: Physician visits prior to treatment for clinically localized prostate cancer. Arch Intern Med 170:440–450, 2010

Jayadevappa R, Malkowicz SB, Chhatre S, et al: The burden of depression in prostate cancer. Psychooncology 21:1338–1345, 2012

Kotwal AA, Schumm P, Mohile SG, et al: The influence of stress, depression, and anxiety on PSA screening rates in a nationally representative sample. Med Care 50:1037–1044, 2012

Kramer BS, Hagerty KL, Justman S, et al: Use of 5-alpha-reductase inhibitors for prostate cancer chemoprevention: American Society of Clinical Oncology/American Urological Association 2008 Clinical Practice Guideline. J Clin Oncol 27:1502–1516, 2009

Lin CY, Lane HY, Chen TT, et al: Inverse association between cancer risks and age in schizophrenic patients: a 12-year nationwide cohort study. Cancer Sci 104:383–390, 2013

Mehnert A, Lehmann C, Graefen M, et al: Depression, anxiety, post-traumatic stress disorder and health-related quality of life and its association with social support in ambulatory prostate cancer patients. Eur J Cancer Care (Engl) 19:736–745, 2010

Mohler J, Armstrong A, Bahnson R: National Comprehensive Cancer Network Guidelines Version 3.2013: Prostate Cancer. Ft. Washington, PA, National Comprehensive Cancer Network, 2013. Available at: http://www.nccn.org/professionals/physician_gls/f_guidelines.asp#prostate. Accessed July 20, 2013.

Mortensen PB: Neuroleptic medication and reduced risk of prostate cancer in schizophrenic patients. Acta Psychiatr Scand 85:390–393, 1992

Moyer VA: Screening for prostate cancer: U.S. Preventive Services Task Force recommendation statement. Ann Intern Med 157:120–134, 2012

Platz EA, Rimm EB, Willett WC, et al: Racial variation in prostate cancer incidence and in hormonal system markers among male health professionals. J Natl Cancer Inst 92:2009–2017, 2000

Qaseem A, Barry MJ, Denberg TD, et al: Screening for prostate cancer: a guidance statement from the Clinical Guidelines Committee of the American College of Physicians. Ann Intern Med 158:761–769, 2013

Raymond VM, Mukherjee B, Wang F, et al: Elevated risk of prostate cancer among men with Lynch syndrome. J Clin Oncol 31:1713–1718, 2013

Risch HA, McLaughlin JR, Cole DE, et al: Population BRCA1 and BRCA2 mutation frequencies and cancer penetrances: a kin-cohort study in Ontario, Canada. J Natl Cancer Inst 98:1694–1706, 2006

Schroder FH, Hugosson J, Roobol MJ, et al: Screening and prostate-cancer mortality in a randomized European study. N Engl J Med 360:1320–1328, 2009

Sharpley CF, Bitsika V, Christie DR: The incidence and causes of different subtypes of depression in prostate cancer patients: implications for cancer care. Eur J Cancer Care (Engl) 22:815–823, 2013

Siegel R, Naishadham D, Jemal A: Cancer statistics, 2013. CA Cancer J Clin 63:11–30, 2013

Stewart SB, Freedland SJ: Influence of obesity on the incidence and treatment of genitourinary malignancies. Urol Oncol 29:476–486, 2011

Theobald DE, Kirsch KL, Holtsclaw E, et al: An open-label, crossover trial of mirtazapine (15 and 30 mg) in cancer patients with pain and other distressing symptoms. J Pain Symptom Manage 23:442–447, 2002

Thompson D, Easton DF: Cancer incidence in BRCA1 mutation carriers. J Natl Cancer Inst 94:1358–1365, 2002

Van Tol-Geerdink JJ, Leer JW, van Lin EN, et al: Depression related to (neo)adjuvant hormonal therapy for prostate cancer. Radiother Oncol 98:203–206, 2011

Williams S, Dale J: The effectiveness of treatment for depression/depressive symptoms in adults with cancer: a systematic review. Br J Cancer 94:372–390, 2006

Wilt T, MacDonald R, Rutks I, et al: Systematic review: comparative effectiveness and harms of treatments for clinically localized prostate cancer. Ann Intern Med 148:435–448, 2008

Wolf AM, Wender RC, Etzioni RB, et al: American Cancer Society guideline for the early detection of prostate cancer: update 2010. CA Cancer J Clin 60:70–98, 2010

CHAPTER 21

Lung Cancer

Craig R. Keenan, M.D.

Case Discussion

Mr. N is a 48-year-old white man with schizophrenia (since age 18), hypertension, and tobacco abuse who presents for follow-up for his medications. His mother was just diagnosed with lung cancer, and Mr. N wonders if he should have a chest X ray. He has no new symptoms and denies shortness of breath, wheezing, chest pain, or hemoptysis. He smokes two packs of cigarettes per day and has done so for 30 years. He takes risperidone, lisinopril, and aspirin. He does not drink alcohol or use illicit substances. He is single and lives with his brother. On physical examination, his blood pressure is 130/78 mmHg and oxygen saturation on room air is 98%. His lungs are clear to auscultation and percussion, and the remainder of his examination is normal.

Clinical Overview

Lung cancer is the leading cancer killer in the United States, accounting for as many deaths in 2012 as the next three most common cancers combined. It is the second most common cancer in both men and women, and the number one killer in both. The American Cancer Society estimates that over 283,000 new lung cancer diagnoses and approximately 159,000 deaths occurred in 2013. Although new diagnoses and deaths have been declining along with smoking rates, lung cancer remains one of the most common and lethal cancers (American Cancer Society 2013).

Lung cancer has one of the worst survival rates after diagnosis among the common cancers. The 5-year survival rate is only 16.3%, compared with 62.5% for colon cancer and 90% for breast cancer. If lung cancer is detected while still localized to the lungs, the survival rate is higher (52.6%). Unfortunately, only 15% of lung cancer cases are diagnosed at such an early stage (American Lung Association 2012).

Lung cancer refers to cancers of the airways or pulmonary parenchyma. Ninety-five percent of these cancers are classified as either small cell lung cancer (SCLC) or non–small cell (squamous cell, bronchoalveolar, adenocarcinoma, large cell) lung cancer (NSCLC), whereas 5% are other rarer cell types. This classification is critical for staging and treatment, and this chapter is limited to discussion of SCLC and NSCLC. Overall, NSCLC accounts for about 75%–80% of cancers, whereas SCLC accounts for 14% (Jett et al. 2013; Rivera et al. 2013).

The most important risk factor for lung cancer by far is cigarette smoking. It is estimated to account for 90% of all lung cancers, and it increases the risk of lung cancer by 20-fold over that of nonsmokers. Cigar and pipe smoking also increase the risk but to a lesser degree. Marijuana smoking has not been definitively associated with lung cancer. Secondhand tobacco smoke exposure increases the risk by about 20%–30% in nonsmokers who live with a smoker. The second leading cause of lung cancer is thought to be radiation exposure from radon gas released from soil and building materials. Asbestos is also a well-established risk factor for lung cancer. Cigarette smoking in conjunction with asbestos and radon exposure leads to synergistic effects and significant increases in lung cancer risk. Exposures to air pollution, tar, soot, arsenic, chromium, nickel, and radiation (e.g., radiation therapy, uranium mining) all increase lung cancer risk. Male sex, older age, acquired lung diseases (e.g., emphysema, pulmonary fibrosis, tuberculosis), HIV infection, and a family history of lung cancer portend an increased risk, whereas fruit intake and moderate to high physical activity are associated with lower lung cancer risk (Alberg et al. 2013). Lung cancer occurs more frequently in poorer and less educated populations; this is felt to be due to the higher rates of smoking and environmental or occupational exposures in these populations. Patients with mental illness are more likely to be in these low socioeconomic groups.

The prognosis for patients with lung cancer is highly dependent on its type and stage (Table 21–1). For NSCLC, survival rate in stage I disease is relatively high but falls precipitously at higher stages. For SCLC, limited-stage disease has a modest 5-year survival rate, whereas extensive-stage disease is almost uniformly fatal by 5 years (Jett et al. 2013; Ramnath et al. 2013).

Little research is available on the incidence of lung cancer or its prognosis in patients with mental illness. Given the higher rates of cigarette smoking in this population, increased lung cancer rates would be expected. Since

TABLE 21–1. **Prognosis in lung cancer: 5-year survival**

Cancer stage	5-year survival rate
Non–small cell lung cancer	
Stage I	60%–80%
Stage II	30%–50%
Stage IIIA	16%
Stage IIIB	3%–7%
Stage IV	2%
Small cell lung cancer	
Limited stage	20%–25%
Extensive stage	0%

the early 1900s, there have been observations of lower cancer incidence in patients with schizophrenia, but this has not been a consistent finding, with some studies finding an increase in rates. Specific to lung cancer, some studies have shown an increase in lung cancer incidence in patients with schizophrenia, whereas others have shown a lower incidence (Barak et al. 2005; Hippisley-Cox et al. 2007; Lichtermann et al. 2001). In a prospective cohort of French patients with schizophrenia, Tran et al. (2009) found a twofold increase in lung cancer mortality in men. Studies of the effects of mental illness on lung cancer are often limited by the inability to account for major potential confounders, especially smoking. Catts et al. (2008) performed a meta-analysis and reported on the standardized incidence ratio (SIR) of cancer (including lung and other cancers) in patients with schizophrenia. In the unadjusted analysis for lung cancer, the SIR was 1.31, indicating an increased risk of lung cancer in these patients compared with the general population. However, with adjustment for smoking rates, the SIR was 0.69, indicating a possible protective effect for schizophrenia. This meta-analysis is limited by significant heterogeneity in the studies. Thus, the data are conflicting as to the effect of schizophrenia on lung cancer.

Studies of the effect of depression on cancer, and lung cancer specifically, have shown disparate results. One Finnish cohort study found that "depressiveness scores," but not clinical depression, were associated with a higher incidence of lung cancer (Knekt et al. 1996). A U.S. cohort study found that depressed mood was associated with cancer development in current smokers but not in nonsmokers (Linkins and Comstock 1990). Patients with depression have higher smoking rates, increased smoking intensity, and lower propensity to quit, and these higher-risk behaviors may be the cause behind the increased cancer rates, rather than the biological effects of the depression itself.

Several researchers have shown that patients with severe mental illness are less likely to get recommended cancer screening, but others have not (Howard et al. 2010). Notably, none of these studies included lung cancer screening. With the new recommendations for lung cancer screening, however, low screening rates in this high-risk, smoking population may be an issue.

Practical Pointers

- Lung cancer is the leading cause of cancer death in men and women.
- Cigarette smoking, which has higher rates in persons with mental illness, is the key risk factor for lung cancer, accounting for 90% of lung cancers.
- Patients with schizophrenia may have a lower risk of cancer compared to the general population; however, patients with depression or schizophrenia may have a higher incidence of lung cancer, especially if they are smokers. Thus, they are prime targets for intensive smoking cessation interventions.
- Lung cancer preventive care primarily is through 1) identifying smokers and helping them to quit (primary prevention), 2) screening for lung cancer for early identification (secondary prevention), and 3) surveillance for recurrence of cancer after treatment (tertiary prevention).

Diagnosis

Until recent screening recommendations were published, most lung cancers were diagnosed in symptomatic patients, and about 10% were found incidentally in asymptomatic patients who had chest radiography for other reasons (e.g., preoperative chest X ray) (Beckles et al. 2003). The symptoms and signs of lung cancer are listed in Table 21–2. Usual symptoms include cough, hemoptysis, chest pain, and shortness of breath. Cough is the most common presenting symptom. Hemoptysis is usually only blood-streaked sputum, which should not be ignored in patients with a smoking history. Chest pain may be from the local tumor, pleural invasion, or tumor invasion into the chest wall. Importantly, patients frequently present with nonspecific symptoms, such as anorexia, weight loss, or fatigue, as opposed to symptoms related to the primary tumor. Occasionally, presenting symptoms may be from extrathoracic metastases or paraneoplastic syndromes. Metastatic disease can cause lymphadenopathy; bony pain from bone involvement; headache, nausea, vomiting, and seizures from central nervous system metastases; and

TABLE 21–2. **Symptoms and signs of lung cancer**

From primary tumor

Cough

Dyspnea

Hemoptysis

Chest pain

From intrathoracic spread

Hoarseness (from recurrent laryngeal nerve palsy)

Phrenic nerve paralysis

Pancoast tumor (pain, skin temperature change, muscle wasting)

Horner syndrome (ptosis, miosis, anhidrosis due to sympathetic nerve chain involvement)

Chest pain (from chest wall or pleural invasion)

Pleural effusion

Superior vena cava obstruction (facial swelling, dilated veins on upper torso and arms, headaches)

Pericardial effusion

Dysphagia (from esophageal compression or invasion by tumor or lymphadenopathy)

From distant metastases

Bone pain or fracture

Lymphadenopathy

Abnormal liver function tests, hepatomegaly, weakness (from liver metastases)

Adrenal insufficiency (from adrenal lesions, rarely clinically evident)

Headache, nausea, vomiting, focal neurological deficits (from brain lesions)

Paralysis, bowel or bladder incontinence, sensory loss (from spinal cord compression by metastases)

From paraneoplastic syndromes

Hypercalcemia (from parathyroid-related peptide or bony metastases)

Hyponatremia (from syndrome of inappropriate antidiuretic hormone)

Cushing syndrome (from ectopic adrenocorticotropic hormone secretion)

Neurological syndromes (e.g., mononeuritis multiplex, encephalomyelitis, peripheral neuropathy, Lambert-Eaton myasthenic syndrome)

Source. Adapted from Beckles et al. 2003.

right upper quadrant pain from liver metastases. Paraneoplastic syndromes include hypercalcemia, hyponatremia due to the syndrome of inappropriate antidiuretic hormone, and neurological syndromes, and are more common in SCLC. Physical examination may reveal evidence of mass or pleural effusion (e.g., dullness to percussion, decreased breath sounds), distant metastases (e.g., cervical lymphadenopathy, hepatomegaly, neurological findings), or clubbing of the digits.

A patient with suspected lung cancer is usually first evaluated with a chest radiograph, which may show a mass (>3 cm), nodule (≤3 cm), pleural effusion, or hilar or mediastinal adenopathy. Suspicious lesions on X ray are usually followed up with a chest computed tomography (CT) scan with contrast. The CT scan can better characterize the suspicious lesion, assess for enlarged lymph nodes suspicious for intrathoracic metastases, and determine the extent of disease. Occasionally, positron emission tomography (PET) imaging is also part of the initial diagnostic pathway.

Once a patient is suspected of having lung cancer, the diagnostic process can be complex, but the next step is a tissue diagnosis. This can be done via sputum cytology, thoracentesis of a pleural effusion with pleural fluid cytology, fine-needle aspiration of supraclavicular lymph node or other suspected metastatic site, bronchoscopy with biopsy, transthoracic CT-guided biopsy, or thoracoscopic or open surgical biopsy (Rivera et al. 2013).

After an initial tissue diagnosis, further tests are often done to determine the lung cancer stage. Staging generally involves a thorough physical examination; laboratory tests; possible further imaging with CT, PET, bone scans, and magnetic resonance imaging of the brain; and/or further tissue biopsies used to look for metastatic disease. For SCLC, the most commonly used staging system is the VA Lung Study Group system (Green et al. 1969), which breaks it down into limited stage (LS-SCLC) and extensive stage (ES-SCLC). For NSCLC, the American Joint Committee on Cancer (2010) classification system defining TNM stages I–IV is used.

Preventive Guidelines

Primary prevention of lung cancer should be the key focus; this involves limiting exposures to known risk factors. Of course, the clinician's foremost goal is to counsel and assist patients to quit smoking cigarettes, pipes, and cigars (see Chapter 8, "Tobacco Dependence"). Avoiding secondhand smoke is also important. Limiting exposure to environmental toxins such as asbestos or radon is also recommended. The Environmental Protection Agency (2012) provides recommendations about radon testing and mitigation. Radon levels can be easily and cheaply measured in the home.

Given that lung cancer is so lethal, often presenting at later stages, and is sometimes curable if found in early stages, it has been a hopeful target for secondary prevention by screening. Unfortunately, multiple trials of chest radiography and/or sputum cytology in the 1950s–1970s found no benefit of screening. In 2011, the results of the National Lung Screening Trial using low-dose CT (LDCT) scanning versus chest radiography in more than 50,000 high-risk smokers were published (National Lung Screening Trial Research Team et al. 2011). Results showed that compared to chest radiography, LDCT screening found more cancers in earlier, more treatable stages. Most importantly, the study found a 20% reduction in lung cancer mortality and a 6.7% reduction in overall mortality in the LDCT screening group. This translates to preventing 1 death for every 320 patients screened with CT. Subsequently, many organizations have recommended adopting screening in a similar population, including the American Cancer Society (Wender et al. 2013) and the American Lung Association (2012). The U.S. Preventive Services Task Force has made the following recommendations for lung cancer screening (Moyer 2013):

- Annual LDCT screening for asymptomatic adults ages 55–80 years with a 30 pack-year smoking history and who currently smoke or who have quit within the past 15 years
- Annual screening until the patient has not smoked for 15 years, develops a health problem that significantly limits life expectancy, or is not able or willing to have curative lung surgery

It is important to recognize that potential harms can come with this screening. There is a significant rate of false-positive LDCT results—95% of all positive results do not lead to a cancer diagnosis. Many of these patients get additional imaging, and some undergo invasive procedures with their inherent risks (e.g., pneumothorax). Patients also experience emotional stress from having a suspicious lesion. Another potential risk is radiation, which can cause cancer from cumulative exposure with annual scans. Lastly, screening cannot prevent most lung-cancer related deaths (Moyer 2013).

Tertiary prevention targets patients after diagnosis and treatment of lung cancer to look for recurrences or new primary lung cancers. This care generally involves history taking, physical examination, and chest CT scans every 4–6 months for the first 2 years, then annually thereafter. Smoking cessation is also an important tertiary preventive treatment for these patients.

Chemoprevention with many different agents for primary prevention in smokers and former smokers or for tertiary prevention for patients with lung cancer has not shown benefit. In fact, a randomized trial of β-carotene and vitamin A supplementation in smokers, former smokers, and persons exposed to asbestos showed a 28% increase in lung cancer development (Omenn et al. 1996). There are no currently recommended chemoprevention agents for lung cancer (Szabo et al. 2013).

Treatment Recommendations

The treatment of lung cancer is complex and usually requires a multidisciplinary approach with pulmonologists, thoracic surgeons, medical oncologists, and radiation oncologists. Treatment is very dependent on the type of lung cancer (NSCLC or SCLC) and the stage. Table 21–3 summarizes current treatment approaches.

For NSCLC, patients with stage I or II disease account for about 25%–30% of cases. If at all possible, these patients should undergo surgical resection with curative intent. If a patient cannot tolerate surgical resection, radiation therapy (RT) or radiofrequency ablation are the usual secondary options. After surgery, adjuvant chemotherapy is recommended for patients with completely resected stage II NSCLC. Postoperative RT may be used in patients with stage I or II disease with positive bronchial margins (Howington et al. 2013).

The treatment of stage III NSCLC patients, who account for about 37% of cases, is complex and controversial. No treatments leave a high probability for cure. In general, patients who can tolerate curative therapy undergo surgical resection followed by chemotherapy and RT (Ramnath et al. 2013). For patients with stage III disease who cannot undergo surgical resection due to comorbidities or the extent of disease, chemotherapy and RT are given. Patients with stage IV disease and good performance status get prolonged survival and improved quality of life with chemotherapeutic agents, biological agents, or newer targeted therapies. Early palliative care also improves duration and quality of life in advanced disease. RT may be used for palliative reasons for regional or distant metastases (e.g., bone or brain metastases) (Ramnath et al. 2013; Socinski et al. 2013).

LS-SCLC is treated with systemic chemotherapy plus thoracic RT. Rare patients with minimal disease may be treated with surgical resection prior to chemotherapy. ES-SCLC is treated with systemic chemotherapy. Prophylactic brain irradiation for possible brain metastases is recommended for both groups if they respond to chemotherapy (Jett et al. 2013).

Lastly, smoking cessation is an important treatment target for lung cancer patients. Quitting smoking has immediate benefits, including improvements in mood, sleep, performance status, and appetite, as well as reduced fatigue and shortness of breath. Continuing to smoke is associated with reduced survival time and efficacy of chemotherapy and RT; increased postoperative, chemotherapy, and RT complications; increased risk of second

TABLE 21–3. Summary of treatment for lung cancer

Cancer stage	Treatment
Non–small cell lung cancer	
Stage I	Surgery ± RT
Stage II	Surgery + chemotherapy ± RT
Resectable stage III	Surgery + chemotherapy + RT
Unresectable stage III	Chemotherapy + RT
Stage IV	Chemotherapy or biologics or new targeted therapies
	RT for palliation
Small cell lung cancer	
Limited stage	Chemotherapy + thoracic RT
	Prophylactic TBI if response to therapy
Extended stage	Chemotherapy
	Prophylactic TBI if response to therapy

Note. RT = radiation therapy; TBI = total brain irradiation.

lung cancers; and decreased quality of life (Cataldo et al. 2009). Chapter 8, "Tobacco Dependence," discusses tobacco abuse and treatment in detail.

When to Refer

- Patients, especially smokers, with symptoms of lung cancer (e.g., chronic cough, shortness of breath, chest pain, unintended weight loss, hoarseness, hemoptysis, bone pain) should be referred to a primary care physician for evaluation.
- Patients with suspicious lesions on chest X ray should be referred to a primary care physician or a pulmonologist for further evaluation.
- Patients with suspicious lesions on screening low-dose CT scan should be seen by a pulmonologist for further evaluation.
- Cigarette smokers who are willing to participate in a formal smoking cessation program should be referred whenever possible due to higher success rates in such programs.

Special Treatment Considerations for the Psychiatric Patient Population

The evaluation for and treatment of lung cancer is highly complex and usually involves multiple modalities, including surgery, chemotherapy, and RT. It can be challenging to navigate the treatment even with ideal support systems. Patients with psychiatric illness face many barriers that may impact their treatment of lung cancer; these may include difficulty with transportation, suboptimal treatment of their psychiatric illness, poor follow-up with appointments, refusal of treatment due to poor understanding, and poor adherence to therapy (Cole and Padmanabhan 2012). Patients with lung cancer and severe mental illness are also likely to have significant comorbid medical illnesses such as emphysema, coronary disease, malnourishment, or obesity, which may make treatment complications more problematic (Howard et al. 2010).

Drug-drug or drug-disease interactions may be important in patients undergoing concomitant chemotherapy and psychopharmacotherapy. Treatment with RT, especially to the head due to the plastic mask that is worn, can be challenging for patients with paranoia or severe anxiety, given the immobilization that is required (Howard et al. 2010). Obtaining informed consent, involving the patient in treatment decisions, and end-of-life planning discussions can also be challenges for some patients with severe mental illness, because they may lack the capacity for decision making. Given the lethality of disease, such discussions are very complex and quite common in treatment of lung cancer patients.

Depression is common after the diagnosis of lung cancer, affecting up to 15% of patients during the year after diagnosis of advanced lung cancer (Akechi et al. 2001; Uchitomi et al. 2000). Depression is associated with poorer survival in patients with metastatic disease (Pirl et al. 2008, 2012). Faller et al. (1999) found that depressive coping and emotional distress were independently associated with survival in lung cancer patients. These data, although not robust, suggest that psychological issues may be important targets of lung cancer treatment.

Also, neuropsychological deficits are frequently seen in SCLC patients, including memory deficits in up to 80%, deficits in frontal lobe executive functions, and impaired motor coordination (Meyers et al. 1995). These problems are often present before treatment. Some studies suggest that neurotoxic chemotherapy and prophylactic brain irradiation used in SCLC may also cause neurocognitive defects in some patients, although prospective studies have not shown this decline (D'Ambrosio et al. 2007).

Having a strong social, psychological, and psychiatric support team is critical for many patients with lung cancer and concomitant mental illness. Anticipating barriers to care, treatment of underlying psychiatric symptoms, and consultation with mental health professionals about medications are important parts of the overall care plan.

Case Discussion (*continued*)

Mr. N meets criteria for LDCT screening, which finds a 5-cm mass in the peripheral left upper lung. Upon seeing this result, his psychiatrist refers him to a pulmonologist, and Mr. N undergoes a CT-guided biopsy, which shows adenocarcinoma. Subsequent CT/PET imaging shows no evidence of enlarged intrathoracic lymph nodes or distant metastases, indicating a stage II NSCLC. The patient begins strong efforts at smoking cessation, including starting bupropion, and undergoes a left upper lobectomy with curative intent. Postoperatively, he undergoes adjuvant chemotherapy. He is doing well 1 year after surgery, with periodic chest CT imaging to look for recurrence or metastatic disease.

Clinical Highlights

- Smoking cessation is the most important preventive measure for reducing lung cancer risk.
- Annual screening for lung cancer with low-dose chest computed tomography is recommended for selected high-risk smokers and ex-smokers between ages 55 and 80 years.
- Treatment is highly dependent on lung cancer type (non–small cell lung cancer [NSCLC] vs. small cell lung cancer [SCLC]) and stage.
- Potentially curable NSCLC is treated with surgical resection, often followed by systemic chemotherapy and/or radiation therapy.
- SCLC has usually metastasized at the time of diagnosis, so it is usually treated with systemic chemotherapy and radiation therapy. Patients who respond well to treatment also undergo prophylactic total brain irradiation for possible brain metastases.
- Smoking cessation is an important treatment even after patients develop lung cancer. It can improve treatment efficacy, improve symptoms and quality of life, and improve survival.
- Treatment of lung cancer can be highly complex, so a multidisciplinary approach by psychiatric and oncological care providers with strong social support assistance is important.

Resources

For Patients

American Lung Association: http://www.lung.org/lung-disease/lung-cancer/
National Cancer Institute: http://www.cancer.gov

For Clinicians

National Cancer Institute: http://www.cancer.gov

National Comprehensive Cancer Network: http://www.nccn.org

References

Akechi T, Okamura H, Nishiwaki Y, et al: Psychiatric disorders and associated and predictive factors in patients with unresectable nonsmall cell lung carcinoma: a longitudinal study. Cancer 92:2609–2622, 2001

Alberg AJ, Brock MV, Ford JG, et al: Epidemiology of lung cancer. Chest 143:e1S–e29S, 2013

American Cancer Society: Cancer Facts and Figures 2013. Atlanta, GA, American Cancer Society, 2013. Available at: http://www.cancer.org/acs/groups/content/@epidemiologysurveilance/documents/document/acspc-036845.pdf. Accessed February 20, 2014.

American Joint Committee on Cancer: Lung, in AJCC Cancer Staging Manual, 7th Edition. Edited by Edge SB, Byrd DR, Compton CC, et al. New York, Springer, 2010, pp 253–270

American Lung Association: Providing Guidance on Lung Cancer Screening to Patients and Physicians 2012. Chicago, IL, American Lung Association, April 23, 2012. Available at: http://www.lung.org/lung-disease/lung-cancer/lung-cancer-screening-guidelines/lung-cancer-screening.pdf. Accessed February 17, 2014.

Barak Y, Achiron A, Mandel M, et al: Reduced cancer incidence among patients with schizophrenia. Cancer 104:2817–2821, 2005

Beckles MA, Spiro SG, Colice GL, et al: Initial evaluation of the patient with lung cancer: symptoms, signs, laboratory tests, and paraneoplastic syndromes. Chest 123:97S–104S, 2003

Cataldo JK, Dubey S, Prochaska JJ: Smoking cessation: an integral part of lung cancer treatment. Oncology 78:289–301, 2009

Catts VS, Catts SV, O'Toole BI, et al: Cancer incidence in patients with schizophrenia and their first-degree relatives—a meta-analysis. Acta Psychiatr Scand 117:325–336, 2008

Cole M, Padmanabhan A: Breast cancer treatment of women with schizophrenia and bipolar disorder from Philadelphia, PA: lessons learned and suggestions for improvement. J Cancer Educ 27:774–779, 2012

D'Ambrosio DJ, Cohen RB, Glass J, et al: Unexpected dementia following prophylactic cranial irradiation for small cell lung cancer: case report. J Neurooncol 85:77–79, 2007

Environmental Protection Agency: A citizen's guide to radon: the guide to protecting yourself and your family from radon. 2012. Available at: http://www.epa.gov/radon/pubs/citguide.html. Accessed July 7, 2014.

Faller H, Bulzebruck H, Drings P, et al: Coping, distress, and survival among patients with lung cancer. Arch Gen Psychiatry 56:756–762, 1999

Green RA, Humphrey E, Close H: Alkylating agents in bronchogenic carcinoma. Am J Med 46:516-525, 1969

Hippisley-Cox J, Vinogradova Y, Coupland C, et al: Risk of malignancy in patients with schizophrenia or bipolar disorder. Arch Gen Psychiatry 643:1368–1376, 2007

Howard LM, Barley EA, Davies E, et al: Cancer diagnosis in people with severe mental illness: practical and ethical issues. Lancet Oncol 11:798–804, 2010

Howington JA, Blum MG, Chang AC, et al: Treatment of stage I and II non-small cell lung cancer: Diagnosis and management of lung cancer, 3rd ed: American College of Chest Physicians evidence-based clinical practice guidelines. Chest 143:e278S–e313S, 2013

Jett JR, Schild SE, Kesler KA, et al: Treatment of small cell lung cancer: diagnosis and management of lung cancer, 3rd ed: American College of Chest Physicians evidence-based clinical practice guidelines. Chest 143:e400S–e419S, 2013

Knekt P, Raitasalo R, Heliovaara M, et al: Elevated lung cancer risk among persons with depressed mood. Am J Epidemiol 144:1096–1103, 1996

Lichtermann D, Ekelund J, Pukkala E, et al: Incidence of cancer among persons with schizophrenia and their relatives. Arch Gen Psychiatry 58:573–578, 2001

Linkins RW, Comstock GW: Depressed mood and development of cancer. Am J Epidemiol 132:962–972, 1990

Meyers CA, Byrne KS, Komaki R: Cognitive deficits in patients with small cell lung cancer before and after chemotherapy. Lung Cancer 12:231–235, 1995

Moyer VA: Screening for Lung Cancer: U.S. Preventive Services Task Force Recommendation Statement. Ann Intern Med December 31, 2013 [Epub ahead of print]

National Lung Screening Trial Research Team; Aberle DR, Adams AM, et al: Reduced lung-cancer mortality with low-dose computed tomographic screening. N Engl J Med 365:395–409, 2011

Omenn GS, Goodman GE, Thornquist MD, et al: Effects of a combination of beta carotene and vitamin A on lung cancer and cardiovascular disease. N Engl J Med 334:1150–1155, 1996

Pirl WF, Temel JS, Billings A, et al: Depression after diagnosis of advanced non–small cell lung cancer and survival: a pilot study. Psychosomatics 49:218–224, 2008

Pirl WF, Greer JA, Traeger L, et al: Depression and survival in metastatic non–small cell lung cancer: effects of early palliative care. J Clin Oncol 30:1310–1315, 2012

Ramnath N, Dilling TJ, Harris LJ, et al: Treatment of stage III non–small cell lung cancer. Chest 143:e314S–e340S, 2013

Rivera MP, Mehta AC, Wahidi MM: Establishing the diagnosis of lung cancer. Chest 143:e400S–e419S, 2013

Socinski MA, Evans T, Gettinger S, et al: Treatment of stage IV non–small cell lung cancer. Chest 143:e342S–e365S, 2013

Szabo E, Mao JT, Lam S, et al: Chemoprevention of lung cancer. Chest 143:e40S–e60S, 2013

Tran E, Rouillon F, Loze J, et al: Cancer mortality in patients with schizophrenia. Cancer 115:3555–3562, 2009

Uchitomi Y, Mikami I, Kugaya A, et al: Depression after successful treatment for nonsmall cell lung carcinoma. Cancer 89:1172–1179, 2000

Wender R, Fontham ET, Barrera E Jr, et al: American Cancer Society lung cancer screening guidelines. CA Cancer J Clin 63(2):107–117, 2013

CHAPTER 22

Colorectal Cancer

Cerrone Cohen, M.D.
Jaesu Han, M.D.

Case Discussion

Ms. J is a 52-year-old black woman with a history of diabetes, generalized anxiety disorder, and major depression who presents for a routine follow-up appointment with her psychiatrist. She has been hospitalized once, 3 years ago, for depression shortly after the death of her younger brother from colon cancer. Her depression and anxiety have been well controlled with a selective serotonin reuptake inhibitor for the past 6 months. During the visit, Ms. J reveals that she has recently had difficulty sleeping due to the recurrent thoughts that she will die from the same disease that her brother died from. On further questioning, she reports that she avoids seeing her primary care doctor so that she will not have to discuss screening examinations. The prospect that she may have cancer is often too much for her to handle. She is otherwise going to work and functioning normally.

Clinical Overview

Colorectal Cancer Incidence and Mortality

Colorectal cancer (CRC) is the third most commonly diagnosed form of cancer in the United States among both men and women and is the second leading cause of cancer-related death. Approximately 1 of every 20 people will develop CRC in his or her lifetime (Siegel et al. 2013). In the United States, the overall incidence of CRC has gradually declined. This decrease has largely been credited to improvements in screening and removal of potentially precancerous lesions (Edwards et al. 2010).

Colorectal Cancer and Psychiatric Illness

Overall incidence and mortality rates for CRC among patients with co-occurring psychiatric illness are unknown. However, individual studies have shown elevated mortality rates for patients with CRC and mental disorders when compared with individuals without a psychiatric diagnosis (Baillargeon et al. 2011). Several reasons may account for the disparity. Compared with individuals without a psychiatric diagnosis, patients with psychiatric illness are more likely to be diagnosed with CRCs already in advanced stages, less likely to receive cancer treatment following diagnosis, and more likely to have a longer delay between diagnosis and initial treatment (Robertson et al. 2004).

Types of Colon Cancers

Most colon cancers evolve from preexisting growths in the lining of the colon or rectum known as *polyps.* Constituting an estimated 96% of all polyps, adenomas are by far the most common form of polyp found in the colon and rectum (Stewart et al. 2006). Autopsy studies show that more than 30% of individuals will develop adenomatous polyps by age 60. Adenomas are neoplastic polyps and are the most common type of polyp to progress to cancer (Bond 2000). This proposed adenoma-carcinoma sequence is not well understood; however, most colon cancers develop slowly over the course of 10–15 years (Kelloff et al. 2004). Although all adenomas have malignant potential, less than 10% of adenomas will evolve to become adenocarcinomas (Levine and Ahnen 2006). A smaller number of CRCs may be attributed to genetic syndromes such as familial adenomatous polyposis or Lynch syndrome. These are inherited conditions that predispose individuals to vastly elevated rates of colon cancer, particularly at younger ages, than in individuals without such a history (Lynch and de la Chapelle 2003).

Risk Factors

Aside from defined heritable syndromes, a positive family history of CRC remains one of the strongest risk factors for developing cancer. Individuals who have a first-degree relative diagnosed with CRC are at 2–3 times greater risk of developing CRC themselves than are individuals without a family history of the disease. This risk increases further if multiple family members are affected or if the relative was diagnosed at a young age (Butterworth et al. 2006; Johns and Houlston 2001). Other nonmodifiable risk factors include a personal history of inflammatory bowel disease, diabetes, male gender, African American ethnicity, and increasing age (American Cancer Society 2011; Ekbom et al. 1990; Yang et al. 2005).

Common modifiable risk factors include obesity, smoking, and alcohol consumption (Botteri et al. 2008; Cho et al. 2004; Larsson and Wolk 2007). A number of dietary factors have also been implicated in studies of modifiable risks, notably consumption of red meat. However, newer data suggest that cooking red meat at high temperatures for long periods of time may be responsible for this correlation rather than the meat itself (Chao et al. 2005; Cross et al. 2010).

Common Presentations and the Role of Screening

CRCs are generally asymptomatic in the early stages. The prognosis is most favorable when CRC is detected in the asymptomatic stage. As the lesion grows, individuals may present with hematochezia, melena, abdominal pain, weight loss, occult anemia, constipation or diarrhea, or changes in stool caliber (Speights et al. 1991). However, these signs and symptoms are not highly specific for colon cancer and may be indicative of other gastrointestinal pathology, including inflammatory bowel disease, diverticulitis, irritable bowel syndrome, infectious colitis, hemorrhoids, and mesenteric ischemia. Screening tests for colon cancers are appropriate only for asymptomatic patients. Evaluation in symptomatic individuals should focus on diagnostic modalities such as colonoscopy rather than screening.

Screening Tests for Colon Cancers

Declines in cancer-related deaths have largely been attributed to improvements in screening. Fecal occult blood tests (FOBTs), flexible sigmoidoscopy, and colonoscopy have the best evidence for benefit. More recently, the fecal immunochemical test has gained wider acceptance because of greater specificity and fewer dietary restrictions than with FOBT. Table 22–1 compares the relative pros and cons for each test.

Practical Pointers

- Colorectal cancer is commonly asymptomatic until it progresses to more advanced stages.
- Fecal occult blood tests are a relatively inexpensive, noninvasive, and effective way to screen for colorectal cancer when samples are collected correctly.

TABLE 22–1. Benefits and limitations of colorectal cancer screening methods

Test	Benefits	Limitations
Fecal occult blood test (FOBT)	Does not require bowel preparation Test completed at home Inexpensive Noninvasive Substantial research exists supporting improvements in cancer mortality	Requires multiple stool samples Poor detection of polyps Higher rate of false-positive results than other tests Pretest dietary limitations Colonoscopy necessary if abnormalities detected
Fecal immunochemical test	Does not require bowel preparation Test completed at home Noninvasive Fewer dietary restrictions than FOBT More specific for human blood than guaiac-based tests	Poor detection of polyps More expensive than traditional FOBT Colonoscopy necessary if abnormalities detected
Stool DNA test	Does not require bowel preparation Test completed at home Noninvasive Usually requires only one stool sample	Poor detection of polyps More costly than other stool tests Still being researched; adequate screening intervals uncertain Colonoscopy necessary if abnormalities detected

TABLE 22–1. Benefits and limitations of colorectal cancer screening methods *(continued)*

Test	Benefits	Limitations
Flexible sigmoidoscopy	Requires minimal bowel preparation Does not require sedation Substantial research exists supporting improvements in cancer mortality Lower risk of complications than colonoscopy	Examines only the distal colon Bowel preparation required May cause discomfort Cannot remove large polyps Small risk of bowel perforation Colonoscopy necessary if abnormalities detected
Colonoscopy	Examines entire colon Polyps can be removed and biopsied Can diagnose other colon pathology Required for abnormal results from all other tests Long interval between screenings	Full bowel cleansing required More expensive than stool testing Requires sedation Patients may have to miss a day of work Highest risk of complications compared with other methods No randomized trials illustrating mortality benefits

TABLE 22–1. Benefits and limitations of colorectal cancer screening methods (*continued*)

Test	Benefits	Limitations
Double-contrast barium enema	Can view entire colon No sedation needed	Largely fallen out of favor as newer methods have developed Full bowel preparation needed Cannot remove polyps and often misses small polyps Exposes patients to radiation Colonoscopy necessary if abnormalities detected
Computed tomographic colonography	Noninvasively examines entire colon Performance is similar to optical colonoscopy for large polyps and invasive cancers Few complications No sedation needed	Full bowel preparation needed Cannot remove polyps Exposes patients to radiation Expensive May not be readily available in smaller centers or rural areas Colonoscopy necessary if abnormalities detected

Source. Adapted from American Cancer Society 2011.

- Screening guidelines vary for patients with a strong family history of colorectal cancer or inflammatory bowel disease, and individuals with genetic syndromes that predispose them to colonic polyp formation.
- Individuals with mental illness may be at increased risk for developing colorectal cancer due to high rates of smoking, alcohol consumption, and other modifiable risk factors.

Diagnosis

Individuals with concerning symptoms for which there is a high suspicion for CRC should not undergo screening examinations. These patients should be directly referred for a diagnostic evaluation. Colonoscopy with biopsy is the current standard for diagnosing CRC. Once a diagnosis is made, individuals should be referred to a specialist to discuss options for treatment. Treatment options largely depend on the stage of the cancer when it is diagnosed.

Multiple organizations have offered guidelines for the routine CRC screening of average-risk patients, including the U.S. Preventive Services Task Force (USPSTF; 2008). The American Cancer Society (ACS) joined with the U.S. Multi-Society Task Force for Colorectal Cancer (MSTF) and the American College of Radiology (ACR) to publish joint screening recommendations in 2008 (Levin et al. 2008). A summary of these two major guidelines is provided in Table 22–2.

The primary differences between these guidelines involve the time frame for discontinuing treatment and the scope of recommended options for screening. Both organizations recommend initiating screening at age 50. The USPSTF limits recommended screening options to FOBT, sigmoidoscopy combined with FOBT, and colonoscopy. The ACS-MSTF-ACR considers additional options and delineates tests as either useful in early cancer detection (i.e., stool-based studies) or useful for cancer prevention (i.e., studies that provide some visualization of the colon whether directly or indirectly). The guidelines differ on when to halt screening, with the ACS-MSTF-ACR basing recommendations on life expectancy rather than specific ages, as recommended by the USPSTF. The recommendations of the American College of Gastroenterology (ACG) are similar to those of the ACS-MSTF-ACR, although ACG recommends earlier screening for African Americans due to increased risk of CRC and considers colonoscopy the preferred screening modality (Rex et al. 2009).

Guidelines vary for high-risk individuals—namely, those with a history of familial adenomatous polyposis or other inherited syndromes associated with colon cancer, those with a history of colon cancer in family members before the age of 50, individuals with a history of radiation exposure, those with prior personal history of colon cancer, patients with inflammatory bowel dis-

TABLE 22–2. Summary of colorectal screening guidelines for individuals

Organization	Initiating screening	Method of screening	Frequency of screening	Discontinuing screening
USPSTF[a]	All adults at age 50	Highly sensitive guaiac FOBT	Annually	Discontinue routine screening sometime between ages 76 and 85, although this decision should be made on an individual basis based on personal risks and health status; no screening beyond age 85
		Combined flexible sigmoidoscopy and highly sensitive guaiac FOBT	Sigmoidoscopy every 5 years, with FOBT every 3 years	
		Colonoscopy	Every 10 years	
		Computed tomographic colonoscopy	Insufficient evidence to support this as a tool for routine screening	
ACS-MSTF-ACR[b]	Average-risk adults at age 50	**Tests for early cancer detection**		Discontinue screening when life expectancy is less than 10 years
		Highly sensitive guaiac FOBT	Annually	
		Fecal immunochemical test	Annually	
		Stool DNA testing	Unknown	

TABLE 22–2. Summary of colorectal screening guidelines for individuals (continued)

Organization	Initiating screening	Method of screening	Frequency of screening	Discontinuing screening
ACS-MSTF-ACR[b] (continued)		**Tests for prevention and early cancer detection**		
		Flexible sigmoidoscopy	Every 5 years	
		Colonoscopy	Every 10 years	
		Computed tomographic colonoscopy	Every 5 years	
		Double-contrast barium enema	Every 5 years	

Note. ACS-MSTF-ACR=American Cancer Society, U.S. Multi-Society Task Force for Colorectal Cancer, and American College of Radiology; FOBT=fecal occult blood test; USPSTF=U.S. Preventive Services Task Force.
[a]Guidelines not meant to apply to patients with inflammatory bowel disease or specific hereditary syndromes such as familial adenomatous polyposis or Lynch syndrome.
[b]Guidelines designed for patients deemed to be at average risk for developing colorectal cancer.
Source. Adapted from guidelines provided by Levin et al. 2008 and U.S. Preventive Services Task Force 2008.

ease, and individuals with multiple first-degree relatives with colon cancers. Individuals in these categories should be referred to a specialist for discussion of the timeline for both initial screening and the subsequent screening intervals.

Preventive Guidelines

Research on primary prevention of CRC has shown that exercise is a protective factor (Wolin et al. 2009). Dietary studies have focused on the role of fiber, diets high in fruits and vegetables, vitamin D, and calcium supplementation in decreasing cancer risks. The data on high-fiber diets and diets high in fruits and vegetables are mixed, with some studies showing decreased cancer incidence and others reporting no benefit (Howe et al. 1997). Calcium supplementation and vitamin D supplementation have each been associated with a decreased risk of developing CRC, although an effective dose has not been established (Weingarten et al. 2008).

Several classes of medication have also been studied for the primary prevention of CRC. There is strong evidence that aspirin and other nonsteroidal anti-inflammatory drugs (NSAIDs) may reduce the risks of CRC; however, they are not routinely recommended due to increased risks of gastrointestinal bleeding and other side effects (Flossmann et al. 2007). The USPSTF specifically recommends against routine use of aspirin or NSAIDs for primary prevention of CRC (U.S. Preventive Services Task Force 2008). Data on the benefit of statins in reducing colon cancers are inconclusive (Coogan et al. 2007; Poynter et al. 2005).

Treatment Recommendations

Patients who have CRC should be referred to surgery. Removal of the malignancy from the colon is often curative and should be followed up with surveillance colonoscopies. For advanced cases, an oncologist should be involved in the care, and chemotherapy and/or radiation therapy may be used, as well.

When to Refer

- Patients with signs and symptoms suspicious for CRC should be referred directly for a diagnostic workup.
- Asymptomatic patients with abnormal results from a screening test should be referred for a diagnostic workup.
- Individuals with a history of a hereditary syndrome associated with colon cancer, radiation exposure, a prior personal history of colon cancer or inflammatory bowel disease, multiple first-degree relatives with CRC,

or a history of colon cancer in young family members should be referred for an individualized timeline for screening.

Special Treatment Considerations for the Psychiatric Patient Population

The potential benefits of colorectal screening are negated if patients are either unable or unwilling to complete the test or undergo timely follow-up of positive results. Thus, it is important to individualize screening recommendations, particularly for individuals with any degree of impairment from mental illness. To date, there are no commonly agreed-on screening guidelines for patients with comorbid mental illness. We recommend that screening for average-risk individuals with co-occurring mental illness begin at age 50. Choice of screening modality should take into account the severity of current psychiatric symptoms, patient preference, and reliability of follow-up.

A suggested algorithm for CRC screening in average-risk individuals with mental illness appears in Figure 22–1. The algorithm is specially adapted from current USPSTF guidelines to fit the needs of psychiatric populations in particular. The provider should begin by assessing the severity of current psychiatric symptoms based on the patient's level of impairment, as described in Table 22–3. We recommend that patients with well-controlled or mild symptoms be screened with stool studies and sigmoidoscopy. Stool studies are safe and noninvasive, and require no bowel preparation. Screening accuracy is increased when stool-based tests are combined with flexible sigmoidoscopy. Unlike colonoscopy, flexible sigmoidoscopy does not involve sedation. For high-functioning patients, this may be appealing. However, because preprocedural anxiety has been shown to correlate to pain and discomfort after flexible sigmoidoscopy, patients with poorly controlled anxiety may be less ideal candidates (Johnson et al. 2008).

For patients with moderate to severe symptoms, the clinician should first try to optimize treatment of the underlying psychiatric condition. If symptom control is likely to improve over the next one to two visits, then it is reasonable to defer screening until symptoms are better controlled and to reassess the patient prior to making specific screening recommendations. However, screening should not be delayed if a significant improvement in symptoms is not expected in the near future, because significant delays may lead to failure in initiating screening at all. We recommend that individuals with persistent moderate to severe symptoms be screened by colonoscopy. The sedation associated with a colonoscopy may be preferred for those with more severe illness and allows for screening and diagnostic biopsy if needed during the same procedure.

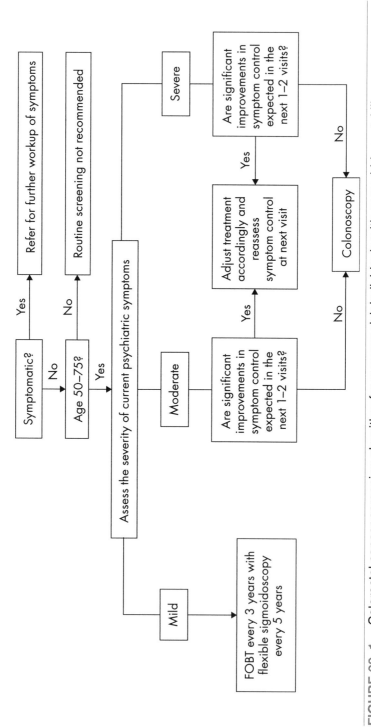

FIGURE 22–1. Colorectal cancer screening algorithm for average-risk individuals with comorbid mental illness.

Note. FOBT = fecal occult blood test.

TABLE 22–3. **Assessing the severity of current psychiatric symptoms based on level of impairment**

Mild	Few or no active psychiatric symptoms are present. If symptoms are present, they do not cause impairment in social, occupational, interpersonal, or cognitive functioning.
Moderate	Several active psychiatric symptoms may be present, causing some mild impairment in social, occupational, interpersonal, or cognitive functioning.
Severe	Symptoms are present that cause serious impairment in social, occupational, interpersonal, or cognitive functioning.

Case Discussion (*continued*)

Ms. J's primary risk factors for developing colon cancer include her age, smoking history, race, and family history. At her current age of 53, all major guidelines would recommend screening for CRC. When discussing screening options, the clinician should take the patient's current anxiety symptoms into account. Her symptoms cause some degree of impairment in functioning in that her anxiety prevents her from being able to see her primary care doctor for her other health concerns. Given her level of anxiety and associated impairment, her symptoms would be classified as moderately severe. She would be considered a poor candidate for stool-based studies given that her uncontrolled anxiety may worsen with false-positive results and may also affect her ability to undergo further testing following positive stool results. After hearing recommendations to improve her anxiety, Ms. J is apprehensive about medication adjustments. Rather than put off screening indefinitely until her symptoms are better controlled, the clinician recommends colonoscopy while simultaneously beginning weekly psychotherapeutic interventions. After hearing a description of the screening, the patient is comforted to find out that she will not be awake during the procedure and may only need repeated screening every 10 years if results are normal. She agrees to colonoscopy and contacts her primary care doctor to schedule the procedure.

Clinical Highlights

- All screening tests for colon cancer, except colonoscopy, are useful for the asymptomatic stage only.
- The decision of when to institute screening and the interval at which to screen should be based on patient risk factors for colorectal cancer (CRC). Most guidelines are designed for individuals at average risk.

- Mental health providers should be active in promoting primary prevention of CRCs.
- The specific screening modality to recommend should be individualized and take into account patient preference, complexity of the procedure and tolerability, likelihood of compliance, and control of current psychiatric symptoms.

Resources

American Cancer Society: http://www.cancer.org

National Cancer Institute: http://www.cancer.gov/cancertopics/types/colon-and-rectal

U.S. Preventive Services Task Force: http://www.uspreventiveservicestaskforce.org

References

American Cancer Society: Colorectal Cancer Facts and Figures 2011–2013. Atlanta, GA, American Cancer Society, 2011. Available at: http://www.cancer.org/acs/groups/content/@epidemiologysurveilance/documents/document/acspc-028312.pdf. Accessed August 12, 2014.

Baillargeon J, Kuo YF, Lin YL, et al: Effect of mental disorders on diagnosis, treatment, and survival of older adults with colon cancer. J Am Geriatr Soc 59:1268–1273, 2011

Bond JH: Polyp guideline: diagnosis, treatment, and surveillance for patients with colorectal polyps. Practice Parameters Committee of the American College of Gastroenterology. Am J Gastroenterol 95:3053–3063, 2000

Botteri E, Iodice S, Bagnardi V, et al: Smoking and colorectal cancer: a meta-analysis. JAMA 300:2765–2778, 2008

Butterworth AS, Higgins JP, Pharoah P: Relative and absolute risk of colorectal cancer for individuals with a family history: a meta-analysis. Eur J Cancer 42:216–227, 2006

Chao A, Thun MJ, Connell CJ, et al: Meat consumption and risk of colorectal cancer. JAMA 293:172–182, 2005

Cho E, Smith-Warner SA, Ritz J, et al: Alcohol intake and colorectal cancer: a pooled analysis of 8 cohort studies. Ann Intern Med 140:603–613, 2004

Coogan PF, Smith J, Rosenberg L: Statin use and risk of colorectal cancer. J Natl Cancer Inst 99:32–40, 2007

Cross AJ, Ferrucci LM, Risch A, et al: A large prospective study of meat consumption and colorectal cancer risk: an investigation of potential mechanisms underlying this association. Cancer Res 70:2406–2414, 2010

Edwards BK, Ward E, Kohler BA, et al: Annual report to the nation on the status of cancer, 1975–2006, featuring colorectal cancer trends and impact of interventions (risk factors, screening, and treatment) to reduce future rates. Cancer 116:544–573, 2010

Ekbom A, Helmick C, Zach M, Adami HO: Ulcerative colitis and colorectal cancer. A population-based study. N Engl J Med 323:1228–1233, 1990

Flossmann E, Rothwell PM; British Doctors Aspirin Trial and the UK-TIA Aspirin Trial: Effect of aspirin on long-term risk of colorectal cancer: consistent evidence from randomised and observational studies. Lancet 369:1603–1613, 2007

Howe GR, Aronson KJ, Benito E, et al: The relationship between dietary fat intake and risk of colorectal cancer: evidence from the combined analysis of 13 case-control studies. Cancer Causes Control 8:215–228, 1997

Johns LE, Houlston RS: A systematic review and meta-analysis of familial colorectal cancer risk. Am J Gastroenterol 96:2992–3003, 2001

Johnson CD, Chen MH, Toledano AY, et al: Accuracy of CT colonography for detection of large adenomas and cancers. N Engl J Med 359:1207–1217, 2008

Kelloff GJ, Schilsky RL, Alberts DS, et al: Colorectal adenomas: a prototype for the use of surrogate end points in the development of cancer prevention drugs. Clin Cancer Res 10:3908–3918, 2004

Larsson SC, Wolk A: Obesity and colon and rectal cancer risk: a meta-analysis of prospective studies. Am J Clin Nutr 86:556–565, 2007

Levin B, Lieberman DA, McFarland B, et al: Screening and surveillance for the early detection of colorectal cancer and adenomatous polyps, 2008: a joint guideline from the American Cancer Society, the U.S. Multi-Society Task Force on Colorectal Cancer, and the American College of Radiology. CA Cancer J Clin 58:130–160, 2008

Levine JS, Ahnen DJ: Clinical practice. Adenomatous polyps of the colon. N Engl J Med 355:2551–2557, 2006

Lynch HT, de la Chapelle A: Hereditary colorectal cancer. N Engl J Med 348:919–932, 2003

Poynter JN, Gruber SB, Higgins PD, et al: Statins and the risk of colorectal cancer. N Engl J Med 352:2184–2192, 2005

Rex DK, Johnson DA, Anderson JC, et al: American College of Gastroenterology guidelines for colorectal cancer screening 2009[corrected]. Am J Gastroenterol 104(3):739–750, 2009

Robertson R, Campbell NC, Smith S, et al: Factors influencing time from presentation to treatment of colorectal and breast cancer in urban and rural areas. Br J Cancer 90:1479–1485, 2004

Siegel R, Naishadham D, Jemal A: Cancer statistics, 2013. CA Cancer J Clin 63:11–30, 2013

Speights VO, Johnson MW, Stoltenberg PH, et al: Colorectal cancer: current trends in initial clinical manifestations. South Med J 84:575–578, 1991

Stewart SL, Wike JM, Kato I, et al: A population-based study of colorectal cancer histology in the United States, 1998–2001. Cancer 107 (suppl 5):1128–1141, 2006

U.S. Preventive Services Task Force: Screening for colorectal cancer: U.S. Preventive Services Task Force recommendation statement. Ann Intern Med 149:627–637, 2008

Weingarten MA, Zalmanovici A, Yaphe J: Dietary calcium supplementation for preventing colorectal cancer and adenomatous polyps. Cochrane Database Syst Rev (1):CD003548, 2008

Wolin KY, Yan Y, Colditz GA: Physical activity and colon cancer prevention: a meta-analysis. Br J Cancer 100:611–616, 2009

Yang YX, Hennessy S, Lewis JD: Type 2 diabetes mellitus and the risk of colorectal cancer. Clin Gastroenterol Hepatol 3:587–594, 2005

CHAPTER 23

Cervical Cancer

Elizabeth Davis, M.D.
Sharad Jain, M.D.

Case Discussion

Ms. C is a 36-year-old woman with schizophrenia and a history of sexual trauma who is followed closely by her psychiatrist and case manager. She has been sexually active with several male partners over the past decade. She has heard of Pap smears but has never had one. She feels "uncomfortable" when going to the doctor and has canceled all recent appointments with primary care providers (PCPs).

Clinical Overview

Improved efforts to screen for cervical cancer have resulted in a significant decrease in the number of patients who have this condition. In 2008, the incidence of cervical cancer was 6.6 per 100,000 women, and the mortality rate was 2.38 per 100,000 women; these rates are about half of what they were 30 years ago (Committee on Practice Bulletins—Gynecology 2012). Also in support of screening, most cases of invasive cervical cancer occur in people who have had inadequate screening or who have not been screened (Committee on Practice Bulletins—Gynecology 2012; Moyer and U.S. Preventive Services Task Force 2012). Cervical cancer takes about 20 years to develop after infection with the human papillomavirus (HPV) (Lin et al. 2013).

In addition to the psychiatric patient population, other high-risk groups include women without regular health care, immigrants, and uninsured women (Committee on Practice Bulletins—Gynecology 2012). Personal factors that increase the risk of cervical cancer relate to the role that HPV, a sexually transmitted infection, plays in the pathogenesis of cervical cancer. The following risk factors increase the risk of becoming infected with HPV or affect the host response to HPV: early onset of intercourse, multiple partners, decreased immune function, poor nutritional status, and cigarette smoking (Moyer and U.S. Preventive Services Task Force 2012). HIV is a strong risk factor for the development of cervical cancer, and frequent HPV screening is highly recommended for patients with HIV.

HPV types 16 and 18 are the most carcinogenic strains of HPV (Committee on Practice Bulletins—Gynecology 2012), although there are several other carcinogenic strains as well. Although the incidence of HPV infection is greatest in women in their 20s, most of these infections are transient and do not progress to neoplasia. The risk of cervical neoplasia is greatest in the third decade of life and decreases thereafter (Moyer and U.S. Preventive Services Task Force 2012). The HPV vaccine is a recent development over the last decade and is leading to lower rates of cervical neoplasia (Gertig et al. 2013). The vaccine is recommended for nonpregnant women who are age 26 or younger.

Prognosis depends on the type of neoplasia found on screening. Low-grade neoplasia, cervical intraepithelial neoplasia-1 (CIN-1), often reflects a transitory response to acute HPV infection. Only 1% of these lesions progress to cervical cancer (Douglas 2011), and 60% revert to normal histology (Committee on Practice Bulletins—Gynecology 2012; Douglas 2011). In contrast, 31% of untreated high-grade neoplasia (CIN-3) will progress to cervical cancer (McCredie et al. 2008). These more severe types of dysplasia typically take 3–7 years to progress to invasive cancer (Committee on Practice Bulletins—Gynecology 2012).

Although cervical cancer screening rates range from 49% to 78% in women over age 18 years, two recent reviews showed that screening rates for cervical cancer are much lower in women with mental illness (20%–30% lower in multiple studies), even when those patients are engaged with primary care (Aggarwal et al. 2013; Happell et al. 2012). History of sexual trauma (Farley et al. 2002) and substance use (Abrams et al. 2012) are also associated with lower cervical cancer screening rates. However, there are also studies that indicate these disparities can be overcome. In a study of veterans with depression and posttraumatic stress disorder, the rates of cervical cancer screening were no different from those in patients without psychiatric diagnoses (Weitlauf et al. 2013). Interestingly, the 75%–77% rate of screening in this Veterans Health Administration study is high compared to nationwide rates, perhaps indicating systemic factors that both increased the baseline rate for all women and removed any disparity. The authors cite lack of financial or insurance barriers and colocation of mental health with primary care as factors contributing to the lack of disparity in screening rates.

Cervical cancer rates may also be higher in women with mental illness. A study of over 70,000 Taiwanese women with schizophrenia showed a rate of cervical cancer 1.6 times higher than in the general population of Taiwan (Lin et al. 2013). Studies in Taiwan and Australia have also shown 30% higher fatality rates in psychiatric patients with malignancies than in the general population (Chou et al. 2011; Kisely et al. 2013).

Practical Pointers

- Patients should be asked about past sexually transmitted infections and history of cervical cancer screening.
- Patients who need cervical cancer screening should be referred to primary care providers.
- Patients who have abnormal screening results should be referred for further diagnostic testing.
- The human papillomavirus (HPV) vaccine should be recommended to female patients who are 26 years or younger who have not been vaccinated and who are not pregnant.
- Patients who have a psychotic or mood disorder should be closely monitored for unsafe sexual practices and increased risk for HPV. Cervical cancer is essentially a sexually transmitted disease, and steps should be taken to prevent it in high-risk groups.

Diagnosis

Cervical screening techniques include cytology and HPV testing. For cytology testing, clinicians can use liquid-based or conventional methodologies. Multiple studies have shown that using a small amount of water-soluble lubricant does not interfere with the results of the cytology testing. There is no difference in the specificity or sensitivity between liquid-based and conventional methodologies. The Bethesda System for reporting cervical cytology results is a standardized format that includes the following components: specimen type, specimen adequacy (i.e., satisfactory for evaluation), general categorization, and interpretation/result (i.e., malignancy or negative for intraepithelial lesion). HPV testing looks for the presence of the most common 13–14 high-risk genotypes (Committee on Practice Bulletins—Gynecology 2012).

For women with positive HPV testing and negative cytology, the American Congress of Obstetricians and Gynecologists (ACOG) recommendations include more specific HPV 16/18 genotyping or retesting in 12 months

(Jin et al. 2013). For women with atypical squamous cells of undetermined significance (ASCUS) and negative HPV testing, the American Society for Colposcopy and Cervical Pathology (ASCCP) recommends repeat cytology at 12 months. Women with repeat ASCUS results or positive HPV serology should undergo colposcopy. Most women with low-grade squamous intraepithelial lesions or high-grade squamous intraepithelial lesions on cytology should undergo colposcopy (Massad et al. 2013).

Preventive Guidelines

The American Cancer Society (Saslow et al. 2012), the U.S. Preventive Services Task Force (Moyer and U.S. Preventive Services Task Force 2012), and the ACOG (Lin et al. 2012) came out with nearly identical guidelines in 2012, all of which recommended less frequent screening and larger emphasis on HPV testing than did prior guidelines. The screening guidelines are illustrated in Figure 23–1. All three guidelines recommend cytology (with no HPV testing) every 3 years between ages 21 and 29, and either cytology screening every 3 years or cytology and HPV cotesting every 5 years after age 30. Screening should stop at age 65 in women who meet two criteria: 1) adequate screening, defined as three negative cytology results or two negative cytology and HPV results in the last 10 years, with the most recent test within the last 5 years, and 2) no history of CIN-2 or higher-grade lesions within the last 20 years. HPV vaccination does not affect screening recommendations. Screening should stop in women who have had a hysterectomy for benign conditions and whose cervix has been removed (Jin et al. 2013). Because women with HIV have higher rates of HPV infection and cervical neoplasia, they should have cytology testing twice in the first year after HIV diagnosis and yearly thereafter.

The most important aspect of applying ACOG guidelines to psychiatric populations is to lower barriers to cervical cancer screening. In a qualitative study interviewing both women with mental illness and their providers, the participants noted communication and collaboration between mental health providers and PCPs as key to increasing rates of cancer screening in women with mental illness (Miller et al. 2007). In another qualitative study of barriers to screening, women with mental illness valued receiving screening from well-known providers and found women's health clinics colocated within mental health clinics to be an effective solution (Owen et al. 2002). Other strategies for improving cervical cancer screening rates that have been successful include group education, patient and provider incentives, and reducing out-of-pocket costs for patients (Community Preventive Services Task Force 2012) (Table 23–1).

Current guidelines do not recommend HPV testing alone because of incomplete data comparing HPV testing alone to cervical cytology with HPV

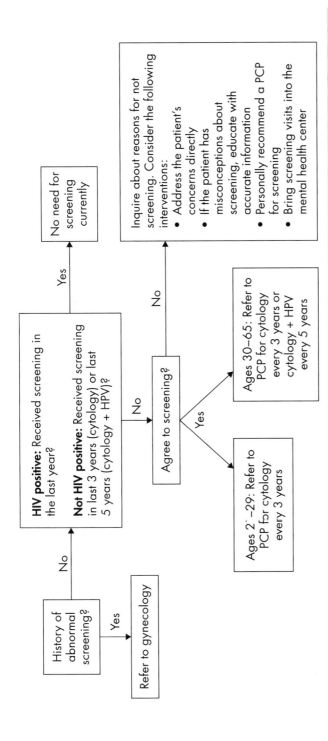

FIGURE 23–1. Screening for cervical cancer.

Note. HPV=human papillomavirus; PCP=primary care provider.

TABLE 23–1. **Methods to improve screening for cervical cancer in those with mental illness**

Colocating primary care and mental health care, with an emphasis on prevention

Peer education and support groups

Decreasing out-of-pocket expenses for patients who need screening

Emphasizing that early detection and treatment often translates to a good long-term prognosis

Referring HIV-positive patients for periodic cervical cancer screening

cotesting (Committee on Practice Bulletins—Gynecology 2012). However, self-collection of cervicovaginal specimens for HPV testing is emerging as a potential method for overcoming barriers for testing of women who decline pelvic examinations. In one study in rural Appalachia, women overdue for cervical cancer screening completed self-collection, and those with abnormal results were much more likely to agree to pelvic examinations than they were prior to receiving self-collection results (Vanderpool et al. 2014).

Treatment Recommendations

Women should have regular cervical cancer screening per guidelines. They should be referred to gynecologists for further evaluation if HPV or cytology testing is abnormal. Further treatment recommendations are based on the colposcopy findings.

The ASCCP developed new guidelines in 2012 to guide the treatment of CIN lesions and adenoma in situ (AIS). Ablation and excision are both effective ways to treat CIN. Young women and pregnant women can be followed with serial colposcopy and cytology. AIS is ideally treated with hysterectomy for women who do not want to have children, but it can also be managed conservatively with excision and close follow-up for women who do want to maintain fertility. The latter option carries a risk of persistent AIS and progression to cervical cancer (Massad et al. 2013).

When to Refer

- The patient should be referred to a PCP for regular cervical cancer screenings.
- The patient should be referred to a gynecologist for further evaluation if HPV or cytology testing is abnormal.

Special Treatment Considerations for the Psychiatric Patient Population

Recommendations for cervical cancer screening for psychiatric patients are essentially the same as for the general population. The literature demonstrates that integration of mental health and primary care services enhances screening rates for patients with psychiatric conditions. Psychiatrists should work with PCPs to ensure that their patients receive appropriate testing and follow-up based on the results of the screening. It is important for patients with certain conditions (e.g., HIV infection, prior abnormal Pap results) to have more frequent screening. In addition, it is worth recommending HPV vaccination to females between ages 9 and 26 who have not been vaccinated and who are not pregnant.

Because colposcopy and treatment for CIN or AIS can cause emotional distress, it is important for mental health providers to coordinate closely with gynecologists. Such coordination can include mental health providers guiding gynecologists with how best to work with their high-risk, mentally ill patients, and gynecologists guiding mental health providers in helping their patients understand the results and the treatment plan.

Case Discussion (*continued*)

Ms. C has a higher than normal risk of cervical cancer because she has never been screened. Her psychiatrist recognizes that although Ms. C has not attended primary care appointments, she feels connected to the mental health center. Ms. C's psychiatrist talks with her about the importance of cervical cancer screening and explains how screening is performed. A PCP comes to the mental health center monthly to provide cervical cancer screening for patients there. Although anxious about having a pelvic exam, Ms. C is reassured by both her psychiatrist and her PCP and agrees to have a Pap smear and HPV testing. Her HPV test is positive, and her cytology shows high-grade squamous intraepithelial lesions. She is referred to a gynecologist, and her psychiatrist, case manager, and gynecologist work together to decrease barriers to further workup and treatment. She is found to have CIN-3 and undergoes an excision. In her follow-up appointments, some of which are conducted at the mental health center, she has no recurrence of cervical neoplasia.

Clinical Highlights

- Cervical cancer rates can be dramatically reduced with effective screening, but rates of screening are lower in populations with mental illness.
- Screening recommendations are as follows:
  - Cytology every 3 years for women ages 21–29.

- Cytology every 3 years or cytology and human papillomavirus (HPV) screening every 5 years for women ages 30–65.
- Women with human immunodeficiency virus (HIV) should be screened twice in the year after diagnosis, and then yearly.
- Screening can stop in women over age 65 who have had adequate screening the previous 10 years and have not had CIN-2 or higher-grade lesions in the last 20 years.
- Abnormal HPV or cytology results should trigger referral to a gynecologist.
- Integrating primary care and mental health by providing cervical cancer screening at mental health centers may help improve screening rates for patients with mental illness.

Resources

For Patients

American College of Obstetricians and Gynecologists: Patient Education Fact Sheet: New Guidelines for Cervical Cancer Screening. Available at: http://www.acog.org/~/media/For%20Patients/pfs004.pdf?dmc=1&ts= 20140814T1517469737.

WomensHealth.gov: Pap Test. Available at: http://www.womenshealth.gov/ publications/our-publications/fact-sheet/pap-test.html.

For Clinicians

Every Woman Counts: Cervical Cancer Facts and Stats. Available at: http:// qap.sdsu.edu/screening/cervicalcancer/facts.html#3.

U.S. Preventive Services Task Force: Screening for Cervical Cancer. Available at: http://www.uspreventiveservicestaskforce.org/3rduspstf/cervcan/ cervcanrr.htm#clinical.

References

Abrams MT, Myers CS, Feldman SM, et al: Cervical cancer screening and acute care visits among Medicaid enrollees with mental and substance use disorders. Psychiatr Serv 63:815–822, 2012

Aggarwal A, Pandurangi A, Smith W: Disparities in breast and cervical cancer screening in women with mental illness: a systematic literature review. Am J Prev Med 44:392–398, 2013

Chou FH, Tsai KY, Su CY, et al: The incidence and relative risk factors for developing cancer among patients with schizophrenia: a nine-year follow-up study. Schizophr Res 129:97–103, 2011

Committee on Practice Bulletins—Gynecology: ACOG Practice Bulletin Number 131: screening for cervical cancer. Obstet Gynecol 120:1222–1238, 2012

Community Preventive Services Task Force: Updated recommendations for client- and provider-oriented interventions to increase breast, cervical, and colorectal cancer screening. Am J Prev Med 43:92–96, 2012

Douglas JM: Papillomavirus, in Goldman's Cecil Medicine, 24th Edition. Edited by Goldman L, Schafer AI. Philadelphia, PA, Saunders, 2011, pp XX–XX

Farley M, Golding JM, Minkoff JR: Is a history of trauma associated with a reduced likelihood of cervical cancer screening? J Fam Pract 51:827–831, 2002

Gertig DM, Brotherton JM, Budd AC, et al: Impact of a population-based HPV vaccination program on cervical abnormalities: a data linkage study. BMC Med 11:227, 2013

Happell B, Scott D, Platania-Phung C: Provision of preventive services for cancer and infectious diseases among individuals with serious mental illness. Arch Psychiatr Nurs 26:192–201, 2012

Jin XW, Lipold L, McKenzie M, Sikon A: Cervical cancer screening: what's new and what's coming? Cleve Clin J Med 80:153–160, 2013

Kisely S, Crowe E, Lawrence D: Cancer-related mortality in people with mental illness. JAMA Psychiatry 70:209–217, 2013

Lin GM, Chen YJ, Kuo DJ, et al: Cancer incidence in patients with schizophrenia or bipolar disorder: a nationwide population-based study in Taiwan, 1997–2009. Schizophr Bull 39:407–416, 2013

Massad LS, Einstein MH, Huh WK, et al: 2012 updated consensus guidelines for the management of abnormal cervical cancer screening tests and cancer precursors. Obstet Gynecol 121:829–846, 2013

McCredie MR, Sharples KJ, Paul C, et al: Natural history of cervical neoplasia and risk of invasive cancer in women with cervical intraepithelial neoplasia 3: a retrospective cohort study. Lancet Oncol 9:425–434, 2008

Miller E, Lasser KE, Becker AE: Breast and cervical cancer screening for women with mental illness: patient and provider perspectives on improving linkages between primary care and mental health. Arch Womens Ment Health 10:189–197, 2007

Moyer VA, U.S. Preventive Services Task Force: Screening for cervical cancer: U.S. Preventive Services Task Force recommendation statement. Ann Intern Med 156(12):880–891, 2012

Owen C, Jessie D, De Vries Robbe M: Barriers to cancer screening amongst women with mental health problems. Health Care Women Int 23:561–566, 2002

Saslow D, Solomon D, Lawson HW, et al: American Cancer Society, American Society for Colposcopy and Cervical Pathology, and American Society for Clinical Pathology screening guidelines for the prevention and early detection of cervical cancer. Am J Clin Pathol 137: 516–542, 2012

Vanderpool RC, Jones MG, Stradtman LR, et al: Self-collecting a cervico-vaginal specimen for cervical cancer screening: an exploratory study of acceptability among medically underserved women in rural Appalachia. Gynecol Oncol 132(suppl):S21–S25, 2014

Weitlauf JC, Jones S, Xu X, et al: Receipt of cervical cancer screening in female veterans: impact of posttraumatic stress disorder and depression. Womens Health Issues 23:e153–e159, 2013

CHAPTER 24

Skin Cancers

Gwendolyn Ho, M.D.
Mamta Parikh, M.D.
Paul Aronowitz, M.D., F.A.C.P.

Case Discussion

Mr. W, a 55-year-old man with a history of schizophrenia and tobacco use who is currently living in transitional housing, presents for follow-up with his psychiatrist. His schizophrenia is well controlled on his current medication regimen, and he provides for himself primarily by working as a laborer with a construction company. On examination, his psychiatrist notes multiple thick dark-pigmented scaly lesions on his skin, notably on his face, nose, and chest. On full skin examination, Mr W is found to have these lesions throughout his skin, primarily in sun-exposed areas.

Clinical Overview

Epidemiology

Skin cancer accounts for one-third of all cancers in the United States, with one in six Americans developing skin cancer at some time in life. Most patients develop nonmelanomatous skin cancers, such as basal or squamous cell carcinoma. Malignant melanoma occurs in about 2% of people during their lifetime but accounts for 75% of all deaths associated with skin cancer (Jerant et al. 2000). There does not appear to be a familial predisposition for the development of skin cancer in those who have psychiatric illness. Moreover, psychotropic medications do not likely increase the risk of any form of skin cancer. Although limited studies have been completed to determine skin cancer–related morbidity and mortality in those with severe mental illness (SMI) compared with the general population, we believe patients who have SMI are less likely to be screened for skin lesions and therefore have a higher overall burden from all types of skin cancer.

Prevention of and Screening for Skin Cancer

Because exposure to ultraviolet (UV) light has been strongly linked to all types of skin cancer, sun protection is critical during childhood and beyond. This is most important in individuals with fair skin or a family or personal history of skin cancer. Regular sunscreen use, even in those with prior history of skin cancer, is beneficial and can reduce the development of premalignant lesions. Avoidance of tanning parlors is also highly recommended (Croswell and Shin 2012).

There is no clear evidence that mass screening for skin cancer is beneficial. There remains controversy about who should be screened, who should perform the screening, and how often the screening should be done. The U.S. Preventive Services Task Force does not recommend for or against routine skin examination but does recommend that physicians be vigilant in identifying potentially malignant lesions when examining patients for other reasons, especially if they have risk factors for melanoma (Wolff et al. 2009). For men and women above age 20 years, the American Cancer Society recommends that during a periodic health examination, a cancer-related checkup should include examination of the skin as well as health counseling about tobacco use, sun exposure, risk factors, and environmental exposures. (Smith et al. 2012). When screening is performed, the examiner should systematically inspect the entire skin surface. We recommend that screening for skin cancer be done in the primary care setting during a routine examination every 1–3 years for those who are fair skinned, have a history of skin cancer, have congenital discrete skin lesion(s), or were frequently sunburned during childhood and beyond.

Practical Pointers

- Patients should be encouraged to use sunscreen regularly and to avoid tanning parlors or excessive sun exposure.
- It is important to be vigilant in identifying potential premalignant and malignant lesions, specifically basal cell carcinoma, actinic keratosis, squamous cell carcinoma, and melanoma, as described in the next section, "Diagnosis and Treatment."

- A definitive diagnosis is established with a skin biopsy.
- The clinician should refer patients to a dermatologist for further evaluation and treatment of suspicious skin lesions.

Diagnosis and Treatment

Basal Cell Carcinoma

Clinical overview. Basal cell carcinoma is the most common malignant neoplasm, comprising about 80% of nonmelanomatous skin cancers, and primarily affects people over age 40. About 99% of cases occur in whites, especially those with fair skin. Other risk factors include UV radiation exposure, particularly UVB (shortwave rays), prior radiation exposure, and chronic skin conditions such as lichen planus or lichen sclerosus.

Diagnosis. BCCs are typically slow growing, are sometimes associated with crusting and bleeding, and are primarily asymptomatic. Because they are slow growing, early detection and treatment is often successful. They usually occur on the face or the backs of hands and spread locally. Metastasis is very rare. There are five distinct BCC histological types: nodular (most common), superficial, micronodular, infiltrating, and morpheaform. About 40% of lesions contain two or more histological types.

Nodular BCC appears mostly as a pearly, translucent papule with telangiectasias. It may also appear pigmented and can be mistaken for melanoma. Superficial BCC occurs mostly on the trunk and extremities and appears scaly, although still with the raised, pearly white borders similar to nodular BCC. Both micronodular and infiltrating BCC appear similar to nodular BCC. Morpheaform BCC is usually a firm, yellow-colored, ill-defined mass. Incisional or excisional biopsy is required for definitive diagnosis (Figure 24–1 and Figure 24–2). While the five histologic types of BCC can be identified by characteristic physical features, the definitive diagnosis is made by incisional or excisional biopsy.

Treatment. Although BCCs typically grow slowly and do not have biological potential for metastasis, they may result in significant tissue destruction and disfigurement if left untreated. Surgical excision can be used for both diagnostic and curative treatment, with cure rates of up to 99% for low-risk lesions (those that are smaller than 1.5 cm in diameter and that are located in nonfacial and superficial areas) (Pariser and Phillips 1994). Treatment with electrodessication and curettage or liquid nitrogen cryotherapy can also be done by the primary care physician, but healing may take weeks. These treatment modalities are not useful in sclerosing or recurrent tumors. Other less commonly used specialized therapies, including radiation therapy, photody-

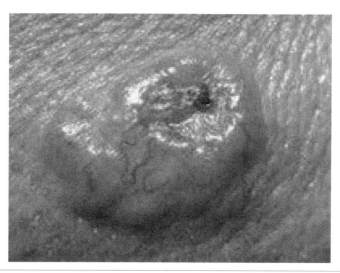

FIGURE 24–1.   Basal cell carcinoma.

namic therapy, and Mohs micrographic surgery, warrant a dermatology referral. This is especially true in patients with large lesions, typically greater
than 1.5 cm, recurrent BCC, or lesions located in difficult-to-treat areas such
as the face.

Squamous Cell Carcinoma

Clinical overview. Squamous cell carcinoma accounts for about 20% of
nonmelanomatous skin cancers. SCC tends to affect males at a slightly increased rate and is more prevalent after age 40 (Alam and Ratner 2001). As
with BCCs, sun exposure or other UV radiation predisposes individuals to
developing this malignancy. For this reason, fair-skinned individuals are
more commonly affected by SCC. However, the presence of actinic keratosis—precancerous lesions due to chronic sun exposure—provides an opportunity for early detection and intervention to prevent progression to SCC.
Exposure to tobacco, chemical carcinogens, therapeutic radiation, and certain human papillomavirus strains (6, 11, 16, and 18) has also been associated
with the development of SCC. Immunosuppressive states independently appear to contribute to SCC development.

Diagnosis. The goal in diagnosis of SCC should be focused on identifying
premalignant lesions whenever possible. Most commonly discovered in
chronically sun-damaged skin areas, actinic keratosis is classically described
as scaly, erythematous macules or papules (Figure 24–3). Areas most commonly affected (lips, ears, and dorsa of the hands) should be thoroughly ex-

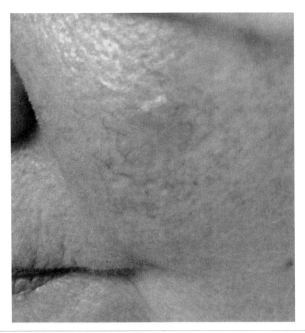

FIGURE 24–2.   Basal cell carcinoma.

amined. SCC should be suspected in patients who are homeless and consistently exposed to the sun.

SCC tends to appear as a firm, smooth, hyperkeratotic papule or plaque with a central ulceration (Figure 24–4). There is also a verrucous form, resembling a wart, which is less common but tends to be more invasive. SCC tumors are faster growing than BCC. Although shave biopsies of the most abnormal appearing skin can help establish the diagnosis of SCC, patients with small tumors that are pigmented may benefit from either full excision or punch biopsy to rule out melanoma (Firnhaber 2012).

Treatment. Treatment of SCC depends on the size and location of the tumor. Actinic keratosis can be treated with electrodessication and curettage, cryotherapy, photodynamic therapy, or topical therapies such as 5-fluorouracil (5%). SCC lesions smaller than 8 mm in diameter should undergo local or surgical excision. Lesions larger than 8 mm in diameter may need multiple therapies, including surgical excision and radiation therapy (Arora and Attwood 2009). Cryotherapy or electrodessication with curettage is also an option for small tumors (<2cm in diameter) and can be done by the primary care physician, although healing can be slow and scarring may result. Other procedures, such as excision, Mohs micrographic surgery, or radiotherapy, warrant referral to a dermatologist.

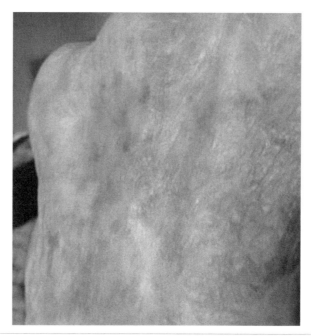

FIGURE 24–3.   Actinic keratosis.

Melanoma

Clinical overview. Although some estimates suggest that melanoma accounts for only about 10% of skin cancers, it poses the greatest risk for mortality. It affects people of all ages. Radiation exposure increases the risk of developing melanoma. Unlike in cases of SCC, intense periods of sun exposure with burning are more highly associated with development of melanoma than is chronic sun exposure or cumulative radiation load. Congenital nevi or multiple nevi increase the risk of development of melanoma, although they are rarely precursor lesions. In addition, there appears to be a hereditary component to the disease; having first- or second-degree relatives with melanoma increases the risk in individuals. In addition, there is a familial syndrome (familial atypical mole–melanoma syndrome) that carries an even stronger risk of developing melanoma (Humphreys 2001).

Diagnosis. Because malignant melanoma is curable, vigilant monitoring for early detection is important. Lesions tend to appear on the trunk in men and on the legs in women. The "ABCDE rules" (Table 24–1) are typically employed to identify superficial spreading melanoma, which is the most common form of the malignancy (Friedman et al. 1985). Superficial spreading melanoma accounts for approximately 70% of melanomas and typically pre-

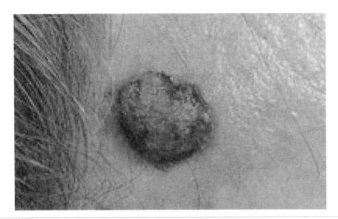

FIGURE 24–4.   Squamous cell carcinoma.

sents as an irregularly pigmented macule or plaque. Lesions are identified by being asymmetric with irregular borders of variegated color and with a diameter greater than 6 mm. There are other subtypes of melanoma. The nodular subtype looks like a dark brown or black papule or nodule (Figure 24–5). Pigmented macules on the head or neck of elderly patients can represent an indolent form of melanoma, called lentigo maligna. The acral-lentiginous type, which makes up 2%–8% of melanomas, may present as discoloration in the fingernails or toenails.

Complete excision of melanomas is important for two reasons: to provide a potentially curative effect and to determine the tumor thickness or depth of invasion. Once melanoma has metastasized, the 5-year survival rate decreases significantly to as low as 5%. Tumor thickness is the variable that best predicts long-term survival.

Treatment.   The first step in treatment of melanoma is proper excisional biopsy, usually done by a dermatologist or a surgeon. Once melanoma has metastasized, the 5-year survival rate decreases significantly (5%). There are multiple new therapies under development for the treatment of metastatic melanoma. One of these treatments, interferon alfa-2b, has shown some success in treating patients with high-risk or metastatic melanoma; however, this treatment has also been found to be associated with adverse neuropsychiatric effects, including manic symptoms and severe depression. In patients receiving this therapy, vigilant monitoring for these symptoms is recommended, and medical treatment with antidepressants and mood stabilizers may be warranted. In some cases when there are severe symptoms, such as severe mania, the therapy may need to be stopped (Greenberg et al. 2000; Raison et al. 2005; Valentine and Meyers 2005).

TABLE 24–1.   **ABCDE rules for identifying melanoma**

Asymmetry	In color or shape
Border	Irregular, notched
Color	Dark, variegated color
Diameter	Rapidly changing size (>6 mm)
Evolving	Evolution or changes in ABCD

When to Refer

Situations warranting referral to a primary care provider and/or dermatologist include the following:

- Presence of widespread symptoms—fever, weight loss, and/or fatigue
- Inability to diagnose skin lesion(s)
- Personal or family history of skin cancer
- Abnormal skin lesion that needs to be biopsied

Special Treatment Considerations for the Psychiatric Patient Population

Although several studies have highlighted the high prevalence of psychiatric disorders among patients with skin disease, little is known about the prevalence of skin cancer in patients with known psychiatric illness. A few single-center studies have found a strong correlation between hospitalized chronic psychiatric patients and skin diseases in general. Because patients with mental illness may be more subjected to poor lifestyle factors, including smoking, poor self-care, and poor housing conditions, they may be at greater risk for skin cancer. One Dutch study found the incidence of skin cancer in patients with psychiatric illness to be 1.4%, compared to 0.13%–0.5% in the general population (Mookhoek et al. 2011). Homeless patients have a high risk of skin cancer due to regular sun exposure, lack of sunscreen use, and low skin cancer screening rates (Chau et al. 2002; Wilde et al. 2013). Although no large studies have evaluated the risk or incidence of skin cancer in patients with mental illness in comparison to other subgroups, these patients may represent a population in which skin cancer screening may be overlooked or neglected because more emphasis is placed on managing their psychiatric illness. It is often difficult to perform a thorough skin examination in a patient who is paranoid, acutely agitated, or severely depressed. Patients with mental illness and substance use are much less likely to use health care maintenance

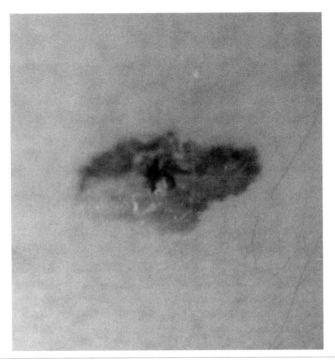

FIGURE 24–5. Melanoma.

and preventive services. Psychiatrists may be these patients' primary access to medical care and are therefore in a unique position to identify potentially malignant lesions and to counsel patients on prevention.

Case Discussion (*continued*)

Given Mr. W's extensive skin lesions, his psychiatrist refers him to a dermatologist, who diagnoses him with actinic keratosis and treats him with cryotherapy. Early detection of this precancerous lesion in this man with significant risk factors (tobacco use, chronic sun exposure) leads to prevention of SCC. Mr. W is advised to stop using any tobacco products, because this increases the risk for SCC. He is also encouraged to follow up with his social worker if he ever becomes homeless again, and he understands that ongoing sun exposure can increase his risk for the development of SCC. This patient is also given a referral to a primary care provider. Given his history of long-term sun exposure, smoking, poor access to primary medical care, and actinic keratosis, he is strongly advised to have skin examinations every 1–3 years.

Clinical Highlights

- Malignant melanoma occurs in about 2% of people during their lifetime but accounts for 75% of all deaths associated with skin cancer.

- Basal cell carcinoma is the most common skin cancer, primarily occurring in whites with fair skin. It is slow growing with low potential for metastasis but can lead to tissue destruction and disfigurement if left untreated.

- Squamous cell carcinoma accounts for approximately 20% of nonmelanomatous skin cancers. Sun exposure poses greatest risk. Therefore, patients with lesions in sun-exposed areas, such as lips, ears, dorsa of the hands, and ears, should be referred to a primary care provider or dermatology for further examination and workup.

- Intense periods of sun exposure with burning are more highly associated with development of melanoma than is chronic sun exposure.

- Superficial spreading melanoma accounts for approximately 70% of melanomas and typically presents as an irregularly pigmented macule or plaque, with asymmetric and irregular borders of variegated color and with a diameter greater than 6 mm.

Resources

American Academy of Dermatology: http://www.aad.org
American Cancer Society: http://www.cancer.org
Skin Cancer Foundation: http://www.skincancer.org

References

Alam M, Ratner D: Cutaneous squamous-cell carcinoma. N Engl J Med 344:975–983, 2001

Arora A, Attwood J: Common skin cancers and their precursors. Surg Clin North Am 89:703–712, 2009

Chau S, Chin M, Chang J, et al: Cancer risk behaviors and screening rates among homeless adults in Los Angeles County. Cancer Epidemiol Biomarkers Prev 11:431–438, 2002

Croswell J, Shin YR: Behavioral counseling to prevent skin cancer. Am Fam Physician 86:773–774, 2012

Firnhaber JM: Diagnosis and treatment of basal cell and squamous cell carcinoma. Am Fam Physician 86:161–168, 2012

Friedman RJ, Rigel DS, Kopf AW: Early detection of malignant melanoma: the role of physician examination and self-examination of the skin. CA Cancer J Clin 35:130–151, 1985

Greenberg DB, Jonasch E, Gadd MA, et al: Adjuvant therapy of melanoma with interferon-alpha-2b is associated with mania and bipolar syndromes. Cancer 89:356–362, 2000

Humphreys TR: Skin cancer: recognition and management. Clin Cornerstone 4:23–32, 2001

Jerant AF, Johnson JT, Sheridan CD, et al: Early detection and treatment of skin cancer. Am Fam Physician 62:357–368, 2000

Mookhoek EJ, van de Kerkhof PC, Hovens JE, et al: Substantial skin disorders in psychiatric illness coincide with diabetes and addiction. J Eur Acad Dermatol Venereol 25:392–397, 2011

Pariser DM, Phillips PK: Basal cell carcinoma: when to treat it yourself, and when to refer. Geriatrics 49:39–44, 1994

Raison CL, Demetrashvili M, Capuron L, et al: Neuropsychiatric adverse effects of interferon-alpha: recognition and management. CNS Drugs 19:105–123, 2005

Valentine AD, Meyers CA: Neurobehavioral effects of interferon therapy. Curr Psychiatry Rep 7:391–395, 2005

Wilde M, Jones B, Lewis BK, et al: Skin cancer screening in the homeless population. Dermatol Online J 19:14, 2013

Wolff T, Tai E, Miller T: Screening for skin cancer: an update of the evidence for the U.S. Preventive Services Task Force. Ann Intern Med 150:194–198, 2009

SECTION VI

Special Topics

CHAPTER 25

Geriatric Preventive Care

Margaret W. Leung, M.D., M.P.H.

Thuan Ong, M.D., M.P.H.

Dilip V. Jeste, M.D.

Case Discussion

Mr. E is a 72-year-old man with a history of poorly controlled diabetes, atrial fibrillation, glaucoma, and major depression with anxiety. He presents to the clinic because his children have found numerous medication bottles unopened, he has fallen twice in the past 2 months, and he has not returned their phone calls. Mr. E has no specific concerns. He feels he can manage his medications independently. He attributes his falls to having left some clothes on the floor. He admits to forgetting to return his children's phone calls but does not want to bother them. His medications include warfarin, aspirin, metoprolol, amiodarone, insulin, citalopram, clonazepam, and latanoprost eyedrops. He lives alone and has hired weekly housekeeping. He continues to drive. He has given his children control of his finances because he does not want to keep up with the bills. On examination, he weighs 5.4 kg (12 lb) less compared with 8 months earlier, wears ill-fitting dentures, has an irregular heart rhythm, has decreased sensation to pinprick on his feet and legs, and has old bruises over his right hip and leg. Mr. E cannot recall two of three words on delayed recall, and his clock drawing is abnormal.

Clinical Overview

Preventive health takes a different tenor when applied to the geriatric population compared with the rest of the general population. Adults age 65 years and older have increased from 35 million in 2000 to 41 million in 2011, and the number is expected to double to 92 million by 2060 (Administration on Aging 2012). The oldest-old—those older than age 84 years—have the highest rate of acute illnesses, chronic disease, and disability, and are expected to triple from nearly 6 million in 2011 to 14 million in 2040. Despite these burgeoning numbers, few studies of preventive medicine include older adults. Guidelines for older adults often extrapolate from guidelines for younger populations, with limited specific consideration given to how they may impact older adults; do not mention upper age limits on care decisions; or fail to acknowledge insufficient evidence.

The unique needs of individuals who are elderly go beyond the standard medical evaluation. Common conditions in the elderly such as falls, frailty, and incontinence are classified as geriatric syndromes. *Geriatric syndromes* are health conditions that are caused by many factors that interact with one another, leading to impairment on multiple levels in an older individual (Inouye et al. 2007), and that do not fit into discrete disease categories. In addition, an evaluation of the physical health of a geriatric patient, comprehensive geriatric assessment includes the assessment of functional independence and psychological, social, and environmental factors (Devons 2002). Psychiatrists are well versed to assess how current function, cognition, mood disorders, and social support impact the well-being of older adults.

Individuals with psychiatric diagnoses are disproportionately affected by medical comorbidities. Psychiatrists, in their diagnosis and treatment of this population, should therefore be mindful of the interaction among psychiatric illness, medical illnesses, and function. Elderly adults with bipolar disorder have an average of three to four medical conditions (Lala and Sajatovic 2012). In older adults, depression affects functional disability, which can improve when depression is treated (Nyunt et al. 2012; Proctor et al. 2003).

The geriatric population is a heterogeneous group, but overall goals often are to maintain high functional capacity and quality of life. The emphasis on functionality in a comprehensive geriatric assessment will help guide the approach to take with preventive health care. A useful guide in considering a preventive clinical approach is to determine which of three populations the geriatric patient best fits: 1) independent function with or without chronic disease and with life expectancy of more than 5 years, 2) dependent function with multiple chronic morbidities and life expectancy of 2–5 years, or 3) life expectancy of less than 2 years (Reuben 2009).

Well elderly who have longer life expectancies with many years of independent living are more likely to benefit from primary and secondary prevention efforts. Primary prevention aims to avoid disease and disability, and secondary prevention attempts to target and to treat asymptomatic older adults who have risk factors or preclinical disease. Frail elderly individuals whose impaired functional capacity, disability, or dependency shortens life expectancy receive most of their medical care through tertiary care efforts. Tertiary prevention involves medical care for established disease and attempts to restore the highest possible functioning, decrease morbidity, and prevent disease-related complications. The American Geriatrics Society's ethics committee recommends detecting illnesses that contribute to symptoms rather than screening for asymptomatic disease in older adults with a shortened life expectancy (American Geriatrics Society 2003).

In this chapter we highlight a preventive approach to evaluating and treating common geriatric syndromes, including falls, sensory impairment, polypharmacy, and malnutrition. Primary and secondary preventive care involving cancer screening, elder abuse, immunizations, and cognitive impairment will also be reviewed.

Practical Pointers

- To help guide the preventive approach, the initial step is for the clinician to determine into which of three groups the elderly patient best fits (Reuben 2009):
  - Independent function, with life expectancy of more than 5 years
  - Dependent function, with multiple chronic morbidities and life expectancy of 2–5 years
  - At the end of life, with life expectancy of less than 2 years

Evaluating and Treating Common Geriatric Syndromes

Falls

Falls in community-dwelling older adults are a treatable geriatric syndrome that is associated with high morbidity and mortality, threatens independence, and impacts quality of life. One in every three individuals over age 65 years will suffer a fall (Hausdorff et al. 2001). Falls are the leading cause of death due to injury among older adults. One in 10 falls results in serious injury, such as fracture or subdural hematoma (Sattin 1992). Even without injury, older adults who fall will often develop a fear of falling and limit their activities, leading to a self-perpetuating cycle of reduced mobility, further loss of physical fitness, and increasing risk of falling (Deshpande et al. 2008; Zijlstra et al. 2007).

As listed in Table 25–1, many risk factors contribute to falls in older adults (Gillespie et al. 2012). The preventive goal is to identify and reduce the impact of risk factors, high-risk activities, and injuries in the event of a fall.

Screening begins with inquiring whether the patient has had a fall in the past year. Patients may not consider their fall as a true fall and often attribute their fall as a "trip" or "slip." More positive screens may result by asking, "In the past year, have you had any fall including a slip or trip in which you lost your balance and landed on the floor or ground or lower level?" (Lamb et al. 2005). A fall history should include the following questions:

- Symptoms: Are there any prodromal symptoms (e.g., palpitations, light-headedness, vertigo)?
- Prior falls: Is there a history of prior falls?
- Location: Where did the fall happen?
- Activity: What were you doing at the time of the fall?
- Timing: What time did it happen?
- Trauma: Are there any injuries and residual functional impairment?

Clinically observed gait or balance abnormalities are the best predictors of future falls (Table 25–2) (Tinetti and Ginter 1988). Action should be taken to remedy any modifiable risk factors to prevent injury once an older adult is identified as a fall risk. It is important to explicitly discuss how older adults will activate medical assistance in the event of a serious injury where phones or help may not be within reach. Proprietary personalized medical emergency systems are available. Placing a small cell phone on a lanyard is a possible solution for some. Injury prevention also includes assessing for fracture risk. Appropriately using mobility assistive devices can increase stability in balance and gait, and thereby reduce likelihood of falls.

Sensory Impairment

Sensory impairment is common in older adults and contributes to common geriatric syndromes such as confusion, falls, and social withdrawal. Estimates of dual sensory loss (i.e., combined vision and hearing loss) range from 7% to 21% in older adults (McDonnall 2009). More than 60% of persons older than age 70 years have hearing loss, with about 30% having moderate to severe levels (Lin et al. 2011). Taking into account the prevalence of cataracts, macular degeneration, and glaucoma, an estimated one in two older adults by 2030 will have some significant visual disorder (Eichenbaum 2012). Sensory loss not only leads to decreased quality of life but also has been as-

TABLE 25–1. Modifiable risk factors for falls in community-dwelling older adults

Risk factor	Intervention
Movement and balance	
Gait abnormality	Group exercise
Muscle weakness	Individualized exercise program
Poor balance	Tai chi
Vitamin D insufficiency	Vitamin D supplementation: ≥800 international units daily, unless deficient
Environmental hazards	Home safety assessment and modification
Cardiac arrhythmia	Cardiac pacemaker or implantable cardioverter defibrillator
Diminished visual acuity	
Cataracts	Cataract removal surgery
Use of multifocal glasses	Single-lens glasses
Medication	
Class of medication	Reduction in and/or gradual withdrawal of medications, including psychotropics, diuretics, antihypertensives, antiarrhythmics, anticonvulsants, and anticholinergics
Number of medications	Four or more medications increase falls

TABLE 25–1. Modifiable risk factors for falls in community-dwelling older adults (*continued*)

Risk factor	Intervention
Podiatric conditions	
Foot pain	Podiatry referral
Poor footwear	Discourage walking in high heels, bare feet, or socks indoors; an ideal shoe has a low heel, a supported heel collar, and a thin, firm, and slip-resistant sole
Postural hypotension	Reduce offending medication(s) that is affecting blood pressure
	Use compression stockings
	Slowly rise, in stages, from supine to seated to standing; perform isometric handgrips when standing; and increase fluid and/or salt intake

Source. Adapted from Gillespie et al. 2012.

TABLE 25–2. Gait components and office-based testing to indicate fall risk in older adults

Test	Abnormality in performance indicating fall risk
Gait observation	Hesitates, stumbles, or grabs or touches objects for support when initiating gait
	Weaves or sways side to side
	Scrapes or shuffles and does not clear floor consistently
	With turning, stops before initiating turn, staggers, has noncontinuous motion, or grabs objects for support
Timed Get Up and Go test	Is unable to rise from chair without use of upper arms, walk 10 feet, turn, and return to seated position in chair in < 10 seconds
One-legged stance	Unable to maintain stance for 5 seconds

Source. Adapted from Tinetti and Ginter 1988.

sociated with depression, anxiety, and dementia (McDonnall 2009; Pacala and Yueh 2012).

Older adults often do not recognize hearing loss or attribute it to normal aging. A change from baseline behavior, loss of interest in hobbies, social withdrawal, depression, anxiety, or cognitive or functional decline should prompt a hearing screen. Patient or family reports of difficulty communicating, confusion in social situations, excessive volume of television or radio, or having to repeat themselves can suggest hearing impairment. Risk factors for hearing loss in adults include noise exposure, family history of hearing loss before age 50 years, age greater than 65 years, smoking, diabetes, and exposure to ototoxic medications.

Recommendations for hearing screens vary with different organizations. The U.S. Preventive Services Task Force (USPSTF; 2013) found insufficient evidence to balance the benefits and harms of screening for hearing loss in asymptomatic adults age 50 years and older. The American Speech-Language-Hearing Association (1997) recommends screening all adults once every decade until age 50 and then every 3 years thereafter. Screening questions and examinations are available (Table 25–3). A positive screen would warrant a referral to an audiologist.

Older adults with visual problems may report difficulty reading fine print, miss exit signs while driving, avoid driving at sunrise or sunset, or complain of

TABLE 25–3. Screening questions and examinations for hearing loss

Questions	Examination
Do you feel you have hearing loss? Would you say you have any difficulty in hearing?	**Whisper test** While patient occludes one ear, examiner stands at arm's length behind patient and whispers 6 letter-number combinations. A positive test is failure to repeat half of the letter-number combinations correctly.
	Finger rub Examiner gently rubs fingers together at a distance of 6 inches from patient's ear. A positive test is failure to identify rub in >2 of 6 attempts.

disruptive headlight glare at night. The four most common causes of visual loss in people who are elderly are macular degeneration, cataract, glaucoma, and diabetic retinopathy (Table 25–4). The early stages of these diseases are often asymptomatic, and early screening is advised. The American Academy of Ophthalmology (2010) recommends an eye examination every 1–2 years for individuals age 65 years and older, even in the absence of symptoms.

Polypharmacy

Adverse drug events are common among older adults and lead to poor outcomes. Age-related pharmacokinetic and pharmacodynamic changes and a greater number of chronic medical conditions necessitating more medications are predisposing risk factors for adverse drug events in older adults. Avoiding the use of inappropriate and high-risk drugs and applying a rational approach to prescribing are important strategies in reducing adverse drug events in older adults. *Polypharmacy* is not defined by a specific number of medications (Hajjar et al. 2007). A more clinically useful definition of *polypharmacy* is the administration of more medications than are clinically indicated (Montamat and Cusack 1992).

Age-related pharmacokinetic changes occur to every organ system (Sera and McPherson 2012). For example, older adults have decreased total body water and volume of distribution, and increased adipose tissue. Consequently, water-soluble medications such as ethanol will have higher serum concentrations, and lipid-soluble drugs such as barbiturates and benzodiazepines will have longer half-lives. The effects of centrally active medications often have greater impact on older adults, thereby requiring smaller doses for equal

TABLE 25–4. Four common causes of visual impairment in elderly patients

Diagnosis	Symptoms	Select risk factors	Preventive intervention
Age-related macular degeneration	Loss of central vision Scotoma (i.e., blind spot) Use of brighter light or magnifying glass for fine visual acuity Distortion of straight lines	Low levels of antioxidants Cigarette smoking	Zinc and antioxidants were beneficial in moderate and advanced cases in decreasing progression, but not for mild cases or primary prevention (Evans 2012).
Cataract	Loss of central vision Difficulty reading in dim light Glare with night driving	Cigarette smoking Excess sunlight exposure Corticosteroid therapy Diabetes	Limited prevention measures
Glaucoma	Loss of peripheral vision Painless unless closed-angle glaucoma	African American race Increased intraocular pressure	Limited prevention measures
Diabetic retinopathy	Decreased visual acuity Floaters Curtain falling	Poorly controlled blood glucose	Glycemic, blood pressure, and lipid control; eye exam at time of type 2 diagnosis and within 5 years of type 1 diagnosis

clinical efficacy. Drug-drug interactions are common because older adults often take multiple medications. Drugs can inhibit or induce the action of hepatic enzymes. Enzyme inhibitors may increase the half-life of drugs that are enzyme substrates and potentially lead to toxic levels. Conversely, enzyme inducers may decrease a substrate's half-life and cause subtherapeutic levels.

Rational prescribing requires, among other things, identifying the therapeutic goal of the drug (Table 25–5). Recognizing potentially inappropriate medications is also important in rational prescribing. To avoid potentially inappropriate medications, the clinician needs to consider therapeutic duplications of medications within the same class or with the same mechanism of action, drug-drug interactions, and high-risk drugs for older adults. The "Beers Criteria for Potentially Inappropriate Medication Use in Older Adults," commonly called the Beers Criteria, are an important quality measure used by the Centers of Medicare and Medicaid Services and the National Committee of Quality Assurance to improve the safety of prescribing medications for older adults to help prevent adverse drug events, hospitalizations, and mortality (American Geriatrics Society 2012). Medications such as antihistamines, antipsychotics, benzodiazepines, and muscle relaxants should be avoided because of adverse drug events in older adults.

Malnutrition

Adequate nutrition is an important determinant of health, physical, and cognitive status. The old adage of a well-balanced diet is not only practical but also clinically important because overt manifestations of malnutrition states emerge from long-standing nutritional deprivation of calories, protein, minerals, fiber, and/or vitamins. The prevalence of malnutrition is high among chronically ill older adults across all health care settings (Kaiser et al. 2010). Advancing age is characterized by loss of lean body mass with a relative increase in fat mass.

Undernutrition and weight loss are common issues in frail older adults. Most nutritionists will recommend that older adults add an iron-free multivitamin with minerals to compensate for common micronutrient deficiencies. Common causes of involuntary weight loss in older adults should be sought when appropriate, although many cases have unknown etiologies (Morley and Silver 1995). Table 25–6 lists common causes of involuntary weight loss in older adults. Clinically significant weight loss is defined as 4.5 kg (10 lb) or greater or 5% or greater of baseline body weight over a 6- to 12-month period. Although cancer is the most common cause of involuntary weight loss, accounting for 16%–36% of cases, involuntary weight loss in older adults may be part of a frailty syndrome related to underlying age-related changes, medical conditions, psychosocial issues, and medication side effects.

TABLE 25–5. **Rational drug prescribing for older adults**

Practical steps to consider in optimizing prescribing to older adults	Comment
Request patients to "brown bag" their medications and bring them to clinical visits.	Ask patients to bring in all their prescription and over-the-counter medicines, supplements, and herbal drugs being taken to accurately reconcile medications.
When starting a new drug, set a 1) therapeutic goal and 2) therapeutic time frame.	Establish a therapeutic goal and time frame to reassess clinically the efficacy for each medication and reduce polypharmacy.
Start low and go slow.	Start medications at low doses and titrate up to the lowest effective dose to limit untoward effects of drugs.
Avoid prescription cascades.	Evaluate whether medications may be causing side effects that are misdiagnosed as symptoms, triggering prescription of additional medication to treat the drug's side effect.
Look for drug-drug and drug-disease interactions, and potentially inappropriate medications.	Refer to the Beers Criteria (American Geriatrics Society 2012) and other pharmacology texts.
Limit medication changes to one or two per clinical encounter.	Avoid too many medication changes at a single visit because of potential miscommunication and/or adverse drug events.
Deprescribe when possible (Bain et al. 2008).	Periodically reassess: ask for patient and/or family preferences, look for clinical indications, review for potential harm, and assess medication utilization.

TABLE 25–6. **Common causes of involuntary weight loss in older adults**

Medications (e.g., diuretics, serotonin reuptake inhibitors, benzodiazepines, β-blockers, metformin)

Psychiatric disorders (e.g., dementia, depression, alcoholism, anorexia nervosa, paranoia)

Difficulty with swallowing or chewing

Endocrinological disorders (e.g., hyperthyroidism, hypothyroidism, hypoparathyroidism)

Gastrointestinal problems (e.g., nausea, malabsorption)

Functional limitations (e.g., inability to feed oneself or obtain food)

Lower socioeconomic status (e.g., availability and amount of food consumed)

Excess consumption of nutrients may lead to negative effects on health and physical and cognitive function. Obesity, an increasing problem in Western societies, can exacerbate age-related decline in physical function and negatively impact quality of life. The American Society for Nutrition and the Obesity Society recommend weight loss therapy to improve physical function, quality of life, and medical complications associated with obesity in older persons (Villareal et al. 2005); they also recommend weight loss therapy for obese older persons to minimize muscle and bone losses or for those who have functional impairments and/or medical complications from obesity.

Calculating the body mass index (BMI) is useful to identify, evaluate, and treat overweight and underweight older adults (Table 25–7). BMI may underestimate body fat in older adults because lean body muscle loss increases with advancing age. There is some evidence that being overweight (BMI 25–29.9) does not confer excess mortality risk in older adults (Heiat et al. 2001). Extremes of BMI or clinically significant weight loss without a clear etiology should warrant a full dietary assessment by a nutritionist.

Primary and Secondary Preventive Care

Cancer Screening

Individualized cancer screening decisions for patients who are elderly should take into account life expectancy, medical comorbidities, functional status, benefits of screening, and patient values and preferences (Walter and Covinsky 2001). Older adults with shorter life expectancy because of advanced age

TABLE 25–7. Body mass index (BMI)

	BMI
Underweight	<18.5
Normal	18.5–24.9
Overweight	25–29.9
Obesity	≥30.0

may not benefit from screening because some may not live long enough and will likely die from other causes. For example, certain types of cancers either are less aggressive in older age or do not demonstrate cancer mortality until 5 years after the start of screening (Walter et al. 2005). Coexisting chronic illnesses in elderly patients are associated with decreased life expectancy after the diagnosis of early-stage colorectal cancer (Gross et al. 2006), raising questions about whether to screen in the first place. A 75-year-old woman with advanced heart failure and Alzheimer's dementia living in a nursing facility will more likely die from cardiovascular complications than from breast cancer, whereas a 75-year-old woman with well-controlled diabetes living independently at home might die from the untreated breast cancer.

The harms of cancer screening also must be weighed against the benefits of screening. Screening can lead to false positives, further diagnostic procedures and complications, psychological distress, and treatment of indolent cancers. In breast cancer, 77–86 per 1,000 women older than age 70 years will have a positive screening mammogram, and 86% of these will be false positives (Welch and Fisher 1998). There is no consensus among various medical societies regarding the upper age at which cancer screenings should stop. A comparison of recommendations by the U.S. Preventive Services Task Force (2013) and the American Geriatrics Society (2000, 2001) is provided in Table 25–8. In general, screening should be avoided in older adults with less than 5-year life expectancies.

Elder Maltreatment

An estimated 1–2 million Americans age 65 and older have experienced elder maltreatment, sometimes known as elder abuse (Bonnie and Wallace 2003). Although no consensus exists on the definition of *elder abuse,* the literature has identified five forms of maltreatment (Table 25–9). The community prevalence of elder abuse, excluding institutional abuses, ranges from 2% to 10% (Acierno et al. 2010; Thomas 2002).

Screening for elder abuse has been controversial due to the lack of a standard screening tool, universal guidance about whom to screen, or actions to

TABLE 25–8. Cancer screening guidelines for elderly patients

Cancer screening	U.S. Preventive Services Task Force (2013)	American Geriatrics Society
Breast	Screen using mammogram biennially women ages 50–74 years Insufficient benefit and harm of screening mammography in women age 75 years or older	Screen using mammogram annually or biennially until age 75 or at least every 3 years thereafter No upper age limit for women with estimated life expectancy of ≥4 years (American Geriatrics Society 2000)
Cervical	Screen with cytology for women ages 21–65 every 3 years, or combination of cytology and human papillomavirus every 5 years Recommend against screening in women older than age 65 years who have had adequate screening and are not otherwise at high risk for cervical cancer	Screen at 1- to 3-year intervals until at least age 60 Beyond age 70, there is little evidence for or against screening women who have been regularly screened in previous years (American Geriatrics Society 2001)
Colon	Screen using fecal occult blood testing, sigmoidoscopy, or colonoscopy for patients ages 50–75 years Recommend against routine screening for patients ages 76–86 but consider individualized assessment Recommend against screening for patients older than 85 years	No specific guidelines
Prostate	Recommend against screening	No specific guidelines

TABLE 25–9. **Types of elder maltreatment**

Form of abuse	Characteristics	Signs and symptoms
Physical	Injuries caused by infliction of pain, inappropriate restraint, or assault (including threats with a weapon)	Bruises, cigarette burn marks, fractures, painful movements
Psychological or emotional	Threatening or coercive behavior such as humiliation, controlling behavior, or threats to institutionalize	Depression, anxiety, self-blame for present situation, impaired mental status
Sexual	Nonconsensual contact, such as fondling; suggestive talk; or forced sexual activity	Bruising or injury around breast or genitalia, bloody or stained underclothing, unexplained sexually transmitted infection
Neglect	Intentional or unintentional failure or refusal by another to meet elder's needs or protect elder from harm, as well as self-neglect by elder	Weight loss, poor hygiene, dehydration, depression, anxiety
Financial	Illegal or improper use of elder's resources for personal profit cr gain	Unexplained change in power of attorney, will, or legal documents

TABLE 25–10. Screening questions for elder maltreatment

Who makes up your social support?

Who makes decisions about your life, such as how you should live or where you should live?

Do you feel uncomfortable with anyone who is taking care of you?

Has anyone forced you to do things you did not want to do?

Has anyone prevented you from getting food, medications, or medical care, or from being with people whom you want to be with?

Have your belongings been taken from you without your permission?

Has anyone close to you hurt you or harmed you recently?

Has someone talked with you who made you feel ashamed or threatened?

take if abuse is identified. The USPSTF found insufficient evidence to recommend for or against screening older adults for abuse and neglect (Moyer and U.S. Preventive Services Task Force 2013). However, the American Medical Association (1992) and the American Academy of Neurology (Schulman and Hohler 2012) recommend that physicians routinely inquire about possible mistreatments of elders.

Psychiatrists may be the first providers to identify abuse through their assessment of the patient's cognitive, behavioral, and medical health. Dementia, cognitive impairment, and psychiatric illnesses such as depression are risk factors for elder abuse (Dyer et al. 2000; Johannesen and LoGiudice 2013). A psychosocial history can identify relational problems between the elder and the caregiver(s), and a history of family violence. Other risk factors include caregiver burden, low social support, poor physical health, and higher functional impairment. Psychiatrists are in an apt position to assess decisional capacity, especially in cases of self-neglect. Despite the lack of a universal screening tool, providers can evaluate older adults by beginning with asking general questions and working toward more direct inquiries (Table 25–10).

Immunizations

The immune system tends to weaken as people age. These immunological changes contribute to older adults being more susceptible to infections, requiring longer durations to convalesce, having poorer prognosis, and experiencing decreased vaccination efficacy compared with younger people. Nevertheless, vaccinations continue to be an important part of preventive health care for all people, regardless of age. The Advisory Committee on Immunization Practices Adult Immunization Work Group et al. (2013) recommend routine vaccinations for older adults (Table 25–11).

TABLE 25–11. **Recommended vaccinations for older adults**

Vaccine	≥65 years old
Influenza	1 dose annually
Tetanus, diphtheria, pertussis (Td/Tdap)	Substitute one-time dose of Tdap for Td booster; then boost with Td every 10 years
Zoster	1 dose (starting at ≥60 years)
Pneumococcal polysaccharide 23	1 dose
Pneumococcal 13-valent conjugate	1 dose

Source. Adapted from Advisory Committee on Immunization Practices Adult Immunization Work Group et al. 2013.

Cognitive Impairment

The global prevalence rate of dementia is projected to increase by over 75% in the next quarter century (Wilmo et al. 2006). Prevention efforts represent a major public intervention, because a delay of disease onset and progression of Alzheimer's disease (AD) by 1 year would result in 9 million fewer cases in 2050 (Brookmeyer et al. 2007). Psychiatrists can play an important role in prevention psychiatry through the life span. Protecting individuals from developing a clinical illness, even in the presence of the underlying risk, is not a futuristic fantasy. Further efforts to expand the spectrum of preventions in psychiatry would be highly beneficial for patients, communities, and societies. A growing body of research on both lifestyle and pharmacological approaches to cognitive impairment indicates that neuroplasticity can occur in aging. This section focuses primarily on prevention of mild neurocognitive disorder and AD.

Risk factors, including hyperlipidemia, diabetes, and smoking, cause oxidative and vascular damage to the brain. Good control of such modifiable risk factors through lifestyle changes and medications can potentially lead to decreased risk for mild neurocognitive disorder and AD. Current smokers have an increased risk compared with never or former smokers (Daviglus et al. 2011). Metabolic syndrome, comprising abdominal obesity, hyperglycemia, hypertension, hypertriglyceridemia, and low high-density lipoprotein levels, accelerates cognitive impairment (Yaffe 2007). The evidence supporting the use of statins to prevent cognitive impairment remains mixed (Cramer et al. 2008; Menezes et al. 2012), and currently there are no diabetes-specific treatments for dementia.

Nonpharmacological approaches such as physical activity and proper nutrition also suggest protective effects. Physical activity, specifically aerobic exercise sufficient to increase heart rate and the body's need for oxygen, has been shown not only to modestly improve cognitive scores but also to increase connectivity of brain cognitive networks and hippocampal volumes, as demonstrated with functional magnetic resonance imaging (Ahlskog et al. 2011). Although increased consumption of vegetables is associated with a lower risk of dementia and slower rate of cognitive decline (Loef and Walach 2012), much of the research has focused on polyunsaturated fats in the diet. Regular fish consumption or omega-3 fatty acid supplemental intake is associated with a decreased risk of all-cause dementia (Barberger-Gateau et al. 2007), and more specifically protects elderly people without dementia but does not prevent or treat those who already have dementia (Fotuhi et al. 2009). Finally, cognitive training, especially when focused on cognitive exercises rather than memory strategies, has a moderate effect on memory-related outcomes (Gates et al. 2011).

Other dietary supplements have not been well supported in clinical trials. *Ginkgo biloba* does not protect against cognitive decline in older adults with normal cognition or mild neurocognitive impairment (Snitz et al. 2009). Other supplements have been studied for their effects on decreasing the level of homocysteine because hyperhomocysteinemia is a risk factor for atherosclerosis and a possible diagnostic marker for AD. Vitamin B_{12}, vitamin B_6, and folic acid have not been found to improve cognitive function in individuals with or without existing cognitive impairment with hyperhomocysteinemia (Balk et al. 2007). Antioxidants such as vitamins E and C are theoretically thought to minimize oxidative stress in AD, but controlled trials have mostly not supported clinical use (Bowman 2012; Farina et al. 2012).

Case Discussion (*continued*)

Mr. E has a complex medical, social, and functional history. He would benefit from a multidisciplinary comprehensive geriatric assessment.

- *Falls:* Mr. E has multiple risk factors for falls, including peripheral neuropathy, sensory impairment, polypharmacy, prior history of falls, and cognitive impairment. His poorly controlled diabetes contributes to his peripheral neuropathy. A referral to podiatry to assess foot pain and prescription for proper-fitting shoes would decrease some risk. A postural blood pressure should be measured. He may benefit from a mobility assistive device such as a walker. A referral to a physical therapist may identify lower extremity weakness that may improve with gait and balance rehabilitation. A home evaluation would identify environmental hazards.
- *Sensory impairment:* Mr. E needs a dilated annual eye examination to evaluate for worsening glaucoma and the presence of diabetic retinopathy, cataracts, and/or macular degeneration. His hearing should also be evaluated.
- *Polypharmacy:* Mr. E has some medications that are listed on the Beers Criteria. Clonazepam should ideally be tapered off because of its impact on

cognition and falls. Amiodarone, used to control atrial fibrillation, interacts with many medications. Metoprolol may cause orthostatic hypotension, causing him to feel light-headed when he stands up too quickly. Citalopram and some antidepressants are associated with falls. Mr. E's visual problems may cause him to draw either too much or too little insulin, contributing to poorly controlled diabetes. Because of the frequent falls, he and his physician will need to decide whether to safely continue warfarin, which would lead to excessive and potentially life-threatening bleeding if a fall occurs.

- *Malnutrition:* Mr. E has lost a clinically significant amount of weight since his previous visit. He will need a workup to determine the cause of his weight loss. His risks for weight loss include denture use, poorly controlled diabetes, medications, and cognitive impairment.
- *Cognitive impairment:* Mr. E tested poorly and therefore needs further evaluation for dementia. He will likely benefit from cognitive training and increased physical activity.
- *Immunizations:* Mr. E needs the following immunizations: pneumococcal polysaccharide vaccine 23, zoster, annual influenza, and tetanus booster if not previously administered.
- *Cancer screening:* Based on the U.S. Preventive Services Task Force's (2013) guidelines, Mr. E should not be screened for prostate cancer. Assuming he does not have dementia, he will need a colonoscopy for colon cancer screening if he has not had one previously. If he is diagnosed with dementia, Mr. E and his physician will need to discuss the risks and benefits of cancer screening, because he may have more complications with comorbid problems related to dementia than from colon cancer itself.
- *Elder maltreatment:* Mr. E has given his children control of his finances, and a screen for financial maltreatment and other forms of maltreatment could identify signs of coercion.

Clinical Highlights

- Preventive geriatric care is multifaceted and addresses the physical, psychological, social, and functional health of an older adult.
- The functional status of an older adult guides the level of preventive care.
- Regular screening for vision and hearing can improve the quality of life in older adults.
- The practice of rational drug prescribing avoids potentially harmful drug interactions related to age-related changes to medications.
- Although there is no specific age at which cancer screenings should be discontinued, the benefits and risks of cancer screenings should be weighed against life expectancy and comorbid medical conditions.
- Increasing research supports lifestyle and pharmacological interventions in the delay and prevention of cognitive impairment.

Resources

For Patients

American Geriatrics Society's Health in Aging Foundation: http://www.healthinaging.org

National Institute on Aging: http://www.nia.nih.gov

For Clinicians

Iowa Geriatric Education Center: Geriatric Assessment Tools. http://www.healthcare.uiowa.edu/igec/tools/

Portal of Geriatrics Online Education: http://www.pogoe.org

References

Acierno R, Hernandez MA, Amstadter AB, et al: Prevalence and correlates of emotional, physical, sexual, and financial abuse and potential neglect in the United States: the National Elder Mistreatment Study. Am J Public Health 199:292–297, 2010

Administration on Aging: A Profile of Older Americans: 2012. Washington, DC, Administration on Aging, 2012. Available at: http://www.aoa.gov/AoARoot/Aging_Statistics/Profile/index.aspx. Accessed May 22, 2013.

Advisory Committee on Immunization Practices Adult Immunization Work Group; Bridges CB, Woods L, et al: Advisory Committee on Immunization Practices (ACIP) recommended immunization schedule for adults aged 19 years and older—United States, 2013. MMWR Surveill Summ 62(suppl):9–19, 2013

Ahlskog JE, Geda YE, Graff-Radford NR, et al: Physical exercise as a preventive or disease-modifying treatment of dementia and brain aging. Mayo Clin Proc 86:876–885, 2011

American Academy of Ophthalmology, Preferred Practice Patterns Committee: Preferred Practice Pattern Guidelines: Comprehensive Adult Medical Eye Evaluation, 2010. San Francisco, CA, American Academy of Ophthalmology, 2010. Available at: www.aao.org/ppp. Accessed July 6, 2014.

American Geriatrics Society: Breast cancer screening in older women. Am J Geriatr Soc 48:842–844, 2000

American Geriatrics Society: Screening for cervical cancer in older women. J Am Geriatr Soc 49:655–657, 2001

American Geriatrics Society: Health screening decisions for older adults: AGS position paper. J Am Geriatr Soc 51:270–271, 2003

American Geriatrics Society: American Geriatrics Society updated Beers Criteria for potentially inappropriate medication use in older adults. J Am Geriatr Soc 60:616–631, 2012

American Medical Association: Diagnostic and Treatment Guidelines on Elder Abuse and Neglect. Chicago, IL, American Medical Association, 1992

American Speech-Language-Hearing Association: Guidelines for audiologic screening, 1997. Available at: http://www.asha.org/docs/pdf/GL1997-00199.pdf. Accessed July 6, 2014.

Bain KT, Holmes HM, Beers MH, et al: Discontinuing medication: a novel approach for revising the prescribing stage of the medication-use process. J Am Geriatr Soc 56:1946–1952, 2008

Balk EM, Raman G, Tatsioni A, et al: Vitamin B6, B12, and folic acid supplementation and cognitive function: a systematic review of randomized trials. Arch Intern Med 167:21–30, 2007

Barberger-Gateau P, Raffaitin C, Letenneur L, et al: Dietary patterns and risk of dementia: the Three-City cohort study. Neurology 69:1921–1930, 2007

Bonnie RJ, Wallace RB (eds): Elder Mistreatment: Abuse, Neglect, and Exploitation in an Aging America. Washington, DC, National Academies Press, 2003, pp 1–8

Bowman GL: Ascorbic acid, cognitive function, and Alzheimer's disease: a current review and future direction. Biofactors 38:114–122, 2012

Brookmeyer R, Johnson E, Ziegler-Graham K, et al: Forecasting the global burden of Alzheimer's disease. Alzheimers Dement 3:1886–1891, 2007

Cramer C, Haan MN, Galea S, et al: Use of statins and incidence of dementia and cognitive impairment without dementia in a cohort study. Neurology 71:344–350, 2008

Daviglus ML, Plassman BL, Pirzada A, et al: Risk factors and preventive interventions for Alzheimer disease. Arch Neurol 68:1185–1190, 2011

Deshpande N, Metter EJ, Lauretani F, et al: Activity restriction induced by fear of falling and objective and subjective measures of physical function: a prospective cohort study. J Am Geriatr Soc 56:615–620, 2008

Devons CAJ: Comprehensive geriatric assessment: making the most of the aging years. Curr Opin Clin Nutr Metab Care 5:19–24, 2002

Dyer CB, Pavlik VN, Murphy KP, et al: The high prevalence of depression and dementia in elder abuse or neglect. J Am Geriatr Soc 48:205–208, 2000

Eichenbaum JW: Geriatric vision loss due to cataracts, macular degeneration, and glaucoma. Mt Sinai J Med 79:276–294, 2012

Evans JR: Antioxidant vitamin and mineral supplements for slowing the progression of age-related macular degeneration. Cochrane Database Syst Rev 11:CD000254, 2012

Farina N, Isaac MG, Clark AR, et al: Vitamin E for Alzheimer's dementia and mild cognitive impairment. Cochrane Database Syst Rev 11:CD002854, 2012

Fotuhi M, Mohassel P, Yaffe K: Fish consumption, long-chain omega-3 fatty acids and risk of cognitive decline or Alzheimer disease: a complex association. Nat Clin Pract Neurol 5:140–152, 2009

Gates NJ, Sachdev PS, Singh MA, et al: Cognitive and memory training in adults at risk of dementia: a systematic review. BMC Geriatrics 11:1–4, 2011

Gillespie LD, Robertson MC, Gillespie WJ, et al: Interventions for preventing falls in older people living in the community. Cochrane Database Syst Rev 9:CD007146, 2012

Gross CP, McAvay GJ, Krumholz HM, et al: The effect of age and chronic illness on life expectancy after a diagnosis of colorectal cancer: implications for screening. Ann Intern Med 145:646–653, 2006

Hajjar ER, Cafiero AC, Hanlon JT: Polypharmacy in elderly patients. Am J Geriatr Pharmacother 5:345–351, 2007

Hausdorff JM, Rios DA, Edelber HK: Gait variability and fall risk in community-living older adults: a 1-year prospective study. Arch Phys Med Rehabil 82:1050–1056, 2001

Heiat A, Vaccarino V, Krumholz HM: An evidence-based assessment of federal guidelines for overweight and obesity as they apply to elderly persons. Arch Intern Med 161:1194–1203, 2001

Inouye SK, Studenski S, Tinetti ME, et al: Geriatric syndromes: clinical, research, and policy implications of a core geriatric concept. J Am Geriatr Soc 55:780–791, 2007

Johannesen M, LoGiudice D: Elder abuse: a systematic review of risk factors in community-dwelling elders. Age Ageing 42:1–7, 2013

Kaiser MJ, Bauer JM, Rämsch C, et al: Frequency of malnutrition in older adults: a multinational perspective using the Mini Nutritional Assessment. J Am Geriatr Soc 58:1734–1738, 2010

Lala SV, Sajatovic M: Medical and psychiatric comorbidities among elderly individuals with bipolar disorder: a literature review. J Geriatr Psychiatry Neurol 25:20–25, 2012

Lamb SE, Jørstad-Stein EC, Hauer K, et al; Prevention of Falls Network Europe and Outcomes Consensus Group: Development of a common outcome data set for fall injury prevention trials: the Prevention of Falls Network Europe consensus. J Am Geriatr Soc 53:1618–1622, 2005

Lin FR, Thorpe R, Gordon-Salant S, et al: Hearing loss prevalence and risk factors among older adults in the United States. J Gerontol A Biol Sci Med Sci 66:582–590, 2011

Loef M, Walach H: Fruits, vegetables and prevention of cognitive decline or dementia: a systematic review of cohort. J Nutr Health Aging 16:626–630, 2012

McDonnall MC: The effects of developing a dual sensory loss on depression in older adults: a longitudinal study. J Aging Health 21:1179–1199, 2009

Menezes A, Lavie CJ, Milani RV, et al: The effects of statins on prevention of stroke and dementia: a review. J Cardiopulm Rehab Prev 32:240–294, 2012

Montamat SC, Cusack B: Overcoming problems with polypharmacy and drug misuse in the elderly. Clin Geriatr Med 8:143–158, 1992

Morley JE, Silver AJ: Nutritional issues in nursing-home care. Ann Intern Med 123:850–859, 1995

Moyer VA; U.S. Preventive Services Task Force: Screening for intimate partner violence and abuse of elderly and vulnerable adults: U.S. Preventive Services Task Force recommendation statement. Ann Intern Med 158:478–486, 2013

Nyunt MS, Lim ML, Yap KB, et al: Changes in depressive symptoms and functional disability among community-dwelling depressive older adults. Int Psychogeriatr 24:1633–1641, 2012

Pacala JT, Yueh B: Hearing deficits in the older patient: "I didn't notice anything." JAMA 307:1185–1194, 2012

Proctor EK, Morrow-Howell NL, Dore P, et al: Comorbid medical conditions among depressed elderly patients discharged home after acute psychiatric care. Am J Geriatr Psychiatry 11:329–338, 2003

Reuben D: Medical care for the final years of life: "When you're 83, it's not going to be 20 years." JAMA 302:2686–2694, 2009

Sattin RW: Falls among older persons: a public health perspective. Annu Rev Public Health 13:489–508, 1992

Schulman EA, Hohler AD: The American Academy of Neurology position statement on abuse and violence. Neurology 78:433–435, 2012

Sera LC, McPherson ML: Pharmacokinetics and pharmacodynamic changes associated with aging and implications for drug therapy. Clin Geriatr Med 28:273–286, 2012

Snitz BE, O'Meara ES, Carlson MC, et al: Ginkgo biloba for preventing cognitive decline in older adults: a randomized trial. JAMA 302:2663–2670, 2009

Thomas C: First national study of elder abuse and neglect: contrast with results from other studies. J Elder Abuse Negl 12:1–14, 2002

Tinetti ME, Ginter SF: Identifying mobility dysfunction in elderly patients. JAMA 259:1190–1193, 1988

U.S. Preventive Services Task Force: Recommendation for Adults. Rockville, MD, U.S. Preventive Services Task Force, 2013. Available at: http://www.uspreventiveservicestaskforce.org/adultrec.htm. Accessed May 25, 2013.

Villareal DT, Apovian CM, Kushner RF, et al: Obesity in older adults: technical review and position statement of the American Society for Nutrition and NAASO, The Obesity Society. Obes Res 13:1849–1863, 2005

Walter LC, Covinsky KE: Cancer screening in elderly patients: a framework for individualized decision making. JAMA 285:2750–2756, 2001

Walter LC, Lewis CL, Barton MB: Screening for colorectal, breast, and cervical cancer in the elderly: a review of the evidence. Am J Med 118:1078–1086, 2005

Welch HG, Fisher ES: Diagnostic testing following screening mammography in the elderly. J Natl Cancer Inst 90:1389–1392, 1998

Wimo A, Jonsson L, Winbald B: An estimate of the worldwide prevalence and direct costs of dementia in 2003. Dementia Geriatr Cogn Disorders 21:175–181, 2006

Yaffe K: Metabolic syndrome and cognitive disorders: is the sum greater than its parts? Alzheimer Dis Assoc Disord 21:167–171, 2007

Zijlstra GA, van Haastregt JC, van Eijk JT, et al: Prevalence and correlates of fear of falling and avoidance of activity in a large random sample of older persons living in the community. Age Ageing 6:304–309, 2007

CHAPTER 26

Child and Adolescent Preventive Care

Anna M. Wehry, B.S.

Robert K. McNamara, Ph.D.

Brooks R. Keeshin, M.D.

Jeffrey R. Strawn, M.D.

Clinical Overview

Psychiatric disorders are prevalent in children and adolescents but are frequently unrecognized and untreated. Accumulating evidence suggests that there are a number of risk factors for pediatric mood disorders, anxiety disorders, attention-deficit/hyperactivity disorder (ADHD), autism spectrum disorders (ASDs), and posttraumatic stress disorder (PTSD). In this chapter we review selected disorders of childhood and adolescence, with special attention focused on risk factors and prevention strategies. However, in addition to reviewing prevention strategies for psychopathology in this population, we discuss interventions directed at preventing morbidity associated with specific psychopharmacological treatments in youths (e.g., second-generation antipsychotics [SGAs]). We also review more general aspects of preventive care in the pediatric population, such as vaccination schedules, prevention of injuries, and substance misuse.

Practical Pointers

- Routine assessment of substance abuse risk early in the course of treatment may facilitate targeted risk-based interventions to prevent substance use disorders in children and adolescents presenting for substance abuse treatment.

- Clinicians should routinely screen pediatric patients treated with second-generation antipsychotics for weight gain and metabolic adverse events and should aggressively treat these complications to decrease associated morbidity.

- Screening for suicidality is critical in the child and adolescent psychiatric population, and clinicians should consider age-specific risk factors when evaluating suicide risk in youths.

Early Recognition and Treatment

Attention-Deficit/Hyperactivity Disorder

ADHD, characterized by symptoms of hyperactivity, impulsivity, and poor sustained attention, is one of the most common psychiatric disorders in children and adolescents. ADHD affects approximately 9% of U.S. adolescents ages 13–18 years (Merikangas et al. 2010). Considerable effort has been directed at identifying risk factors for ADHD; studies have generally focused on genetic, environmental, and psychosocial risk factors. Regarding genetic risk for ADHD, pooled analyses of 20 twin studies suggest that the heritability of ADHD may be as high as 76%, suggesting a strong genetic component to the disorder (Faraone et al. 2005). However, the genetic architecture of ADHD is remarkably complex and likely polyallelic; no genome-wide association studies have identified gene variants at a statistically significant level, despite the identification of multiple candidate genes. In addition to genetic risk factors for ADHD, multiple environmental risk factors have also emerged. In one sample of 2,588 U.S. children, prenatal tobacco exposure was associated with ADHD (odds ratio [OR] = 2.4) (Froehlich et al. 2009), a finding that has been replicated in other large samples (Braun et al. 2006). Additionally, prenatal lead exposure is associated with an increased risk of ADHD (OR = 2.3) (Froehlich et al. 2009); this finding has also been replicated in other samples (Braun et al. 2006; Nigg et al. 2009). Finally, psychosocial adversity, including low income and high levels of family dysfunction, has been associated with more severe forms of ADHD (Scahill et al. 1999). Thus, the extant risk literature suggests that the risk of ADHD in offspring may be reduced through early interventions, such as smoking cessation, particularly by pregnant mothers; screening for lead exposure; and reduction of early psychosocial stressors.

Autism Spectrum Disorders

ASDs, which include several chronic neurodevelopmental disorders, are characterized by impairment of both social interaction and communication, as well as stereotyped interests and behaviors that emerge before age 3 years. The prevalence of ASDs is estimated to be approximately 1 in 88 children (Autism and Developmental Disabilities Monitoring Network Surveillance Year 2008 Principal Investigators 2012). To date, both genetic and environmental factors have been associated with an increased risk of ASDs. A study of 277 twin pairs in the United States found pairwise ASD concordance rates to be 88% and 31% for monozygotic and dizygotic twin pairs, respectively (Rosenberg et al. 2009). Regarding genetic risk factors, whole-genome screens have implicated nearly a dozen genes in ASDs, with a specific chromosomal region at 7q31–q33 showing the strongest linkage (Muhle et al. 2004). However, although ASDs have a strong genetic basis, environmental risk factors appear to play a significant role as well. Prenatal and perinatal risk factors include paternal and maternal age, low birth weight, gestational age, newborn hypoxia, and maternal exposure to valproate (Christensen et al. 2013). Finally, despite significant attention in the lay literature, no relationship has been found between specific foods or vaccines and the risk of autism.

Accumulating evidence suggests that prenatal folic acid supplementation, 0.4 mg daily, may reduce the risk of ASDs. One large prospective study examined the association between periconception supplementation with folic acid and risk of ASDs (Suren et al. 2013). In this study—the Norwegian Mother and Child Cohort Study—0.1% of children whose mothers received folic acid supplementation developed autism compared to 0.21% of those youths whose mothers did not receive folic acid supplementation. Additionally, case-control studies suggest a similar relationship between the risk of ASD and prenatal folic acid intake. In addition to the rationale for folic acid supplementation in pregnancy for prevention of neural tube defects, folic acid supplementation may also have salutary effects for prevention of ASDs. Accordingly, the American College of Obstetricians and Gynecologists recommends supplementation with 0.4 mg/day of folic acid for women of reproductive age.

Posttraumatic Stress Disorder

PTSD, a condition associated with the experience of extraordinary stress, is characterized by intrusive thoughts or memories (e.g., nightmares and flashbacks); avoidance of thoughts or reminders associated with the trauma; negative alterations in cognition; and alterations in arousal and reactivity. These symptoms can appear with or without clinically significant symptoms of dissociation. In youths, PTSD is associated with significant morbidity, including an increased risk for suicide attempts; co-occurring depression; and substance misuse disorders. Although a considerable amount of evidence supports the use of psychotherapeutic interventions for children with PTSD, there is a dearth of data to guide psychopharmacological or psychotherapeutic interventions for youths to prevent the onset of PTSD (Strawn et al. 2010). Although few medications have been investigated to prevent PTSD in children, some proposed medications include those that modify the stress response systems (e.g., sympathetic nervous system), a primary example of which is propranolol.

Propranolol received attention as a means of secondary prevention of PTSD after Famularo et al. (1988) reported improvement in children with child abuse–related PTSD. To date, two published double-blind controlled trials of propranolol for the secondary prevention of PTSD in adults have demonstrated efficacy (Nugent et al. 2010). However, pediatric studies have not observed effectiveness in PTSD prevention. We routinely recommend cognitive-behavioral therapy with a specific trauma component for children and adolescents who have PTSD, and dyadic, caregiver-child interventions for young children with PTSD. Psychotropic medication should be used sparingly and only in severe and treatment-refractory situations.

Prevention of Cardiometabolic Side Effects Related to Second-Generation Antipsychotics

SGAs are frequently used for the treatment of acute manic and psychotic symptoms in pediatric and adolescent patients (Fraguas et al. 2011). Risperidone and aripiprazole are approved for the treatment of irritability associated with ASDs. With the increased availability of data on the efficacy and safety of these agents in youths, there has been a sixfold increase in SGA prescription rates in patients younger than 18 years over the last decade (Olfson et al. 2010).

Despite the efficacy of these medications, several prospective studies indicate that SGAs are associated with significant weight gain, obesity, metabolic syndrome, and elevated overall cardiovascular risk in the majority of previously SGA-naïve pediatric and adolescent patients undergoing first-episode treatment (Correll et al. 2009). In one of the largest prospective studies conducted to date, pediatric and adolescent patients treated with SGAs exhibited significant elevations in body weight, fat mass, waist circumference, and body mass index (BMI) after 4 weeks of exposure. These metabolic parameters, as well as triglyceride levels, continued to increase at 8 and 12 weeks (Correll et al. 2009). Children and adolescents may be at greater risk than adult patients for SGA-induced weight gain. Together, these and other data suggest that exposure to SGAs precipitates clinically significant weight gain and lipid dysregulation in a large subset of pediatric and adolescent patients. Despite consensus and label recommendations for metabolic screening and monitoring for all patients receiving these SGAs (American Diabetes Association et al. 2004), the majority of youths starting SGAs do not receive regular glucose or lipid screening and monitoring in clinical practice at recommended intervals (Table 26–1) (Morrato et al. 2010). These data highlight an urgent and unmet need to identify and address modifiable risk factors.

Lifestyle Modification

Mental health providers should closely monitor BMI for all patients and coordinate treatment with the primary care provider. When an SGA is used, the treating psychiatrist should make sure that appropriate labs are ordered and metabolic derangements are addressed.

When patients present with greater than 7% weight gain due to psychotropic medications or have obesity (i.e., greater than 85th percentile for BMI), the primary care provider should be urgently alerted and a care plan should be developed with the patient and the mental health provider. All patients who are school age should eat a balanced diet and participate in a consistent exercise plan, as outlined in Table 26–2.

Metformin, Topiramate, and the Prevention of SGA-Related Cardiometabolic Side Effects

Two open-label studies suggest that metformin may be efficacious in attenuating weight gain associated with SGA treatment in children and adolescents (Klein et al. 2006; Morrison et al. 2002). In both studies, patients who had experienced antipsychotic-induced weight gain while being treated with olanzapine, risperidone, or quetiapine were treated with metformin. In both samples, the mean decreases in weight and BMI were statistically significant for patients given metformin compared with those given placebo. It is important to note that when used for the treatment of diabetes, metformin is generally considered a "weight-neutral" medication. Metformin should not routinely be used for the treatment of SGA-induced weight gain, but it can be an option for patients who are severely affected and resistant to lifestyle modification.

Topiramate is an antiepileptic indicated for the treatment of complex partial seizures and for the prophylaxis of migraine headaches. It may also be effective in the treatment and prevention of SGA-facilitated or SGA-induced weight gain. In one open-label trial, adolescents with bipolar disorder who

TABLE 26–1. Metabolic monitoring in pediatric patients treated with second-generation antipsychotics

	Baseline	Each visit	3 months	6 months	Annually
Personal and family medical history	X				X
HbA$_{1c}$, fasting blood glucose	X		X[a]		
Waist circumference	X	X			
Weight[b]	X	X			
BMI	X	X			
Blood pressure	X		X[a]		
Lipid profile	X		X[a]		

Note. BMI=body mass index; HbA$_{1c}$=hemoglobin A$_{1c}$.
[a]After 3 months, follow-up every 6 months.
[b]Percentile.
Source. Adapted from Correll CU: "Monitoring and Management of Antipsychotic-Related Metabolic and Endocrine Adverse Events in Pediatric Patients." *International Review of Psychiatry* 20:195–201, 2008.

TABLE 26–2. **General diet and exercise plans for all child and adolescent patients**

Diet

Patients should be encouraged to avoid drinking sodas and to limit intake of fruit drinks that are high in sugar.

Patients should be discouraged from eating fast food that may be high in fat, calories, or salt.

A balanced diet should include vegetables at most meals.

Patients should limit their intake of sugar.

Patients' weight should be monitored at each doctor visit, and patients should make dietary changes well before the body mass index reaches the 85th percentile.

The safest and most effective way to lose weight is to decrease caloric intake, per direction of a primary care provider. Medications such as metformin and topiramate are less effective, often have side effects, and should only rarely be used in treatment-refractory cases.

Exercise

All patients should be encouraged to exercise on a daily basis.

Sedentary activities outside of school should be limited (e.g., watching TV, using the computer, playing video games).

When available, group activities or team-based sports should be encouraged.

---

had experienced weight gain following treatment with a mood stabilizer or SGA were treated with flexibly dosed topiramate (dose range: 25–150 mg/day; mean dose: 112.5 mg/day), and significant decreases in body weight were observed over the course of an 11-week treatment period (Tramontina et al. 2007). A double-blind, placebo-controlled trial also suggested that topiramate was more effective than placebo in attenuating olanzapine-induced weight gain in youths with bipolar disorder (DelBello 2009).

These results suggest that metformin or topiramate could be used as a means of weight control in overweight adolescents being treated with an SGA when lifestyle modification alone is not effective. Further studies are needed to investigate the effectiveness of these drugs if prescribed at the initiation of SGA treatment, as well as to identify risk factors associated with cardio-metabolic side effects in youths. Additional information regarding recommended dosing and common adverse effects of these two medications is provided in Table 26–3.

TABLE 26–3. Guidelines for prevention of cardiometabolic side effects of second-generation antipsychotics in youths

Drug	Beginning dose	Target dosage	Common side effects
Metformin	250 mg bid	850–1,000 mg bid	Diarrhea, abdominal cramping
Topiramate	12.5 mg, increased by 12.5 mg every 7 days until target dose	100 mg bid	Cognitive dulling, paresthesias, dysesthesias (distal extremities), weight loss, appetite suppression, nephrolithiasis

Prevention of Early Childhood Adversity as a Means to Prevent Pediatric Mental Illness

One of the greatest risk factors for future adversity is the experience of prior adversity. Youths who have experienced childhood adversity are significantly more likely than other children to experience multiple adversities or abuses. A greater number of adversities experienced during childhood progressively increases the risk of mental health morbidity. Using data from the National Comorbidity Survey, which involved a nationally representative sample of adults, Green et al. (2010) examined correlations between childhood adversity and the development of mental illness in childhood and adulthood and observed that childhood adversities were associated with nearly half of all childhood-onset psychiatric disorders. In multivariate analyses, physical abuse and sexual abuse during childhood were independently associated with statistically significant increases in mood, anxiety, substance use, and disruptive behavior disorders, accounting for between 50% and 100% increased risk of a specific cluster of psychiatric illnesses.

Currently, many evidence-based models focus on child abuse prevention and the promotion of child well-being. These models generally target families with younger children and can be delivered in the home, in the primary care setting, or through parent training programs. These programs measure outcomes based on subsequent rates of recidivism or abuse. However, it is likely that by decreasing the childhood psychosocial stressors or adversities experienced within the family, a reduction in psychiatric morbidity may result from these and other child abuse prevention programs.

A number of validated measures can be useful for the detection of childhood adversity. The clinician should choose measures that assess the history of different types of adversity as well as symptoms associated with those events. A measure such as the University of California at Los Angeles Posttraumatic Stress Disorder Reaction Index (Pynoos et al. 1998) is an excellent and freely available structured measure, available in both parent and child/adolescent versions, that allows the clinician to systematically evaluate patients for clinically significant adversity.

Prevention of Suicide

Suicide is a significant cause of mortality in the pediatric population. The annual rate of suicide in children ages 10–14 years is 0.9 per 100,000, whereas the rate in adolescents increases to 6.9 per 100,000 (Centers for Disease Control and Prevention 2014). The prevention of suicide may involve either primary prevention of psychiatric disorders associated with increased risk for suicidal behavior (e.g., bipolar disorder, major depressive disorder, anxiety disorders) or secondary prevention strategies that focus on identification of at-risk patients. Clinicians should screen patients for suicidal ideation at all psychiatric visits as well as recognize significant risk factors for suicidal behavior. Risk factors for suicide in children and adolescents are, with several exceptions, similar to risk factors for suicide in adults (Table 26–4). Additionally, in the pediatric population, family cohesion is especially important, with family conflict having the potential to amplify risks in certain individuals. Also, contagion effects are more pronounced in the pediatric population, and awareness of this phenomenon suggests a role for more intensive screening of individuals who have had a peer commit suicide, have attended school with someone who committed suicide, and so forth.

In relation to suicide in children and adolescents, the U.S. Food and Drug Administration's black box warnings regarding suicidality and use of antidepressants in the pediatric population warrant additional discussion. A meta-analysis of treatment-emergent suicidality in pediatric patients suggests that this phenomenon may be more pronounced for patients treated for depressive disorders than for those treated for anxiety disorders. Bridge et al. (2007) found that the number needed to harm in terms of treatment-emergent suicidality was 112 in youths with depressive disorders versus 143 in youths with anxiety disorders. However, regardless of the indication for antidepressant treatment, providers should remain vigilant while monitoring adolescents and young adults who are taking antidepressants. It is also important to discuss the risk of suicide by those taking antidepressants with the patient and parents or guardians.

TABLE 26–4. Risk factors for suicide in children and adolescents

Previous history of suicide attempts

Recent exposure to a suicide or suicide attempt

High levels of anxiety

Hopelessness

History of substance misuse

Access to a gun

Command hallucinations

Contagion (i.e., having exposure to or knowledge of a suicide by a peer, classmate, etc.)

Physical or sexual abuse

Screening for Substance Use in Children and Adolescents

Screening for substance use or misuse is a standard part of well-child checkups for all adolescents; however, more comprehensive screening may be warranted for at-risk adolescents. Risk factors for substance use include the presence of earlier behavior difficulties, a diagnosis of ADHD, and male sex. Pediatricians may refer to the CRAFFT questionnaire for the screening of substance use or abuse in the pediatric population (Table 26–5; Knight et al. 2002). This instrument, which has been endorsed by the American Academy of Pediatrics' Committee on Substance Abuse for use with adolescents and young adults to age 21 years, consists of six questions aimed at detecting high-risk alcohol use and other drug use disorders. The CRAFFT is short and designed to determine the degree to which a more in-depth examination of use, frequency, and risks and consequences of alcohol and other drug use is indicated.

Prevention of Infectious Diseases and Immunoprophylaxis

Immunoprophylaxis represents a cornerstone in the prevention of many serious illnesses in the pediatric population. Despite this, parents or caregivers may experience anxiety in regard to immunizations because of injection-related pain or perceived risks of potential neuropsychiatric illness. As with many interventions used with the pediatric population, anticipatory guidance by physicians can be remarkably effective in reducing the anxiety of the child and the parent.

TABLE 26–5. **The CRAFFT questionnaire for screening adolescents for substance abuse or misuse**

C—Have you ever ridden in a CAR driven by someone (including yourself) who was "high" or had been using alcohol or drugs?

R—Do you ever use alcohol or drugs to RELAX, feel better about yourself, or fit in?

A—Do you ever use alcohol or drugs while you are ALONE?

F—Do your family or FRIENDS ever tell you that you should cut down on drinking or drug use?

F—Do you ever FORGET things you did while using alcohol or drugs?

T—Have you ever gotten into TROUBLE while you were using alcohol or drugs?

One positive answer suggests a need for more evaluation, while more than two affirmative responses suggest a significant problem.

Source. Knight et al. 2002.

Recommendations regarding immunization in the United States frequently change in response to emerging data and are frequently updated by the Centers for Disease Control and Prevention (CDC). The current vaccination schedule for pediatric patients ages 0–18 years is published annually by the CDC (see "Resources: For Clinicians" section below). Several significant changes have been made with regard to vaccinations in the pediatric population over the past decade. First, the human papillomavirus (HPV) vaccine—a quadrivalent vaccine against HPV types 6, 11, 16, and 18—has been approved for females ages 9–26 years and will likely decrease the incidence of genital warts, abnormal cervical cytology, and cervical cancer. Second, vaccination against meningococcal disease is now recommended for adolescents between ages 11 and 12 years, with a booster dose at age 16 years. At present, there are two vaccines against *Neisseria meningitidis:* meningococcal polysaccharide vaccine (MPSV4) and a conjugate polysaccharide vaccine (MCV4). Both are tetravalent and therefore confer protection against A, C, Y, and W-135 serotypes. Third, recommendations regarding vaccination for influenza have changed over this period as well. In fact, since 2008, the American Academy of Pediatrics has recommended annual influenza vaccination for patients ages 6 months to 18 years. Currently, two types are available: a live attenuated influenza vaccine and a trivalent inactivated influenza vaccine. Clinicians should consider several clinical factors prior to administering the live attenuated influenza vaccine. Specifically, this vaccine is approved only for healthy individuals without chronic medical conditions (e.g., chronic heart or lung disease) or a compromised immune system (Brigham and Goldstein 2009).

Prevention of Accidents and Injuries in the Pediatric Population

Unintentional injuries are the leading cause of death for children and adolescents. Although these often-preventable unintentional injuries and accidents vary by age, the most common unintentional injuries in this population include motor vehicle accidents, suffocation, poisonings, and gun violence. Regarding prevention, particularly in the primary care setting, active and passive interventions are frequently recommended by pediatricians to reduce the risk of accidental injuries. Screening for seat belt use is recommended at well-child visits, and patients should be advised to wear seat belts during every car trip. Additionally, for young children, safety seats are recommended; these seats reduce the risk of fatality in motor vehicle accidents by 50%–70% (Centers for Disease Control and Prevention 2014). Similarly, placing a child in the backseat reduces risk of fatality by 40%, and current recommendations are that children should be seated in the backseat away from the airbag until they are older than age 13 years. For infants, suffocation represents the leading cause of mortality, with choking-related injuries most often caused by coins, food, and toys. Thus, small objects and potentially poisonous materials should be kept out of the environment of small children. Health care professionals may provide counseling and education to parents about these risks as well as participate in prevention programs in the community.

Clinical Highlights

- Pediatric patients treated with SGAs should receive screening for changes in hemoglobin A_{1c} levels, blood pressure, and lipid profile at 3 months and then at 6-month intervals following initiation of SGA treatment. Weight and BMI (as well as weight and BMI percentiles) should be monitored at each follow-up visit.
- Fetal exposure to environmental toxins (e.g., tobacco smoke, lead) increases the risk of developing ADHD and therefore may be a target of primary prevention strategies.
- Prenatal folic acid supplementation at a dose of 0.4 mg daily may reduce the risk of ASD.
- Clinicians should remain vigilant in screening for child maltreatment or childhood adversity and may use psychosocial interventions or social services accordingly, given that prevention of

early childhood adversity likely has pleiotropic effects on multiple mental health outcomes in children and adolescents, which often persist into adulthood.

Resources

For Patients

American Academy of Child and Adolescent Psychiatry: Facts for Families. Available at: http://www.aacap.org/aacap/Families_and_Youth/Facts_for_Families/Home.aspx.

For Clinicians

American Academy of Child and Adolescent Psychiatry: http://www.aacap.org.

Centers for Disease Control and Prevention: Growth charts. Available at: http://www.cdc.gov/growthcharts.

Centers for Disease Control and Prevention: Immunization Schedules. Available at: http://www.cdc.gov/vaccines/schedules.

References

American Diabetes Association, American Psychiatric Association, American Association of Clinical Endocrinologists, et al: Consensus development conference on antipsychotic drugs and obesity and diabetes. Diabetes Care 27:596–601, 2004

Autism and Developmental Disabilities Monitoring Network Surveillance Year 2008 Principal Investigators, Centers for Disease Control and Prevention: Prevalence of autism spectrum disorders—Autism and Developmental Disabilities Monitoring Network, 14 sites, United States, 2008. MMWR Surveill Summ 61:1–19, 2012

Braun JM, Kahn RS, Froehlich T, et al: Exposures to environmental toxicants and attention deficit hyperactivity disorder in U.S. children. Environ Health Perspect 114:1904–1909, 2006

Bridge JA, Iyengar S, Salary CB, et al: Clinical response and risk for reported suicidal ideation and suicide attempts in pediatric antidepressant treatment: a meta-analysis of randomized controlled trials. JAMA 297:1683–1696, 2007

Brigham KS, Goldstein MA: Adolescent immunizations. Pediatr Rev 30:47–55, 2009

Centers for Disease Control and Prevention: National Center for Injury Prevention and Control Web-Based Injury Statistics Query and Reporting System (WISQARS). Atlanta, GA, Centers for Disease Control and Prevention, January 27, 2014. Available at: http://www.cdc.gov/injury/wisqars/index.html. Accessed February 21, 2014.

Christensen J, Gronborg TK, Sorensen MJ, et al: Prenatal valproate exposure and risk of autism spectrum disorders and childhood autism. JAMA 309:1696–1703, 2013

Correll CU, Manu P, Olshanskiy V, et al: Cardiometabolic risk of second-generation antipsychotic medications during first-time use in children and adolescents. JAMA 302:1765–1773, 2009

DelBello MP: Topiramate for weight gain in bipolar youth treated with olanzapine. Paper presented at the 56th annual meeting of the American Academy of Child and Adolescent Psychiatry, Honolulu, Hawaii, October 2009

Famularo R, Kinscherff R, Fenton T: Propranolol treatment for childhood posttraumatic stress disorder, acute type. A pilot study. Am J Dis Child 142:1244–1247, 1988

Faraone SV, Perlis RH, Doyle AE, et al: Molecular genetics of attention-deficit/hyperactivity disorder. Biol Psychiatry 57:1313–1323, 2005

Fraguas D, Correll CU, Merchán-Naranjo J, et al: Efficacy and safety of second-generation antipsychotics in children and adolescents with psychotic and bipolar spectrum disorders: comprehensive review of prospective head-to-head and placebo-controlled comparisons. Eur Neuropsychopharmacol 21:621–645, 2011

Froehlich TE, Lanphear BP, Auinger P, et al: Association of tobacco and lead exposures with attention-deficit/hyperactivity disorder. Pediatrics 124:1054–1063, 2009

Green JG, McLaughlin KA, Berglund PA, et al: Childhood adversities and adult psychiatric disorders in the National Comorbidity Survey Replication I: associations with first onset of DSM-IV disorders. Arch Gen Psychiatry 67:113–123, 2010

Klein DJ, Cottingham EM, Sorter M, et al: A randomized, double-blind, placebo-controlled trial of metformin treatment of weight gain associated with initiation of atypical antipsychotic therapy in children and adolescents. Am J Psychiatry 163:2072–2079, 2006

Knight JR, Sherritt L, Shrier LA, et al: Validity of the CRAFFT substance abuse screening test among adolescent clinic patients. Arch Pediatr Adolesc Med 156:607–614, 2002

Merikangas KR, He JP, Burstein M, et al: Lifetime prevalence of mental disorders in U.S. adolescents: results from the National Comorbidity Survey Replication—Adolescent Supplement (NCS-A). J Am Acad Child Adolesc Psychiatry 49:980–989, 2010

Morrato EH, Druss B, Hartung DM, et al: Metabolic testing rates in 3 state Medicaid programs after FDA warnings and ADA/APA recommendations for second-generation antipsychotic drugs. Arch Gen Psychiatry 67:17–24, 2010

Morrison JA, Cottingham EM, Barton BA: Metformin for weight loss in pediatric patients taking psychotropic drugs. Am J Psychiatry 159:655–657, 2002

Muhle R, Trentacoste SV, Rapin I: The genetics of autism. Pediatrics 113:472–486, 2004

Nigg JT, Nikolas M, Knottnerus MG, et al: Confirmation and extension of association of blood lead with attention-deficit/hyperactivity disorder (ADHD) and ADHD symptom domains at population-typical exposure levels. J Child Psychol Psychiatry 51:58–65, 2009

Nugent NR, Christopher NC, Crow JP, et al: The efficacy of early propranolol administration at reducing PTSD symptoms in pediatric injury patients: a pilot study. J Trauma Stress 23:282–287, 2010

Olfson M, Crystal S, Huang C, et al: Trends in antipsychotic drug use by very young, privately insured children. J Am Acad Child Adolesc Psychiatry 49:13–23, 2010

Pynoos R, Rodriguez N, Steinberg A, et al: The University of California at Los Angeles Posttraumatic Stress Disorder Reaction Index (UCLA-PTSD RI) for DSM-IV (Revision 1). Los Angeles, CA, UCLA Trauma Psychiatry Program, 1998

Rosenberg RE, Law JK, Yenokyan G, et al: Characteristics and concordance of autism spectrum disorders among 277 twin pairs. Arch Pediatr Adolesc Med 163:907–914, 2009

Scahill L, Schwab-Stone M, Merikangas KR, et al: Psychosocial and clinical correlates of ADHD in a community sample of school-age children. J Am Acad Child Adolesc Psychiatry 38:976–984, 1999

Strawn JR, Keeshin BR, Geracioti TD, et al: Psychopharmacologic treatment of posttraumatic stress disorder in children and adolescents. J Clin Psychiatry 71:932–941, 2010

Suren P, Roth C, Bresnahan M, et al: Association between maternal use of folic acid supplements and risk of autism spectrum disorders in children. JAMA 309:570–577, 2013

Tramontina S, Zeni CP, Pheula G, et al: Topiramate in adolescents with juvenile bipolar disorder presenting weight gain due to atypical antipsychotics or mood stabilizers: an open clinical trial. J Child Adolesc Psychopharmacol 17:129–134, 2007

CHAPTER 27

Pain Medicine in the Psychiatric Patient Population

Kristin Bennett, D.O.
Gagan Mahajan, M.D.

Clinical Overview

Chronic pain is a global epidemic, with, in the United States, an annual national economic cost of over $600 billion (Institute of Medicine Committee on Advancing Pain Research, Care, and Education 2011). Many clinicians feel apprehensive and frustrated when confronted with the task of managing chronic pain in a patient. The chronic patient population often presents unique challenges to mental health clinicians; these patients can be demanding, ambivalent, despondent, passive-aggressive, or unmotivated, and can arouse many unpleasant emotions and responses from care providers. As difficult as the chronic pain population can be, this group of patients needs a health care provider who can listen to all of their complaints, organize their symptoms, and develop a structured care plan that addresses not only pain issues but also general physical and emotional comorbidities. Furthermore, the hazards of chronic opioid therapy are becoming more apparent as more research uncovers the long-term adverse effects. This chapter is intended to help the reader focus on assessing the patient in pain, developing a comprehensive treatment strategy, and determining appropriateness for prescribing opioids.

Practical Pointers

- People with chronic pain are more likely to suffer from depression and anxiety. Psychiatrists are well positioned to address both the emotional and physical pain.

- Use of cognitive-behavioral therapy can be effective in the treatment of many pain disorders, including somatic symptom disorder.

- Psychiatrists can use the AMPS approach to psychiatric assessment when working with patients who complain of chronic pain.

- Use of opioids can increase risk for accidental death, and psychiatrists can help educate patients to minimize this risk.

Evaluating the Patient in Pain

When initially faced with a patient who has a pain complaint, the clinician needs to obtain a thorough history and physical examination. Many practitioners become overwhelmed by this complex patient population and may miss important examination findings or critical past medical history. For example, poorly controlled hypertension and diabetes may worsen headaches and neuropathy, respectively. If only the pain complaint is addressed, the clinician might miss the underlying cause of the painful condition. Inadequately controlled systemic disease will make pain control difficult. Another prime example is thyroid disease: hypothyroidism can lead to worsening fatigue, daytime somnolence, weight gain, poor motivation and concentration, depression, and generalized myofascial pain, whereas hyperthyroidism can cause irritability, anxiety, palpitations, and insomnia. These thyroid irregularities can be easily evaluated with lab work and usually treated with medication. If not evaluated and addressed, thyroid dysfunction can lead to inappropriate treatment and symptom-driven polypharmacy, because many of the symptoms of thyroid disease coexist in a chronic pain patient. Rheumatological disorders, autoimmune disease, and various malignancies often present as progressive systemic illnesses with numerous associated painful conditions. It is important to know a patient's disease burden and prognosis, because this information will provide a broader understanding of how a pain condition may impact a patient's life.

Obtaining a Pain History

After a thorough past medical history has been obtained, an organized approach to a painful condition includes provocation, quality, radiation, severity, and timing of the pain (Figure 27–1). As simple and rudimentary as this initial assessment seems, many clinicians fail to obtain this valuable information. Assessing location helps to divide localized and generalized conditions. For example, causes for arm pain can be numerous, such as trauma; nerve en-

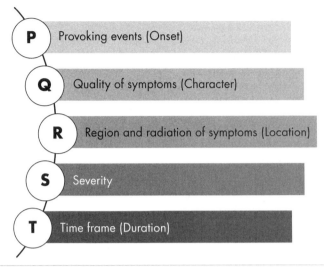

FIGURE 27–1.   PQRST assessment for pain symptoms.

trapment; radicular, myofascial, or degenerative change; and so forth. However, when the question of location is considered, the differential diagnoses may change once the clinician knows whether the pain is unilateral or bilateral, anatomically limited or diffusely distributed, and so on. For example, radiating pain down a single leg may be due to spinal nerve encroachment, with subsequent inflammation stemming from pathology of the lumbar spine such as a disc herniation, bony degenerative change, and/or ligamentous hypertrophy. A similar radiating pattern into both legs may also be caused by the same abnormalities, but the astute clinician will also want to consider spondylolisthesis (displacement of one vertebra over another); this condition commonly presents with bilateral symptoms and can lead to spinal instability, which may warrant a more streamlined treatment plan, including a magnetic resonance imaging or computed tomography scan of the lumbar spine, dynamic lumbar spine X rays, and a spine surgery consultation.

Pain character is another descriptor that is valuable in determining possible diagnoses, recommended additional assessment, and appropriate treatment options. Character descriptors help differentiate between the two general pain categories: *nociceptive* (somatic or visceral) and *neuropathic.* Nociceptive pain is caused by primary afferent nerve injury or inflammation in the periphery. Examples include cutting or burning the skin, fracturing a bone, slamming a finger in a door, and arthritis. Tingling, numbness, pins-and-needles, shooting, or electric-like sensations suggest neuropathic pain conditions. Neuropathic pain results from ongoing nerve stimulation or abnormal messaging in the nervous system and can be peripherally or centrally mediated (Berry et al. 2001). Examples of neuropathic pain include spinal nerve irritation from a herniated disc, carpal tunnel syndrome, and poorly controlled diabetes. Descriptors such as *dull, aching, pressure,* and *sharp* are consistent with somatic pain processes. Visceral pain is usually poorly localized and difficult for patients to describe, such as abdominal pain from intestinal dilation secondary to obstruction. Referred somatic pain is not uncommon with a visceral pain generator. The classic example of this is acute appendicitis; initial symptoms include a dull, achy, poorly localized periumbilical pain that, over time, becomes localized to the right lower abdominal quadrant as ongoing appendiceal obstruction (visceral component) causes peritoneal irritation and inflammation (somatic component). Thus, there should be a low index of suspicion to perform general lab work and imaging to aid in the diagnosis of the underlying disease process.

Duration is an extremely important and often overlooked historical fact that carries crucial information concerning diagnosis. Acute pain is likely due to a temporally related event for which there is a normal progression of pain as the body recovers. Acute pain is usually nociceptive but can be neuropathic (Berry et al. 2001). In contrast to chronic pain, acute pain serves an important biological function of protection from ongoing tissue injury. However, if acute pain persists beyond the natural course of the disease, a pathological metamorphosis may ensue as the acute pain transforms into chronic pain. *Chronic pain* is defined as pain that extends 3–6 months beyond the expected healing process. From a physiological standpoint, chronic pain serves no protective function or adaptive purpose and can degrade health, function, and quality of life (Berry et al. 2001). Distinguishing between acute pain and chronic pain is important, because treatment strategies will vary.

Functional status—or the ability to perform activities of daily living, work or go to school, exercise, and socialize with friends—is one of the most important outcome measures in determining disability and appropriate treatments for a patient. A patient undergoing chronic opioid therapy who only gets out of bed or off the couch to eat, who states that opioids only help to "take the edge off" the pain, and who is not interested in physical therapy because "it just hurts too much and does not help" is a poorly functioning patient whose current pain management plan is suboptimal. Poor functional status does not necessarily indicate disability. For some individuals, secondary gain (e.g., time off from work, financial reward, litigation, increased emotional support if the sick role is maintained and pain continues to be disabling) may be driving a persistent painful condition and lack of interest in getting better. If secondary gain is suspected, most treatment strategies will be minimally effective, because the patient does not want to get better. Psychological counseling and assessment for depression and anxiety should be considered for these patients.

Poor functionality and inadequate pain control can also be the result of poor quality and quantity of sleep. More often than not, patients with chronic pain also suffer from insomnia. Asking the simple question "How do you sleep at night?" is paramount in any pain assessment, because addressing the sleep disturbance can also impact pain severity. Information about sleep may also guide medication selection, because the side effects of several classes of drugs used to treat chronic pain cause sedation. This side-effect profile can be useful in efforts to reduce pain and improve sleep. Before selecting any medication as a sleep aid, the clinician first needs to investigate why a patient may suffer from suboptimal sleep.

Assessment of Sleep

Sleep disturbance can be due to a myriad of factors, including poor sleep hygiene, worsened pain at night, lack of mobility, mechanical issues due to inadequate body or head support from the bed or pillow, ruminating thoughts, anxiety, and anatomical abnormalities. A common cause of sleep disturbance that should be thoroughly evaluated prior to consideration of potentially sedating medications is obstructive or central sleep apnea, an underappreciated life-threatening disease. Nighttime hypoxia leads to frequent bouts of sleep arousal, which lead to daytime somnolence, irritability, headaches, poor concentration, depression, memory impairment, and increased existing pain severity. Although obesity is the most common risk factor for obstructive sleep apnea secondary to airway obstruction, anyone can develop sleep apnea. Thus, a risk assessment should be performed on all patients with chronic pain if poor sleep history is reported. The STOP-BANG Questionnaire is a simple and quick screening tool that uncovers the important sleep apnea risk factors (Figure 27–2). Answers of "yes" to more than three of eight screening items suggest that the patient is at high risk for having sleep apnea (Chung and Elsaid 2009; Chung et al. 2008). Patients at high risk for sleep apnea should have additional evaluation, including polysomnography or referral to a sleep specialist. Undiagnosed sleep apnea combined with opioids and/or benzodiazepines leads to increased morbidity and mortality.

Assessment of Psychiatric Illness

Psychiatric illness should also be evaluated and addressed prior to the initiation of any medication or interventional procedure. Although depression and chronic pain commonly coexist, it is not always clear whether the pain caused the depression or vice versa. Remembering the simple acronym AMPS will help the clinician ask the vital questions pertaining to **A**nxiety, **M**ood, **P**sychosis, and **S**ubstance abuse (McCarron et al. 2009) (Figure 27–3). Any psychiatric condition that has a direct adverse effect on chronic pain is labeled

SNORE: Do you snore loudly enough to be heard through closed doors?	Yes/No
TIRED: Do you often feel tired, without energy, and sleepy during the day?	Yes/No
OBSERVED: Have you been observed to stop breathing while you were sleeping?	Yes/No
PRESSURE: Do you have or are you being treated for high blood pressure?	Yes/No
BODY MASS INDEX (BMI): What is your BMI? Is it >35?	Yes/No
AGE: Is your age over 50 years old?	Yes/No
NECK GIRTH: Do you have a neck circumference >40 cm (male), >35 cm (female)?	Yes/No
GENDER: Are you a male?	Yes/No

FIGURE 27–2. STOP-BANG Questionnaire: a tool to screen for obstructive sleep apnea (OSA) risk.

Note. High risk of OSA with ≥3 answers of "yes." Additional workup by a sleep specialist or by polysomnography is indicated.
Low risk of OSA with <3 answers of "yes."
Source. Adapted from STOP Questionnaire (Chung and Elsaid 2009).

a "psychiatric pain generator." Untreated anxiety, depression, mania, psychosis, or substance misuse can be a tremendous amplifier of any pain condition. Anxiety propagates a vicious cycle of intensified sympathetic response that, if left untreated, will maintain the pain and undermine the treatment plan. Ruminating thoughts also factor into the web of anxiety and pain, often leading to poor sleep. Mood gives the clinician general information about the underlying canvas of each patient. If the patient is depressed, hopeless, suicidal, or sad, this mood disorder will need treatment prior to a direct attempt at effectively addressing the painful condition.

Nonopioid Pharmacological Therapies for the Treatment of Pain

Following the full evaluation of a patient's pain condition, a clinician can more accurately determine whether an opioid trial may benefit the patient. Categorizing suspected pain conditions based on the history, physical examination, and selective laboratory and imaging data will assist a provider in discerning which drug classes are best suited for treating the patient. For ex-

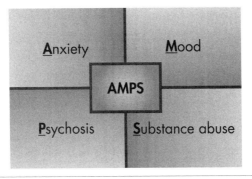

FIGURE 27–3.   AMPS psychiatric assessment.
Source.   Adapted from McCarron et al. 2009.

ample, pain conditions with a significant somatic or visceral component may respond to nonsteroidal anti-inflammatory drugs (NSAIDs) or acetaminophen. The first-line treatment of neuropathic pain almost always involves the use of nonopioid medications, such as tricyclic antidepressants, anticonvulsants, and serotonin-norepinephrine reuptake inhibitors. The selection of which class to start depends on the patient's age and medical comorbidities, because each class can be used for more than one indication and each presents its own side-effect profile.

For those patients in whom a trial of nonopioid analgesics is unsuccessful, a trial of opioids can be considered. Risk stratification, however, should be done prior to initiating an opioid trial. In patients with neuropathic pain as opposed to somatic pain, larger doses of opioids are typically required to determine responsiveness, thereby increasing the likelihood of side effects and tolerance. Inflammatory pain usually responds well to NSAIDs, such as ibuprofen, naproxen, or diclofenac, or even a steroid burst and taper. Myofascial pain and fibromyalgia are examples of pain conditions that respond poorly to opioid therapy because these states can have deep seated psychiatric, deconditioning, or poor coping undertones. Most chronic pain patients have a multifactorial picture with characteristics that fall into several categories, and thus several different classes of medications can be tried in a stepwise fashion to globally decrease pain, increase functionality, and ultimately improve quality of life.

Chronic Opioid Therapy for the Treatment of Pain

One of the most challenging and anxiety-provoking treatment regimen considerations a clinician faces is how to risk-stratify patients who are being con-

TABLE 27–1. **Important considerations before starting opioid therapy for nonmalignant pain**

Assess need for opioids based on *functional status* and not solely on a numerical value that represents severity of pain.

Do not continue to prescribe opioids if there is little to no functional improvement.

Complete a physical examination at each clinical encounter.

Check the state's prescription drug monitoring program.

Make sure there is only one opioid prescriber.

Monitor risk for accidental death in patients taking opioids by

Limiting or eliminating use of sedatives or anxiolytics.

Assessing for sleep apnea.

Assessing for opioids obtained from other sources or for use of illicit drugs (check urine drug test).

Educate the patient about inherent risk associated with long-term opioid treatment.

sidered for chronic opioid therapy for nonmalignant pain (Table 27–1). Common questions include the following: 1) Who should be prescribed opioids? 2) How does one safely monitor patients taking opioids? 3) How does one evaluate efficacy of opioid treatment? and 4) How does one screen for opioid misuse, abuse, and diversion? When considering chronic opioid therapy for a patient, the clinician must first establish a physical diagnosis after a comprehensive history and physical examination. It should be emphasized that if opioid prescribing is considered, both the clinician and the patient should understand that chronic opioid therapy should always be viewed in the context of an extended trial such that the clinician's decision on whether to continue prescribing is based on an ongoing assessment of functional benefit versus risk (Zackaroff et al. 2010).

Screening patients for potential opioid misuse prior to the initiation of chronic opioid therapy should be standard practice (Manchikanti et al. 2012). Screening includes a thorough assessment of a patient's substance abuse history (past and present), substances used (tobacco, alcohol, scheduled drugs, and illicit drugs), arrests or other legal infractions, and substance abuse–related hospitalizations or treatment programs. If a patient has been in a rehabilitation program, important considerations are whether the patient is still attending meetings to facilitate maintenance of sobriety and whether the patient has a sponsor or strong social support network. Several opioid risk screening tools are available that can be completed by the patient or clini-

TABLE 27–2. **Pain and risk assessment tools**

Sample resources available	Web site
Pain assessment	
McGill Pain Questionnaire	http://www.ama-cmeonline.com/ pain_mgmt/pdf/mcgill.pdf
Brief Pain Inventory	http://www.partnersagainstpain.com/ printouts/A7012AS8.pdf
Opioid assessment and screening	
SOAPP (Screener and Opioid Assessment for Patients With Pain)	http://www.PainEdu.org
Current Opioid Misuse Measure	http://www.PainEdu.org

Note. There are many available resources that may be useful in pain and opioid assessment. The tools are to be used as a guide as part of a comprehensive evaluation. No tool or resource used alone is fully validated.

cian (Table 27–2), but none of these tools has been fully validated. All of this information helps a clinician recognize individual risk factors for opioid abuse and may guide treatment strategies. This information should not be used to deny a patient opioid therapy, but it should be used for risk stratification and determining the intensity and frequency of monitoring.

Because patient reporting is subjective, the clinician can use other information as a supplement to guide clinical decision making when initiating or continuing chronic opioid therapy. For example, the clinician can obtain a random urine drug test (UDT), review the state's prescription drug monitoring program (PDMP), and interview third parties (i.e., significant other, spouse, other family member, or roommate) who are present at the time of the patient's clinic visit. A UDT and review of the PDMP database, if available, provide easily attainable, noninvasive, inexpensive, and objective data to demonstrate patient compliance with prescribed opioid treatment.

A UDT can detect most drugs for 1–3 days after use. Within the limits of threshold of detectability, a UDT can document the presence of prescribed and nonprescribed drugs and their metabolites as well as illicit substances and their metabolites. Prior to asking the patient to provide a urine sample for drug testing, the clinician should ask the patient the following questions and document the responses: What opioid(s) are you taking? What is the strength? How often are you taking it? When did you last take the medication? Are you using any nonprescribed medications? Are you using any illegal substances? Having a priori responses to these questions should help minimize potential challenges in interpreting unexpected results. If a provider is uncertain as to how to interpret a result, especially because false positives and false negatives can occur, the provider should contact the testing laboratory for assistance. Adapting a protocol for urine drug testing in all patients undergoing opioid therapy and adhering to an algorithmic approach are recommended (Christo et al. 2011). The protocol, for example, can include obtaining a UDT prior to the initiation of chronic opioid therapy, when taking over this therapy from another provider, and randomly at subsequent follow-up visits (Figure 27–4). The frequency of obtaining subsequent random UDTs, however, may depend on the risk category assigned to the patient. Unexpected UDT results can potentially trigger an unpleasant interaction with the patient. It is important for the clinician to resist the reaction of using a UDT as a "gotcha moment" or firing the patient for transgressions. Instead, the clinician can use this as an opportunity for intervention when the patient has a dual diagnosis of chronic pain and a substance abuse problem. Treatment of one without the other will lead to a suboptimal outcome. In general, having a universal approach to UDTs ensures that all patients receive the same care while avoiding the stigma of stereotyping or profiling.

The protocol used for UDT can also incorporate a review of the database for the PDMP that has been implemented in the majority of states. The database can demonstrate objective evidence about when and where a patient filled a prescription, what medications were prescribed, which provider prescribed the medication, and what dose and amount were given. Red flags may be multiple provider prescriptions, frequent emergency room prescriptions, filling of medications the patient did not report, or early prescription refills. Another example of a red flag is more frequent refilling of prescriptions. For example, a patient may report taking oxycodone 10 mg every 6 hours and is prescribed 120 tablets per month to cover this usage. After checking the PDMP, however, the clinician notes that the patient got a refill of this prescription 2 weeks earlier but now states that he is out of medication and denies that the medication was stolen or lost. The clinician should avoid passing judgment, but extra scrutiny is warranted because this patient may be taking more than reported, someone else may be taking the medication, or there may be diversion. Although there are many potential explanations for discrepancy, it is the prescribing provider's responsibility to be aware of how opioids are being used.

Medical necessity for opioids should follow the World Health Organization (WHO) ladder for analgesic treatment (Figure 27–5). The WHO ladder has guided clinicians around the world for nearly 30 years in the treatment of cancer and noncancer pain. The ladder is a stepwise pain management schematic that helps clinicians maneuver medication escalation (World Health Organization 1996).

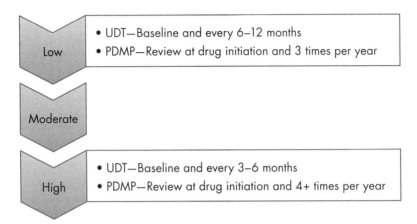

FIGURE 27–4.   Monitoring based on risk stratification.

Once a patient is stratified as low, moderate, or high risk, the above chart can be used to guide a clinician in adherence monitoring. Urine drug test (UDT) should be random. Patients displaying any aberrant behaviors should be counseled and likely tapered off opioids entirely.

PDMP = prescription drug monitoring program.

Source.   Adapted from Manchikanti et al. 2012.

The first step of the ladder is for mild to moderate pain, rated by the patient as less than 5. Treatment should start with a nonopioid medication such as an NSAID or acetaminophen. Before a medication is dismissed as a failure, the patient should take the appropriate dose on a scheduled interval for at least a 2-week trial, barring significant side effects. The first step also includes adding adjuvant treatments, which may include antidepressants, anticonvulsants, topical agents, anxiolytics, antipsychotics, muscle relaxants, and so on, when indicated. If an appropriate nonopioid trial has been unsuccessful and pain persists without functional improvement, movement to the second WHO ladder step is warranted.

The second step involves treatment of moderate to severe pain, rated by the patient as 5–7, that is inadequately managed by nonopioid pharmacotherapy. If a patient has failed nonopioid medication such as NSAIDs, acetaminophen, and other adjuvants combined with physician-ordered physical therapy and a structured exercise program, a trial of opioid medication may be warranted. When considering use of a short-acting opioid such as hydrocodone or codeine, the clinician should educate the patient on opioid risks: *Physical dependence* is a state of adaptation that is manifested by a withdrawal syndrome that can be produced with abrupt cessation, rapid dose reduction, decreasing blood level of the drug, or administration of an antagonist; it is *not* the same as addiction. *Tolerance* is decreased duration of analgesia and then

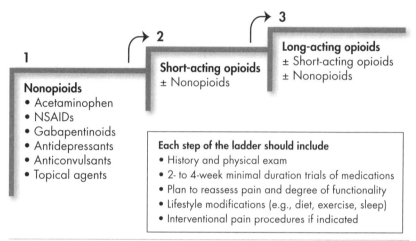

FIGURE 27–5. Three-step analgesic ladder.

NSAID = nonsteroidal anti-inflammatory drug.

Source. Adapted from World Health Organization 1996.

eventual decreased effectiveness. *Addiction* is another possible complication and is described as compulsive use of and preoccupation with the drug and its supply, inability to consistently control the quantity used, craving of the psychological effects of the drug, and continued use despite adverse effects from the drug. Other common side effects include sedation, respiratory depression, impaired judgment, impaired coordination, constipation, nausea, accelerated loss of bone mineral density, and opioid-induced hyperalgesia (a syndrome of increased sensitivity to painful stimuli, worsening pain despite increasing doses of opioids, and pain that extends beyond the distribution of preexisting pain). *Accidental death* is the most serious consideration. Risk of opioid-related accidental death is amplified when opioids are combined with other medications, such as benzodiazepines, that have concomitant side effects of sedation and respiratory impairment.

The patient should be told that the prescribing of an opioid constitutes a "trial" that requires interval evaluations to assess functional status for as long as the patient is taking the opioid. A trial sets certain expectations that long-term chronic opioid treatment is not automatic and not necessarily expected. Trials can be done over a 4- to 6-week time frame, with active participation by the patient in keeping a log of day-to-day activities. Patients should understand that the ultimate goal of opioid therapy is increased function, including physical exercise, healthy weight maintenance, activity participation, control of underlying disease, and ultimately improved quality of life. A clinical tool for mental health providers may aid in assessing and documenting the relevant domains that need attention for each patient undergo-

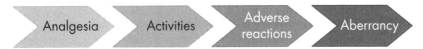

FIGURE 27–6.   Assessment of opioid management with the "4 A's."

The 4 A's is a simple method to monitor outcomes once a patient begins opioid therapy. These factors should be assessed at every office visit to help guide ongoing treatment.

ing chronic opioid treatment (Figure 27–6) (Passik and Wienreb 2000). Appropriate opioid therapy should provide analgesia to allow for improved functional activity with minimal side effects.

Ongoing assessment concerning efficacy of any treatment plan for patients with chronic pain should focus on improved functional outcomes. Questions for the patient concerning opioid efficacy should focus not merely on VAS scores but also on improved ability to care for oneself, exercise, participate in social functions, return to work, and experience improved quality of life. Functional goals will vary from patient to patient and should be constructed with small milestones along the way to remind patients of functional improvement. Attainable goals should be documented at the initiation of therapy and periodically revisited to instill hope and a sense of achievement. If no functional benefit is demonstrated with a particular management strategy, especially with opioids, a slow taper or discontinuation of the unsuccessful therapy should take place with exploration into an alternative care plan.

Nonpharmacological Therapy for the Treatment of Pain

Almost all comprehensive treatment programs should involve a trial of nonpharmacological modalities in conjunction with pharmacological therapy. Nonpharmacological therapies include physical therapy, nutritional assessment, weight loss guidance for those who are overweight, massage, transcutaneous electrical nerve stimulation, acupuncture, yoga, meditation, cognitive-behavioral therapy, hypnosis, and interventional procedures (e.g., soft tissue injections, spine injections, joint injections). Being familiar with indications for some of the common interventional procedures will aid the clinician in making appropriate referrals and in establishing a good relationship with the pain specialist. For example, patients who have radicular spine pain may benefit from an epidural steroid injection; this radiating pattern suggests nerve root impingement from either a disc herniation or stenosis, and the pain is often described as electrical, burning, or shooting in nature.

The clinician should keep in mind, however, that epidural steroid injections are more likely to be helpful for the radicular pain than for the back pain itself.

Patients with axial low back pain that may or may not radiate as far distally as the posterior thigh may benefit from radiofrequency ablation of the medial branch nerves innervating the arthritic facet joints suspected of contributing to the patient's pain. Like the major joints in the appendicular skeleton, facet joints can undergo considerable degeneration from aging, trauma, or one's occupation.

Pain specialists routinely perform trigger point injections. Many patients have myofascial tenderness to palpation, but much of this local tenderness is not categorized as trigger points. A true trigger point is a focal "hyperirritable spot" within a taut muscle band that usually causes a radiating referral pattern or motor or autonomic dysfunction. Many treatments are available for trigger points, including physical therapy, massage, ultrasound, and needle injection with local anesthetic, corticosteroid, or botulinum toxin, or simply dry needling. Discussion of various pain interventions is beyond the scope of this chapter, but the above-noted procedures may provide guidance for the more common indications for referral to a pain interventionist.

Final Thoughts

Chronic pain management involves work with a challenging patient population and encompasses a myriad of layers, including physical, psychosocial, and behavioral issues; substance misuse; and variable family dynamics, motivations, and goals for treatment. Each of these layers requires assessment prior to engaging the core of each individual's pain condition. Treating chronic pain can be stressful, difficult, frustrating, and emotional for the patient and the practitioner. However, as each layer is addressed and treated, it can be very rewarding to see debilitated pain patients transform into successful, independent, functional people who have gained an improved quality of life.

Resources

Screener and Opioid Assessment for Patients in Pain (SOAPP): www.painEDU.org
  SOAPP) is a brief paper-and-pencil tool to facilitate assessment and planning for chronic pain patients being considered for long-term opioid treatment. Can also be found at www.opioidrisk.com under risk assessment tools.
Current Opioid Misuse Measure (COMM): www.PainEdu.org
  COMM will help clinicians identify whether a patient, currently on long-term opioid therapy, may be exhibiting aberrant behaviors associated with

misuse of opioid medications. Can also be found at www.opioidrisk.com under risk assessment tools.

References

Berry PH, Covington EC, Dahl JL, et al (eds): Pain: Current Understanding of Assessment, Management, and Treatments. Glenview, IL, American Pain Society, 2001

Christo PJ, Manchikanti L, Ruan X, et al: Urine drug testing in chronic pain. Pain Physician 14:123–143, 2011

Chung F, Elsaid H: Screening for obstructive sleep apnea before surgery: why is it important? Curr Opin Anaesthesiol 22(3):405–411, 2009

Chung F, Yegneswaran B, Liao P, et al: STOP questionnaire: a tool to screen patients for obstructive sleep apnea. Anesthesiology 108:812–822, 2008

Institute of Medicine Committee on Advancing Pain Research, Care, and Education: Relieving Pain in America: A Blueprint for Transforming Prevention, Care, Education, and Research. Washington, DC, National Academies Press, 2011

Manchikanti L, Abdi S, Alturi S, et al: American Society of Interventional Pain Physicians (ASIPP) guidelines for responsible opioid prescribing in chronic non-cancer pain. Pain Physician 15:S1–S116, 2012

McCarron RM, Xiong GL, Bourgeois J: Lippincott's Primary Care Psychiatry: For Primary Care Clinicians and Trainees, Medical Specialists, Neurologists, Emergency Medical Professionals, Mental Health Providers, and Trainees. Philadelphia, PA, Lippincott Williams & Wilkins, 2009

Passik SD, Wienreb HJ: Managing chronic nonmalignant pain: overcoming obstacles to the use of opioids. Adv Ther 17:70–83, 2000

World Health Organization: Cancer Pain Relief: With a Guide to Opioid Availability, 2nd Edition. Geneva, Switzerland, World Health Organization, 1996

Zackaroff KL, McCarberg BH, Reisner L, et al: Managing Chronic Pain With Opioids in Primary Care, 2nd Edition. Newton, MA, Inflexxion, 2010

Appendix

Preventive Medicine in Psychiatry (PMaP) Guideline

U.S. Preventive Services Task Force guidelines are used when recommendations vary. http://www.uspreventiveservicestaskforce.org; last accessed February 28, 2014.

	Recommendation based on age group (years)				Special considerations for psychiatric populations
	18–39	40–49	50–64	>65	
Cancer screening					
Colorectal cancer			Start screening after age 50; interval depends on method and risk stratification		
Skin cancer	Insufficient evidence for or against routine screening				Frequent monitoring of the homeless and excessively sun-exposed patients
Breast cancer		Screening mammography, with or without clinical breast examination, every 1–2 years	Screening mammography every 2 years for ages 50–74 years; insufficient evidence for screening for age >74		
Cervical cancer	Screen 3 years after sexual activity or at age >21, and then every 3 years			Not recommended if adequate recent screening and no additional risk	People with a history of bipolar, psychotic, or substance use disorder are more likely to acquire sexually transmitted infections

	Recommendation based on age group (years)				Special considerations for psychiatric populations
	18–39	40–49	50–64	>65	
Cancer screening *(continued)*					
Prostate cancer			Routine prostate-specific antigen screening is not recommended; benefits and risks of screening should be discussed prior to testing		
Lung cancer			Screen annually with low-dose computed tomography for ages 55–80, with 30 pack-year smoking history and smoking within past 15 years		Patients with psychiatric (particularly psychotic) disorders are generally more likely to smoke and should be monitored carefully by the health care team
Oral cancer	Insufficient evidence for or against screening				Low threshold to screen for those who have severe mental illness and an extensive history of smoking

	Recommendation based on age group (years)				Special considerations for psychiatric populations[a]
	18–39	40–49	50–64	>65	Schedule for patients taking antipsychotics[a]
Metabolic screening					
Body mass index	Screening is recommended, although interval is uncertain; refer patient to intensive, multicomponent behavioral interventions for BMI >30				Screen 1) at baseline, 4 weeks, 8 weeks, and 12 weeks, every 3 months, then annually or 2) at every visit—whichever is more frequent
Blood pressure	Screen every 2 years with BP <120/80 mmHg, or every year with systolic BP 120–139 mmHg and diastolic BP 80–90 mmHg				Screen 1) at baseline, 12 weeks, and 1 year after starting an antipsychotic, then annually, or 2) at every visit—whichever is more frequent
Lipid panel	Every 3–5 years; more frequent if high risk				Non–high-density lipoprotein may be more reliable and does not require fasting Screen at baseline, 12 weeks, and 1 year and every 5 years after starting an antipsychotic
Fasting glucose/ hemoglobin A₁c			Screening at age >45 or in those with BMI >25 and risk factors		Screen at baseline, 12 weeks, and 1 year after starting an

	Recommendation based on age group (years)				Special considerations for psychiatric populations
	18–39	40–49	50–64	>65	
Infectious diseases					
Sexually transmitted infections (chlamydia, gonorrhea)	Annual screening for all sexually active women age <25				Testing depends on risk factors and recent exposure (e.g., bipolar, psychotic, or substance use disorders)
HIV	Test once in lifetime; annual screening in persons with high-risk behaviors (unsafe sexual practices, injection drug use)				Testing depends on risk factors and recent exposure (e.g., bipolar, psychotic, or substance use disorders)
Hepatitis B	One-time screen for persons born in Asia or Pacific Islands or anyone born in the United States who was not vaccinated at birth and who has at least one parent born in Asia or Pacific Islands (excluding Japan, New Zealand, Australia) Screen high-risk persons: sexual partners of persons infected with hepatitis B, HIV patients, men who have sex with men, injection drug users, people born in countries with prevalence >2%, persons receiving immunosuppressive therapy				Testing depends on risk factors and recent exposure (e.g., bipolar, psychotic, or substance use disorders)
Hepatitis C	One-time screen for persons born between 1945 and 1965 Screen high-risk persons: injection drug users, persons with recognizable exposure such as needle stick, persons who received blood transfusions before 1992, patients with medical conditions with exposure (e.g., long-term dialysis)				Testing depends on risk factors and recent exposure (e.g., bipolar, psychotic, or substance use disorders)

Immunizations[b]	Recommendation based on age group (years)				Special considerations for psychiatric populations
	18–39	40–49	50–64	>65	
Tetanus-diphtheria (Td)[c]	One dose each of DTaP (combined diphtheria, tetanus, and pertussis) at 2 months, 4 months, and 6 months. A fourth dose at 15–18 months and a fifth dose at 4–6 years of age. Children should get a booster vaccine at age 11 or 12 years. Adults need the booster Td every 10 years and should also receive a one-time shot of TDaP vaccine in place of one Td shot.				
Influenza	Annually				
Pneumococcus	Chronic medical illness, active smoking, alcohol misuse, and high-risk environment			Age >65	Recommend if living in psychiatric residential care facility
Varicella zoster			Age >60		
Human papillomavirus[c]	Ages 9–26 years; three-dose series at 0, 2, 6 months; do not give if pregnant)				Those with a history of mania or psychosis may be more likely to acquire virus
Hepatitis A	Based on individual risks (e.g., chronic liver disease, occupation, travel to endemic areas)				Recommended for people with illicit substance use
Hepatitis B	All children; adults without prior vaccination, based on individual risks (e.g., chronic liver disease, occupation, travel to endemic areas, Asian/Pacific Islander)				Recommended for people with illicit substance use
Other					Live vaccination not recommended for people with impaired cell-mediated immunity (e.g., clozapine-induced leukopenia/

| | Recommendation based on age group (years) | | | | Special considerations for psychiatric populations |
	18–39	40–49	50–64	>65	
Sensory screenings					
Vision	Insufficient evidence			Snellen visual acuity chart is recommended	
Hearing	Insufficient evidence			Periodically ask about hearing	
Diabetes					
Retinopathy screening	Annually dilated eye examination by optometrist or ophthalmologist				
Nephropathy screening	Annual spot urine creatinine and microalbumin				
Neuropathy screening	Annual monofilament sensory examination, pulse examination				
Hemoglobin A_{1c}	Every 6 months; 3 months after treatment adjustment				
Hyperlipidemia	Annually; 6 weeks after treatment adjustment; patients should be considered for statin therapy unless contraindicated				
Blood pressure	Checked at each visit; goal blood pressure <140/90 mmHg				

Other	Recommendation based on age group (years)				Special considerations for psychiatric populations
	18–39	40–49	50–64	>65	
Smoking cessation	Screen and recommend cessation counseling and pharmacological treatments, evoking and building motivation				Metabolism of tricyclic antidepressants and antipsychotics may increase with smoking cessation
Osteoporosis			Women >60 with increased risk	Women >65 years	
Aspirin (81 mg)			Men ages 45–79; women ages 55–79 (if low risk of gastrointestinal bleeding); insufficient evidence for age >79		
Thyroid-stimulating hormone	Insufficient evidence to make a recommendation				Screen as part of depression and dementia workup in high-risk groups
Abdominal aortic aneurysm				One-time screening ultrasound for men ages 65–75 who are current or former smokers	

Note.   BMI=body mass index; BP=blood pressure.

[a]Based on American Diabetes Association, American Psychiatric Association, American Association of Clinical Endocrinologists, and North American Association for the Study of Obesity and Diabetes Consensus Guidelines (2004).

[b]"The USPSTF recognizes the importance of immunizations in primary disease prevention. However, the USPSTF does not wish to duplicate the significant investment of resources made by others to review new evidence on immunizations in a timely fashion and make recommendations. The USPSTF therefore will not update its 1996 recommendations. The Centers for Disease Control and Prevention's (CDC) Advisory Committee on Immunization Practices (ACIP) publishes recommendations on immunizations for children and adults. The methods used by the ACIP to review evidence on immunizations may differ from the methods used by the USPSTF. For the ACIP current

Index

*Page numbers printed in **boldface** type refer to tables or figures.*